Pocketbook of Neurological Physiotherapy

Sheila would like to dedicate this book to the memory of her Mum, Chris.

Commissioning Editor: Rita-Demetriou Swanwick
Development Editor: Veronika Watkins/Catherine Jackson
Project Manager: Morven Dean/Jane Dingwall
Text Design: Thomas Gravemaker
Cover Design: Stewart Larking
Illustrator: Richard Morris
Illustration Manager: Merlyn Harvey

Pocketbook of Neurological Physiotherapy

Edited by

Sheila Lennon PhD MSc BSc MCSP

Senior Lecturer (Physiotherapy), School of Health Sciences and Health & Rehabilitation Research Institute, University of Ulster

Maria Stokes PhD MSCP

Professor of Neuromuscular Rehabilitation, School of Health Sciences, University of Southampton

CHURCHILL LIVINGSTONE

ELSEVIER

Edinburgh London New York Oxford Philadelphia St Louis Sydney Toronto 2009

CHURCHILL
LIVINGSTONE
ELSEVIER

© 2009, Elsevier Limited. All rights reserved.

No part of this publication may be reproduced or transmitted in any form or by any means, electronic or mechanical, including photocopying, recording, or any information storage and retrieval system, without permission in writing from the publisher. Permissions may be sought directly from Elsevier's Rights Department: phone: (+1) 215 239 3804 (US) or (+44) 1865 843830 (UK); fax: (+44) 1865 853333; e-mail: healthpermissions@elsevier.com. You may also complete your request on-line via the Elsevier website at http://www.elsevier.com/permissions.

First published 2009

ISBN: 978-0-443-06854-6

British Library Cataloguing in Publication Data
A catalogue record for this book is available from the British Library

Library of Congress Cataloging in Publication Data
A catalog record for this book is available from the Library of Congress

Notice

Knowledge and best practice in this field are constantly changing. As new research and experience broaden our knowledge, changes in practice, treatment and drug therapy may become necessary or appropriate. Readers are advised to check the most current information provided (i) on procedures featured or (ii) by the manufacturer of each product to be administered, to verify the recommended dose or formula, the method and duration of administration, and contraindications. It is the responsibility of the practitioner, relying on their own experience and knowledge of the patient, to make diagnoses, to determine dosages and the best treatment for each individual patient, and to take all appropriate safety precautions. To the fullest extent of the law, neither the Publisher nor the Editors assumes any liability for any injury and/or damage to persons or property arising out or related to any use of the material contained in this book.

Neither the Publisher nor the Editors assume any responsibility for any loss or injury and/or damage to persons or property arising out of or related to any use of the material contained in this book. It is the responsibility of the treating practitioner, relying on independent expertise and knowledge of the patient, to determine the best treatment and method of application for the patient.

The Publisher

ELSEVIER
your source for books,
journals and multimedia
in the health sciences

www.elsevierhealth.com

Working together to grow
libraries in developing countries

www.elsevier.com | www.bookaid.org | www.sabre.org

ELSEVIER   BOOK AID International   Sabre Foundation

The
publisher's
policy is to use
**paper manufactured
from sustainable forests**

Printed in China

Louise Ada BSc GradDipPhty MA PhD
Associate Professor, Discipline of Physiotherapy, The University of Sydney, Lidcombe, Australia

Linda Armstrong BA BSc PGCert(Care of the Elderly) PhD
Consultant Speech and Language Therapist, Speech and Language Therapy Department, Perth Royal Infirmary, Perth, Scotland, UK

Clare Bassile EdD PT
Assistant Professor of Clinical Physical Therapy, Program in Physical Therapy, Columbia University, New York, NY, USA

Patricia Bate PhD MAppSci BAppSci(Phty)
22 Marine Parade, Seacliff 5049, Australia

Julie Bernhardt PhD BSc(Physio)
Director, AVERT Very Early Rehabilitation Stroke Research Program, National Stroke Research Institute, Heidelberg Heights, Victoria; Associate Professor, School of Physiotherapy, La Trobe University, Bundoora, Victoria, Australia

Colleen G Canning BPhty MA PhD
Senior Lecturer, Discipline of Physiotherapy, The University of Sydney, Lidcombe, Australia

Adrian Capp BHSc MSc MCSP
Clinical Specialist Physiotherapist – Neurosurgery/Neurological Care, The National Hospital for Neurology and Neurosurgery, London, UK

Elizabeth Cassidy MSc MCSP
Lecturer in Physiotherapy, School of Health Sciences and Social Care, Brunel University West London, Uxbridge, UK

Paul T Charlton MSc MBAPO SROrt
Senior Orthotist, Peacocks Medical Group, Benfield Business Park, Newcastle upon Tyne, UK

Jennifer A Freeman BAppSci PhD MCSP
Reader in Physiotherapy and Rehabilitation, School of Health Professions, Faculty of Health and Social Work, Plymouth University, Devon, UK; Lecturer, Institute of Neurology, Department of Clinical Neurology (Neurorehabilitation), Queen Square, London, UK

Karen Whalley Hammell PhD MSc OT(C) DipCOT
Honorary Research Associate, Department of Occupational Science and Occupational Therapy, Faculty of Medicine, University of British Columbia, Vancouver, BC, Canada

Fiona Jones PhD MSc MCSP
Principal Lecturer (Physiotherapy), Faculty of Health and Social Care Sciences, St George's University of London, UK

Christopher Kennard PhD FRCP FRCOphth
Professor and Head of Division of Neuroscience and Psychological Medicine Imperial College School of Medicine, Charing Cross Hospital, London, UK

Madhu Khanderia PhD BSc MRPharmS
Chief Pharmacist, Royal Hospital for Neuro-disability, West Hill, Putney, London, UK

Cherry Kilbride PhD MSc MCSP
Lecturer in Physiotherapy, Brunel University West London, Uxbridge, UK

Jeffrey A Kleim PhD
Research Health Scientist, Brain Rehabilitation Research Center, Malcolm Randall VA Hospital, Gainesville, Florida, USA; Associate Professor, Dept of Neuroscience, McKnight Brain Institute, University of Florida Gainesville, Florida, USA

Anne Marie Laverty MSc BMedSc CertEd
Clinical Lead for Stroke, Northumbria Healthcare NHS Foundation, Alnwick Infirmary, Alnwick, Northumberland, UK

Lynn Legg MPH DipCOT
Manager Stroke Therapy Evaluation Project (STEP) (funded by the Big Lottery Fund) and Chief Scientist Office Scotland Health Services Research Fellow, UK

Sheila Lennon PhD MSc BSc MCSP
Senior Lecturer (Physiotherapy), School of Health Sciences and Health &
Rehabilitation Research Institute, University of Ulster, Newtownabbey, Northern
Ireland, UK

Zena Jones PGCert(Res) BPhil(Ed) CertEd RN
Patient, Carer and Public Involvement Manager, UK Stroke Research Network,
Royal Victoria Infirmary, Newcastle upon Tyne, UK

Sue Paddison MCSP Grad Dip Phys
Superintendent Physiotherapist/Clinical Specialist in Spinal Cord Injury,
Royal National Orthopaedic Hospital NHS Trust, Stanmore, UK

Helen Rodgers MBChB FRCP
Reader in Stroke Medicine, School of Clinical Medical Sciences University of
Newcastle upon Tyne, Medical School, Newcastle upon Tyne, UK

Susan Ryerson ScD MA PT
Making Progress, Adult Neurologic Rehabilitation, Alexandria, VA USA;
Research Scientist, Center for Applied Biomechanics and Rehabilitation Research,
National Rehabilitation Hospital, Washington DC, USA

Emma Stack PhD MSc GradDipPhys
Senior Research Fellow, Southampton General Hospital, Southampton, UK

Emma K Stokes BSc(Physio) MSc PhD
Senior Lecturer, School of Physiotherapy, Trinity College Dublin, Ireland

Maria Stokes PhD MSCP
Professor of Neuromuscular Rehabilitation, School of Health Sciences, University of
Southampton, Highfield Campus, Southampton, UK

F Colin Wilson BSc(Hons) MMedSc DClinPsych
Consultant Clinical Neuropsychologist, Regional Acquired Brain Injury Unit,
Musgrave Park Hospital, Belfast, Northern Ireland, UK

Firstly, we thank the authors for generously sharing their knowledge and expertise. We are also grateful to colleagues who provided feedback on the outline structure and peer reviewed chapters: Ann Ashburn, Joy Conway, Judy Deutsch, Sue Edwards, Terri Ellis, Nicola Hancock, JoAnn Kluzik, Margaret Mayston, Karl Schurr, Martha Sliwinski, Mark Smith and Shelagh Tittle. We thank the team at Elsevier who assisted us in producing this book, in particular Heidi Allen, Veronika Watkins, Rita Demetriou-Swanwick, Jane Dingwall and Alison Breewood.

A special thank you goes to our families and friends for their support, encouragement and patience throughout this project. Specifically, Sheila Lennon would like to thank Maria, her co-editor, for her constant support and guidance – it has been fun (sort of!) – and her husband Ian for putting up with being ignored during many evenings and weekends. She would also like to thank the Leverhulme Trust for the award of a Study Abroad Fellowship relating to this pocketbook. Maria Stokes would like to thank Dr KP Asante for arguing convincingly that a pocketbook is a valuable clinical tool and that she should not hesitate to get involved in producing one!

Sheila Lennon, Belfast
Maria Stokes, Southampton
2008

This pocketbook is intended to provide both students and qualified physiotherapists with a basic overview of the physiotherapy management of people with neurological disability. The summarized format designed for quick and easy reference should serve as a useful teaching tool for undergraduate students, as well as a helpful aid for revision. All chapters refer to the scientific and experimental evidence that underlies clinical practice.

Some of the text is based on the book edited by Stokes (2004), particularly Chapter 6 on 'Common neurological conditions' but this pocketbook involves many new authors offering an international perspective on issues that influence clinical practice. The text comprises four sections: Section 1 on 'Background Knowledge' covers basic information on neurological conditions and principles of clinical practice in neurorehabilitation; Section 2 on 'Clinical Decision Making' covers areas relating to dealing with people with neurological conditions, ranging from assessment to treatment approaches; Section 3 deals with 'Other Considerations', including respiratory, communication and cognitive aspects and orthotic management; Section 4 consists of appendices covering topics that the physiotherapist needs to understand but is not directly involved with: medical investigations and drug treatments. The glossary of terms and abbreviations are not exhaustive and include those which are commonly encountered by physiotherapists.

This pocketbook sums up core concepts that are applicable to all physiotherapists working in neurological environments. Working in neurology can be a daunting experience. This concise guide represents our wish list of things you always wanted to know about neurological physiotherapy but were afraid to ask. Well now you don't need to ask – just consult this pocketbook instead!

Sheila Lennon, Belfast
Maria Stokes, Southampton
2008

Reference

Stokes M (ed) 2004 Physical management in neurological rehabilitation. London: Elsevier.

BACKGROUND KNOWLEDGE

CHAPTER 1

Evidence-based practice

Julie Bernhardt and Lynn Legg

INTRODUCTION

Evidence-based practice is every physiotherapist's professional responsibility. In this chapter, we aim to explain what is meant by evidence-based practice, and to provide suggestions about how to ask the right questions, then find and rate evidence and use it to help you make the best decision about patient care. We will focus on stroke as the example for the chapter, but the information provided will be applicable to other neurological conditions.

What is evidence-based practice?

Evidence-based practice (EBP) is a systematic process for finding, appraising and applying current best evidence to inform clinical practice.

Current best evidence is 'up-to-date information from relevant, valid research about the effects of different forms of health care, the potential for harm from exposure to particular agents, the accuracy of diagnostic tests, and the predictive power of prognostic factors' (NIPH, Oslo, 1996).

The aim of evidence-based practice is to enable practitioners to make well-formed decisions about clinical practice based on the 'conscientious, explicit, and judicious use of current best evidence' (Sackett et al 1996). The practice of evidence-based physiotherapy means integrating current best research evidence with clinical expertise and patient values (Haynes et al 2002).

Why should we care about EBP?

There are important reasons why clinicians need to be evidence-based practitioners. Figure 1.1 outlines a range of drivers of EBP. These may vary from health system to health system. However, the concept of 'evidence-based purchasing' (Long & Harrison 1996) is now common, even in countries with health systems that are predominantly government funded.

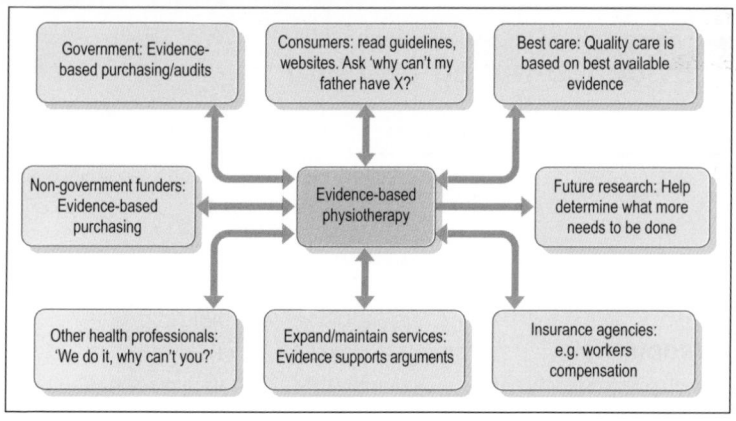

Figure 1.1
Drivers of evidence-based physiotherapy.

EVIDENCE-BASED PHYSIOTHERAPY

Questions and doubts about treatment decisions or usual practices are a normal part of clinical practice. You can begin the process of using evidence to guide practice by asking the following types of questions:

- What is the best way to assess this problem?
- What is the best way to treat this problem?
- What is the rationale for this practice?
- Could the treatment I deliver be done better, more efficiently, or more cost-effectively?
- Can I deliver the best treatment with the resources I have (e.g. facilities, expertise)?
- What evidence supports my decision?
- What are the clinical implications of delivering this treatment?
- Have I overlooked an important treatment?

Having the confidence and ability to ask and answer these types of questions moves you towards improving the efficiency and effectiveness of clinical practice.

Getting started

The practice of evidence-based health care is usually triggered when a healthcare professional is faced with a patient. There are six distinct sequential stages of EBP (Table 1.1):

Table 1.1 The stages of evidence-based practice (EBP).

Stage	Description
1	Formulate a clear clinical question
2	Search the literature for research-derived evidence
3	Appraise the evidence for its validity and usefulness
4	Seek and incorporate the patient's values and preferences (Greenhalgh et al 2003)
5	Implement findings in clinical practice
6	Evaluate effectiveness

Formulating a clear question

As a physiotherapist's time is limited, searching for the best available evidence needs to be efficient and this requires learning the art of building the well-structured question. Physiotherapists' clinical questions are likely to fall into one of the following categories (see Table 1.2).

The PICO framework is useful for formulating a clear question. This framework identifies and defines the essential elements of a well-structured question. It is important to note that a clear question addresses only one problem at any given time.

Patient population or problem of interest

Intervention of interest

Comparison intervention (if applicable)

Outcome

Table 1.3 provides examples of using the PICO framework to develop a well-structured question.

Now that you have formed a clear clinical question you need to find the best evidence to answer your question.

Finding the best evidence

There are many resources you might use to answer questions; personal experience, reasoning and intuition, asking a colleague, consulting a textbook, reading a relevant scientific paper from a personal reprint collection, using a bibliographic database, e.g. Medline or Embase, or consulting the pre-appraised or evidence-based healthcare literature, or clinical practice guidelines (see below).

The problem with relying solely on personal experience and opinion is that sometimes we 'don't know that we don't know', and therefore we may not be

1

Table 1.2 Categories of evidence-based practice (EBP) questions with examples (adapted from Sackett DL et al 1997, with permission).

Categories of EBP question	Description	Example
Diagnosis/assessment	What information should I gather, what is the best way to collect that information and how should I interpret the findings?	What is the best way to assess arm function in stroke patients?
Aetiology	How do I identify the possible causes of a problem?	What is the cause of pain in a patient with post stroke shoulder pain?
Differential diagnosis	When symptoms indicate several potential diagnoses, how do I decide which diagnosis is the most likely?	In a young woman presenting with knee swelling, stiffness, pain, crepitus, quadriceps atrophy on examination, pain on compression and resisted extension, what is the most likely cause – chondromalacia patella or osteoarthritis of the patellofemoral joint?
Prognosis	What is the pattern of recovery over time and are complications likely?	My patient had a stroke six days ago. When will they be able to walk?
Therapy	What intervention is going to produce the best result for my patient? And is it worth the cost and effort involved?	What are the effects of physiotherapy based on the Bobath concept for post stroke patients compared to other physiotherapy treatment approaches across a range of outcomes?
Prevention	How can I prevent new problems or secondary conditions occurring? How can I improve my patient's health?	What is the best method to prevent shoulder pain in patients after stroke?
Self-improvement	How can I continue to be an efficient and effective physiotherapist/manager?	What are the effects of different activities to improve my own knowledge, attitude or skills?
The patient's experience/perceptions	How can I better understand my patient?	What factors motivate or deter individuals from using outpatient physiotherapy services?

Table 1.3 Using the PICO framework to develop a clear question.

	Patient, Population or Problem	Intervention	Comparison	Outcome
	What is the disease/condition that I am interested in?	Which intervention, therapy, treatment, test, procedure, am I interested in?	What is the alternative to the intervention (e.g. different therapy approach, placebo, drug)?	What can I hope to measure, accomplish, improve or affect?
Example	A 57-year-old man with post stroke shoulder pain	Transcutaneous Electrical Stimulation (TENS)	Non-steroidal anti-inflammatory drugs	Reduction in the intensity of pain experienced

The clinical question from this example would be:
'Is TENS better than non-steroidal anti-inflammatory drugs at reducing the intensity of post stroke shoulder pain?'

providing the most efficient, effective and cost-effective treatment. Asking an experienced colleague can be the most efficient method particularly when the question is related to a one-off situation. Textbooks are only as up to date as the most recent reference cited and therefore should be consulted with caution, as often they are out of date before they are published (Oxman et al 1993). Scientific articles found lying around the office may only provide half the story and are unlikely to be tailored towards meeting required information needs. It is only by concentrating on evidence published in bibliographic databases or the evidence-based health-care literature that ineffective, harmful or costly interventions can be identified and reduced, and more efficient and effective physiotherapy interventions can be retained or introduced.

The type of evidence that you want to search for will depend on the focus of your question. Developing an understanding of the different types of research will help you retrieve the highest level of evidence for your particular clinical question.

LEVELS OF SCIENTIFIC EVIDENCE

'Levels of scientific evidence' are classification systems for research designs. According to the type of intervention being assessed (e.g. prognosis, diagnosis, aetiology, therapy etc.) research designs are assessed and ranked according to their reliability i.e. ability to protect a study against bias, a systematic deviation from the truth

1

that can distort the result of the research (Sitthi–amorn & Poashyachinda 1993), and error.

Systematic reviews and meta-analysis of randomized controlled trials and evidence-based clinical practice guidelines (CPGs) are generally considered to be the strongest level of evidence on which to base clinical decisions about treatment. The weakest level of evidence is generally agreed to be expert opinion (i.e. without explicit and objective appraisal of the relevant research) e.g. reports from expert committees. For access to information on levels of evidence, see 'Other resources' below.

Practical resources to support evidence-based practice

There are numerous resources to support evidence-based practice. Clinicians should start with the highest level resource available (see Figure 1.2).

If all else fails and searching the primary literature is the only option to try and answer your question, it is worthwhile recruiting the services of an information specialist (librarian). They are skilled in the art of searching and have extensive knowledge of the structure of the biomedical literature.

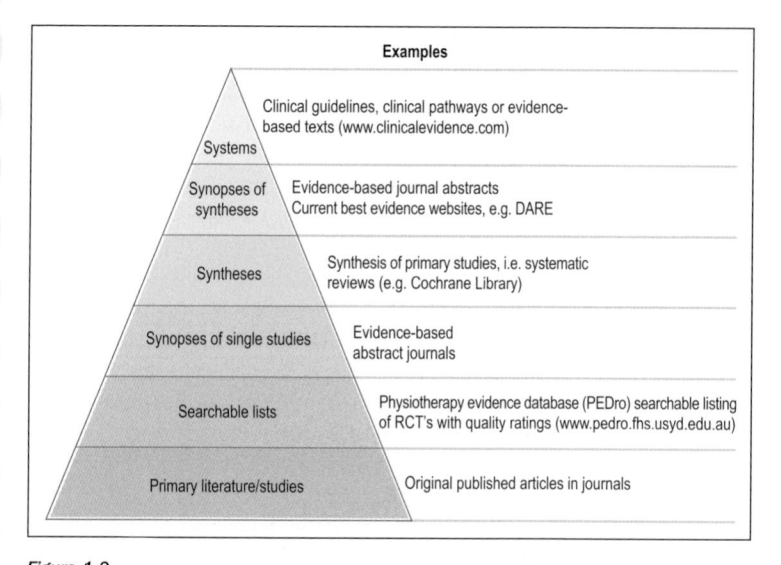

Examples

Level	Examples
Systems	Clinical guidelines, clinical pathways or evidence-based texts (www.clinicalevidence.com)
Synopses of syntheses	Evidence-based journal abstracts. Current best evidence websites, e.g. DARE
Syntheses	Synthesis of primary studies, i.e. systematic reviews (e.g. Cochrane Library)
Synopses of single studies	Evidence-based abstract journals
Searchable lists	Physiotherapy evidence database (PEDro) searchable listing of RCT's with quality ratings (www.pedro.fhs.usyd.edu.au)
Primary literature/studies	Original published articles in journals

Figure 1.2
Levels of organization of evidence from research (adapted from Haynes 2001, with permission). DARE = Database of abstracts of reviews of effects; RCT = randomized controlled trial.

Clinical practice guidelines (CPG) represent the consensus opinion of experts based on explicit and objective reviews of the scientific literature. CPGs are generally developed with the aid of expert panels containing both researchers and expert clinicians and usually conform to national standards for guideline production. They have the advantage of providing clinicians (and often consumers) with an all-in-one reference source of the most up-to-date evidence. A disadvantage of CPGs is that they are time consuming to produce, and therefore often fail to keep pace with new evidence (see 'Other resources' below for links to CPGs). The difference between systematic reviews (a synthesis of primary studies) and CPGs are that CPGs give recommendations to guide clinical practice. Synopses of individual studies or systematic reviews encapsulate the key methodological details and results required to apply the evidence to individual patient care (Haynes 2001, Mulrow 1994; also see 'Other resources' below).

PRIMARY LITERATURE – RESEARCH DESIGNS

There are two broad approaches to research design or methodology; qualitative and quantitative. Both can be rigorous and help answer important questions (Portney & Watkins 2000, Marshall & Rossman 2006; www.sign.ac.uk). It is becoming increasingly accepted that mixed methodologies, using both quantitative and qualitative designs within the same study, are most beneficial – particularly for large trials to evaluate practice.

Quantitative studies

Quantitative studies (for example clinical trials, comparative studies and epidemiological investigations) aim to test a hypothesis concerning pre-determined variables. These studies are used to answer questions about *whether*? (e.g. the PT treatment did more good than harm) or *how much*? (e.g. how strong is the relationship between a particular risk factor (immobility) for the development of a particular disease or condition (pressure sores) (Giacomini & Cook 2000). For further reading see Altman & Bland (1999), Day & Altman (2000), Doust & Del Mar (2001), Kunz & Oxman (1998) and Roberts et al (1998).

Qualitative studies

Qualitative studies, for example, in-depth interviews and focus group work aim to explore and obtain insight into 'social, emotional and experiential phenomena' relating to health and health care. Qualitative studies are used to explore the 'how', 'what' and 'why' questions (Giacomini & Cook 2000). Examples would include exploration of the meaning of the experience of stroke to survivors and families, or the value of patient exercise groups to the users, or the attitudes of physiotherapists and patients towards physiotherapy working patterns and availability of therapy. For further reading, see Green & Britten (1998), Greenhalgh & Taylor (1997), Lambert & McKevitt (2002), Mays & Pope (2000), Meyer (2000), Pope et al (2000) and Strauss & Corbin (1998).

Critical appraisal

Critical appraisal is an essential component of EBP and is the process of methodically examining research evidence to assess its validity, importance and applicability to clinical practice (Greenhalgh 1997). It is important to note that different research designs have different methodological validity, i.e. how these results can be applied in a given clinical setting. For more help on: the types of critical appraisal question to ask for different kinds of research; and evaluating the quality of primary research of systematic reviews, see 'Other resources' below.

IMPLEMENTING EVIDENCE-BASED PRACTICE

Implementing best practice is not easy. Recognizing the barriers to implementation at your site can help you develop a more effective strategy, and improve your chances of success (Grimshaw et al 2001). Common barriers to implementing EBP are shown in Table 1.4.

Many implementation methods have been tried with varying degrees of success. This issue is so important that a branch of the Cochrane Collaboration is devoted to reviewing the most effective ways to implement evidence and change clinical practice (http://www.epoc.uottawa.ca/index.htm). In 2001, Gross and colleagues reviewed the evidence for implementation strategies (see Table 1.5 for a summary).

Table 1.4 Barriers to implementing evidence-based practice (adapted with permission from Grimshaw 2003).

Barrier	Example
Structural	Financial disincentives, policies
Organizational	Inappropriate staff skills, poor facilities or lack of equipment
Peer group	Local standard of care not in line with current practice, folklore well established
Individual	Wrong knowledge, attitudes or skills
Professional–patient interaction	Problems with information processing
Consumers	Wrong information

Table 1.5 Effectiveness of implementation strategies (summarized from Gross et al 2001).

Generally ineffective	Variably effective	Generally effective
Passive guideline dissemination	Audit and feedback	Reminders to clinicians
Publication of research findings	Local opinion leaders	Educational outreach, one-to-one teaching
Didactic (lecture style) education	Local consensus conferences	Interactive education
	Consumer education	Barrier-oriented interventions
	Involving patients in decision making	Multi-faceted interventions (using several of above strategies)

Practical ideas for implementing evidence into everyday practice

In the following section we list some strategies to get you started.

When you have guidelines: The idea of implementing evidence can seem daunting, so as a first step, start small. The most important thing is to start!

● Check – are clinical practice guidelines, or databases of synthesized evidence available in your area of interest?
● Choose one or two clinical questions of interest.
● Examine whether you/your team comply with current best evidence.
● No? What barriers can you identify? How might you overcome them?
● Can you identify champions and opinion leaders from other disciplines to help you break down barriers and make change happen?
● Have a go at implementing change.
● Evaluate whether your implementation has worked (see Table 1.1).

When no guidelines/synthesized evidence are available:
● Get a team of interested people together.
● Start with a burning question about best practice care in your area.
● Ask a librarian to help you conduct a search (look for systematic reviews).
● Use an evaluation tool to help you appraise the literature.
● What recommendations can you make?
● Present this to your peers/team.
● Workshop how you might implement recommendations, then follow the steps in the above section.
● Check – were you successful in making change happen?

*A **word on critical appraisal groups:*** Critical appraisal groups can help clinicians gain confidence in finding and appraising literature, but used alone they are unlikely to lead to changes in clinical practice. Targeted efforts to change in response to a specific question are, in our experience, a much more fruitful endeavour.

Tips for keeping up to date

A final challenge in this fast paced world, is finding ways to keep up with new evidence.

- Look for critically appraised papers or evidence summaries in journals (e.g. professional physiotherapy journals).
- Schedule searches for new literature in your area of interest and run them.
- Set up journal e-mail alerts when relevant articles in your field are published.
- Make a roster for scheduled checks of evidence updates from key sources and distribute the results to team members by e-mail.

Breaking down the clinician/researcher divide

Often there is a real or perceived divide between physiotherapy researchers and clinicians. If clinicians do not feel that research is tackling important clinical questions, they will be less inclined to seek out evidence and less willing to apply it. Bridging the clinician/researcher divide should therefore be an important goal for the physiotherapy profession. The following can help and should be perused if available:

- Clinical research secondments (Pomeroy et al 2003).
- Undergraduate student research placements.
- Training EBP leaders within hospitals.
- Increasing the number of research physiotherapists employed in clinical environments.
- Supporting strategic, clinician-driven, research priorities (Research Committee 1999).

CONCLUSION

Evidence-based practice requires a commitment to providing our patients with the best possible care. In a busy clinical environment, knowing where to find the most up-to-date and appropriate evidence, in the most accessible format, is the first step toward successful evidence-based practice. Having the confidence and desire to change practice in light of the evidence is crucial. Often you may not find the answer you need to help inform your practice. It is important to remember that lack of evidence of effectiveness is not evidence of lack of effect. Experience of not finding evidence should not prevent us from engaging in the evidence-based process, rather it should help stimulate new research to find the evidence we need. As you read this book, research is underway to help fill the gaps in knowledge that we know currently exist.

References

Altman DG, Bland MJ 1999 Treatment allocation in controlled trials: why randomise? BMJ 181:209.

Day JD, Altman DG 2000 Statistics notes: blinding in clinical trials and other studies. BMJ 321:504.

Doust J, Del Mar C 2001 Why do doctors use treatments that do not work? BMJ 328:474–475.

Giacomini M, Cook DJ 2000 Users' Guides to the Medical Literature: XXIII. Qualitative Research in Health Care. A. Are the results of the study valid? JAMA 284:357–362.

Green J, Britten N 1998 Qualitative research and evidence based medicine. BMJ 316:1230–1232.

Greenhalgh T 1997 How to read a paper: papers that summarise other papers (systematic reviews and meta-analyses). BMJ 315:672–675.

Greenhalgh T, Taylor R 1997 How to read a paper: papers that go beyond numbers (qualitative research). BMJ 315:740–743.

Greenhalgh T, Toon P, Russell J et al 2003 Transferability of principles of evidence based medicine to improve educational quality: systematic review and case study of an online course in primary health care. BMJ 326:142–145.

Grimshaw JM 2003 Changing professional behaviour: empirical, theoretical and pragmantic perspectives. Australasian Cochrane Collaboration Course. Sydney, Australia.

Grimshaw JM, Shirran L, Thomas R et al 2001 Changing provider behaviour: an overview of systematic reviews of interventions. Medical Care 39(8):II-2–II-45.

Gross PA, Greenflield S, Cretin S et al 2001 Optimal methods for guideline implementation: conclusions from Leeds Castle meeting. Medical Care 39(8):II-85–II-92.

Haynes RB 2001 Of studies, syntheses, synopses, and systems: the '4S' evolution of services for finding current best evidence. ACP Journal Club Mar–Apr 134:A11–A13.

Haynes RB, Devereaux PT, Guyatt GH 2002 Clinical expertise in the era of evidence based medicine and patient choice. Evidence-based Medicine 7:36–38.

Kunz R, Oxman A 1998 The unpredictability of the paradox: review of empirical comparisons of randomised and non-randomised clinical trials. BMJ 317:1185–1190.

Lambert H, McKevitt K 2002 Anthropology in health research: from qualitative methods to multidisciplinarity. BMJ 325:210–213.

Long A, Harrison S 1996 The balance of evidence. Health Services Journal, Health Management Guide.

Marshall DC, Rossman DB 2006 Designing qualitative research. Thousand Oaks CA, Sage Publications.

Mays N, Pope C 2000 Assessing quality in qualitative research. BMJ 320:50–52.

Meyer J 2000 Using qualitative methods in health related action research. BMJ 320:178–181.

Mulrow CD 1994 Systematic reviews: rationale for systematic reviews. BMJ 309:597–599.

National Institute of Public Health (NIPH) 1996 First Annual Nordic Workshop on how to critically appraise and use evidence in decisions about healthcare. Oslo, Norway.

Oxman AD, Sackett DL, Guyatt GH 1993 Users' guide to the medical literature. I. How to get started. JAMA 270 (17):2093–2095.

Pomeroy VM, Tallis RC, Stitt E 2003 Dismantling some barriers to evidence-based rehabilitation with 'hands-on' clinical research secondments. Physiotherapy 89(5):266–275.

Pope C, Ziebland S, Mays, N 2000 Analysing qualitative data. BMJ 320:114–116.

Portney LG, Watkins MP (eds) 2000 Foundations of clinical research: applications to practice. 2nd edn. London, Prentice-Hall Health.

Roberts C, Torgerson D 1998 Randomisation methods in controlled trials. BMJ 317: 1301.

Research Committee (Victorian Branch) of the Australian Physiotherapy Association. 1999 Evidence-based practice. Australian Journal of Physiotherapy 45:167–171.

Sackett DL, Rosenberg WMC, Gray JAM, Richardson WS 1996 Evidence based medicine: what it is and what it isn't. BMJ 312:71–72.

Sackett DL, Richardson WS, Rosenberg WMC, Haynes RB 1997 Evidence-based medicine: how to practice and teach EBM. London, Churchill-Livingstone.

Sitthi–amorn C, Poashyachinda V 1993 Bias. Lancet 342(2):286–288.

Strauss A, Corbin J 1998 Basics of qualitative research. Thousand Oaks CA, Sage Publications.

Other resources

Clinical guidelines

See National Guidelines for the Therapeutic Management of Disease States (http://www.ukmicentral.nhs.uk)

Critical appraisal questions for different types of research

www.cebm.net/critical_appraisal.asp.

Effective health care bulletins

Implementation of evidence discussions http://www.york.ac.uk/inst/crd/ehcb.htm

Evaluating quality of primary research of systematic reviews

http://www.phru.nhs.uk/casp/critical_appraisal_tools.htm#s/reviews

Evidence-based texts

http://www.clinicalevidence.com
http://www.EffectiveStrokeCare.org

How to find the evidence – the basics in a 90-minute tutorial

http://www.shef.ac.uk/scharr/reswce/reswce3.htm

Nursing and allied health tutorial – what is evidence-based practice?
http://www.mdx.ac.uk/www/rctsh/ebp/main.htm

Levels of evidence
Centre for Evidence Based Medicine: www.cebm.net/levels_of_evidence.asp
Scottish Intercollegiate Guidelines Network (SIGN):
www.sign.ac.uk/guidelines/fulltext/50/index.html

OVID – How to search using OVID – an online tutorial
http://www.mclibrary.duke.edu/training/ovid

Synopses
See Centre for Review and Dissemination (www.crd.york.ac.uk/crdweb), including:
DARE (Database of abstracts of reviews of effects)
NHS Economic evaluation database (NHS EED)
Health technology assessment (HTA) database
American College of Physicians (ACP) Journal Club

Synthesis of primary studies (systematic reviews)
See The Cochrane Library: http://www.cochrane.org/reviews
Physiotherapy evidence database (PEDro). (http://www.pedro.fhs.usyd.edu.au/)

CHAPTER 2

Ensuring patient- and carer-centred care

Anne-Marie Laverty, Zena Jones and Helen Rodgers

INTRODUCTION

Patient and carer involvement is a key component of high quality neurological rehabilitation with benefits to patients, carers, therapists and health services (Department of Health 1999) (Box 2.1). Participation of patients and carers enables the planning, development, delivery and evaluation of services that are effective and responsive to diverse needs (Commission for Health Improvement 2004). The opinions and ideas of patients and carers should be taken into account in order to optimize rehabilitation and support. Enabling patients and carers to be actively involved in these activities is a core skill for neurological physiotherapists and the rehabilitation team.

Although this chapter uses examples from stroke rehabilitation, the general principles and best practice described apply to all patients and carers regardless of the underlying condition.

THEORETICAL FRAMEWORK FOR SERVICE USER PARTICIPATION

There are a range of approaches to patient and carer involvement, for example Wilcox (1994) describes five key levels of participation (Box 2.2). Other theoretical frameworks see patient and carer involvement as a continuum from simply providing information/explanation to consultation through to partnership and service user control (Hickey & Kipping 1998).

These frameworks suggest that different types of involvement are appropriate to different situations, and that one type is not inherently better than another. In a therapist- or service-centred perspective, patients and carers are encouraged to feedback ideas but control lies with the therapist or organization who ultimately decides if, and how the information is used. In a person-centred perspective, power is shifted away from the therapist or organization to the service user who is directly involved in decision making and planning.

Box 2.1 The benefits of patient and carer involvement (extracted from Department of Health 1999, with permission).

● The individual's perspective

'... patients and carers are the 'experts' in how they feel and what it is like to live with or care for someone with a particular illness or condition. ... It lies at the heart of providing quality services.'

● Improving services

'Involving service users and carers is an important part of improving service quality in the NHS. ... Such approaches have often helped to make services both more responsive and cost effective.

By involving users and carers during planning and development, there is less risk of providing inappropriate services and more chance of services being provided in the way people want them.'

● Improving public understanding

'Greater openness, accountability and involvement of the public should all help to create a better understanding of complex NHS and health issues. Effective public consultation and engagement can help to strengthen public confidence in the NHS.'

● Improving health

'When people are involved in and can influence decisions, which directly affect their lives, their self-esteem and self-confidence increases and this in turn improves health and well-being.'

PROMOTING INVOLVEMENT IN CARE

Patient-centred care has various definitions and represents an approach which is sensitive to the needs, expectations and wishes of patients and carers (Verwey & Crystal 1998). The views and values of patients and carers need to be considered alongside clinical evidence and professional judgement. (See Fig. 2.1.)

The rehabilitation team, patient and carer aim to find common ground about an issue and potential treatments or solutions. Although patient-centred care is not a new concept, it is increasingly evidence based, with studies showing improvements in quality of life and satisfaction with care, increased engagement, and reduced anxiety (Stewart 2001). An approach which recognizes the values of the patient and their family, and enables them to express their wishes, is likely to result in a plan of care which will have the best outcomes for all concerned (Department of Health 2004).

Box 2.2 Levels of patient and carer involvement (modified from Wilcox 1994 with permission; see reference for online source).

---

1. Supporting independent initiatives

The physiotherapist/rehabilitation team help patients and carers to achieve what they want perhaps within a framework of professional advice, support and grants.

2. Acting together

Patients, carers and the physiotherapist/rehabilitation team decide together what is best and form a partnership to carry it out.

3. Deciding together

The physiotherapist/rehabilitation team encourage patients and carers to provide some additional ideas and options, and join in deciding the best way forward.

4. Consultation

The physiotherapist/rehabilitation team offer a number of options and listen to the feedback.

5. Information

The physiotherapist/rehabilitation team tell patients and carers what is planned.

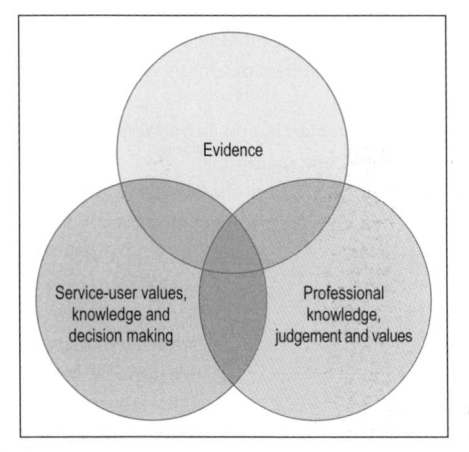

Figure 2.1
Concepts in patient-centred care.

Patient involvement in goal setting

'We need and want to monitor our own health. We need an annual review to help us do this and to look at things like blood pressure, and mobility. This yearly review should be comprehensive and take into account financial pressures and emotional strain' (a carer from a Stroke Patient Reference Group, 2006).

Collaborative communication and involvement of patients and caregivers in deciding on treatment priorities, and setting their own rehabilitation goals, leads to improvements in self care and satisfaction with services (Blair 1995, Huby et al 2004). Although neurological therapists support the principle of patient and carer involvement in goal setting and believe that outcomes will be improved with increased participation, a UK survey found that the shift from a passive patient role to one of true partnership is not embedded in everyday practice: a little over half of the neurological rehabilitation therapists provided patients with a record of their treatment goals, and 30% did not routinely involve patients in the evaluation process (Holliday et al 2005). The 2004 National Sentinel Audit for Stroke found that 67% of patients had rehabilitation goals agreed by a multidisciplinary team (Hoffman et al 2004). It is clear that more needs to be done to enable therapists to actively involve those patients and carers who wish to participate in the goal-setting process. Good practice in goal setting has been identified in Box 2.3 (Sobel et al 1998).

Enabling meaningful discussion and involvement in care

Clinician style is one of the most powerful predictors of motivation for behaviour change. It is important that all members of the rehabilitation team are aware that their behaviour has an impact on the individual patient's motivation both positively and negatively (Maclean et al 2002).

Active patient and carer involvement in rehabilitation involves the therapist being collaborative, enquiring, respectful and non judgemental about the views of the patient and their family and flexible in their approach (see also Chapter 3). The 2006 Commission for Healthcare Audit and Inspection report on stroke found that nearly 20% of patients felt that they had not been involved at all about decisions in their care and treatment.

The importance of information provision: an example from stroke care

Patients and carers consistently identify poor information provision and lack of appreciation of the emotional consequences of stroke as issues which stroke services need to address (Rodgers et al 2001). Information provision is often based upon what professionals think patients and carers want to know rather than what patients and carers believe is important. Passive provision of information, e.g. giving patients and carers leaflets, is widely used in clinical practice but is not

Box 2.3 Good practice in patient-centred goal setting (Sobel et al 1998, with permission). Copyright © 1996, 1998 by David Sobel MD and Robert Ornstein PhD, Mind & Body Health Handbook (Los Altos, CA: DRx).

√ Establish how the individual wishes to participate in goal setting and action planning.

√ Explore all options available.

√ Focus on the individual's concerns and interests.

√ Elicit the patient's perspective; e.g. 'What do you think may be causing this problem?'.

√ Collaborate with the patient, carer, family and others to agree goals that the individual wants and is ready to do.

√ Explore ambivalence: 'What might be some reasons not to change that?'

√ Present choices: 'There are several options – which one do you prefer?'

√ Identify reasonable goals i.e. something they could expect to do that week.

√ Enhance confidence by selecting goals that promote successful actions.

√ Be specific – goals that can answer the questions What? How much? When? How often?

√ Explain/explore additional goals not mentioned by the patient that may be relevant.

√ State goals and teach back: 'So that I am sure I have explained myself properly, can you tell me what you are going to do next?'

√ Provide a record of agreed goals in a manner that is consistent with their level of understanding.

√ Check results – involve the service user in the evaluative process.

√ Use problem solving to overcome obstacles.

√ Adjust as needed to ensure success.

associated with improved outcomes, yet an educational approach based upon the principles of adult learning where patients and carers are helped to develop problem-solving and practical skills may be effective (Forster et al 2001). Box 2.4 identifies key features to consider when preparing information.

In addition to unmet information needs, carers may feel poorly prepared for their new role and experience social isolation and reduced self care (Robinson et al 2005). The 2004 National Sentinel Audit for Stroke found that clinicians did not give sufficient time and care to involving patients and carers in their treatment; less than half of carers had their needs assessed separately (Hoffman et al 2004). One suggestion is to provide carers with skills training. Kalra et al (2004) has demonstrated that a structured training programme for carers to enable them to

Box 2.4 Features of quality information provision (adapted from Skills for Health 2006, with permission). The following is taken from a workshop held by Skills for Health (SFH) and the Patient Information Forum (PiF) in 2006 to inform development of National Occupational Standards for Patient Education.

- All service users and their carers should receive information, repeated as often as necessary, that is consistent with their:
  - level of understanding
  - culture and background
  - preferred method of communicating
  - needs.
- Support verbal information with written information or diagrammatic material, with adherence to health literacy guidelines.
- Consult with service users and their carers on the relevance, suitability and completeness of materials to meet their individual needs.
- Make information freely available to individuals and their families in a variety of languages and formats specific to needs.
- Determine the optimum methods, and locations for these materials ensuring availability of access.
- Service users and their carers should be offered the opportunity to attend education programmes to assist them in adapting to their new roles.
- Improve and increase provision of training and education for all staff (e.g. in facilitating communication, information provision and disability and diversity training).
- All staff involved in patient education should be able to demonstrate the relevant skills and competencies for effective communication/information provision.

have the skills needed to look after someone with a stroke, reduced carers' anxiety and depression and improved patients' psychological outcomes.

INVOLVE: an example of good practice

Patients and carers have tended to be viewed as passive recipients rather than as active participants who can make a valuable contribution to care (see Chapter 3 for more information). INVOLVE (see www.invo.org.uk) aims to improve patient, carer and public involvement in research. INVOLVE has produced guidelines and examples of best practice for researchers (Hanley et al 2003) and for members of the public (Royle et al 2001). It offers advice for researchers in involving the public at different stages of the research process on a range of issues: identifying and prioritizing topics, commissioning, designing research, interpretation, dissemination and evaluation of results.

A review by Oliver et al (2004) concluded that barriers to purposeful consumer involvement in research could 'largely be overcome with good leadership, purposeful outreach to consumers, investing time and effort in good communication, training and support and thereby building good working relationships and building on experience.' One example of surmounting these types of barriers is the ACT NoW study on communication therapy after stroke (Young et al 2007) which developed a research users' group to promote patient and carer involvement at all levels. A similar approach could be adopted for service delivery issues.

KEY CLINICAL MESSAGES

- Patient and carer involvement is valued by service users and improves clinical outcomes.
- Active involvement should be encouraged at all levels and at all stages of the rehabilitation process including research and service development.
- The perspective of the majority of patients and carers is 'nothing about us without us'.
- Health professionals, including neurological physiotherapists, need skills and training to ensure they can provide this vital component of health care.

References

Blair C 1995 Combining behaviour management and mutual goal setting to reduce physical dependency in nursing home residents. Nursing Research 44:160–165.

Commission for Healthcare Audit and Inspection 2006 Caring for people after they have had a stroke. A follow up survey of patients. London.

Commission for Health Improvement (CHI) 2004 Sharing the learning on patient and public involvement from CHI's work: i2i involvement to improvement. London: Commission for Health Improvement.

Department of Health 1999 Patient and public involvement in the new NHS London: HMSO.

Department of Health 2004 Patient and public involvement in health: the evidence for policy implementation. London: HMSO.

Forster A, Smith J, Young J et al 2001 Information provision for stroke patients and their caregivers. Cochrane Database of Systematic Reviews (3):CD001919.

Hanley B, Bradburn J, Barnes M et al 2003 Involving the public in NHS, public health and social care research: briefing notes for researchers (second edition). INVOLVE. Online. Available: http://www.invo.org.uk/pdfs/Briefing%20Note%20Final.dat.pdf.

Hickey G, Kipping C 1998 Exploring the concept of user involvement in mental health through a participation continuum. Journal of Clinical Nursing 7:83–88.

Hoffman A, Lowe D, Rudd A et al 2004 National Sentinel Stroke Audit. London: Royal College of Physicians.

Holliday R, Antoun M, Playford E D 2005 A survey of goal-setting methods used in rehabilitation. Neurorehabilitation and Neural Repair 19:228–231.

Huby G, Stewart J, Tierney A, Rogers W 2004 Planning older people's discharge from acute hospital care: linking risk management and patient participation in decision-making. Health, Risk and Society 6:115–132.

Kalra L, Evans A, Perez I et al 2004 Training carers of stroke patients: randomised controlled trial. British Medical Journal 328:1099–1104.

Maclean N, Pound P, Wolfe C et al 2002 The concept of patient motivation: a qualitative analysis of stroke professionals' attitudes. Stroke 33:444–448.

Oliver S, Clarke-Jones L, Rees R et al 2004 Involving consumers in research and development agenda setting for the NHS: developing an evidence-based approach. London: NHS R&D HTA Programme.

Robinson L, Francis J, James P et al 2005 Caring for carers of people with stroke: developing a complex intervention following the Medical Research Council framework. Clinical Rehabilitation 19:560–571.

Rodgers H, Bond S, Curless R 2001 Inadequacies in the provision of information to stroke patients and their families. Age and Ageing 30:129–133.

Royle J, Steel R, Hanley B et al 2001 Getting involved in research: a guide for consumers. Online. Available: http://www.invo.org.uk/pdfs/UserCon_Rptfinal%20web081205.pdf.

Skills for Health 2006 Available htpp://www.skillsforhealth.org.uk.

Sobel D, Ornstein R 1998 Mind and Body Health Handbook. Los Altos, CA: DRx.

Stewart M 2001 Towards a global definition of patient-centred care. British Medical Journal 322:444–445.

Verwey S, Crystal A 1998 A patient-centred approach to health care communication: the role of health communication. Communication 24:31–42.

Wilcox D 1994 The guide to effective participation project. Joseph Rowntree Foundation. Online. Available: http://www.partnerships.org.uk/guide

Young A, Pearl G, Lee J et al 2007 Assessing the effectiveness of communication therapy in the North West. Interim report. Online. Available: http://www.uksrn.ac.uk/images/files/involving_service_users_in_research.pdf.

The wider context of neurorehabilitation

Karen Whalley Hammell

INTRODUCTION

Research demonstrates that clients often perceive rehabilitation to be meaningless (Abberley 1995), decontextualized (French 2004) and irrelevant to their lives (Johnson 1993). This chapter examines how a client-centred approach to practice that is informed by both meaning and context can make rehabilitation relevant and useful to the lives of those with neurological impairments. Chapter 3 builds on concepts of evidence-based practice (Chapter 1) and of patient/carer perspectives (Chapter 2). It has two key aims:

- to explore the relevance of context and meaning to the neurorehabilitation process and to client-centred care;
- to explain the concept of client-centred care and its relevance to the rehabilitation process.

Should we refer to 'clients' or 'patients' in the context of rehabilitation? The term 'patients' suggests passivity and conveys the idea of recipients of treatments that are done to them (Hammell 2006). 'Client' is used throughout this chapter, in the absence of a more appropriate word.

THE CONCEPT AND RELEVANCE OF CONTEXT

This chapter is grounded in the belief that rehabilitation is a process of learning to live well with impairments in the context of one's own environment. Physiotherapists recognize that movement always occurs within a context (Cott et al 1995); the environmental context has many dimensions (CAOT 2002; see Box 3.1). The physical environment, for example, stimulates us to move; cultural values may prohibit the use of certain mobility aids; and the presence of family members in the physiotherapy department may induce a client to strive harder than when therapy is undertaken in social isolation.

The importance of context to human health and well-being, and the dynamic interactions that occur between people and their environments, have been acknowledged by the World Health Organization in the 'ICF': the International Classification of Functioning, Disability and Health (WHO 2001; see Box 3.2).

Box 3.1

Dimensions of the environment
- Physical (the natural and constructed environment).
- Cultural (the norms, values and practices arising from one's culture).
- Social (priorities and values associated with relationships).
- Economic (wealth distribution, financial priorities and supports).
- Legal (laws and legal services).
- Political (legislation, government services and policies).
- Institutional (organizational practices, policies and procedures).

Box 3.2

ICF Terminology
- Body functions and body structures
  Impairments are problems in body functions or structures
- Activities: the execution of a task or action by an individual
  Activity limitations are difficulties in executing a task or action
- Participation: involvement in a life situation
  Participation restrictions are problems an individual may have in involvement in life situations

---

The WHO developed the ICF to provide a framework for classifying human function that would enable the interactions between human ability and environmental context to be identified.

Because of the emphasis of the ICF (www.who.int/icf) on *activity* and *participation*, this model has been embraced by many therapists, who value its acknowledgement of issues that are central to rehabilitation. However, the ICF is just one model of health and disability (and not necessarily the one best suited to rehabilitation), but its widespread use internationally requires that all those engaged in the provision of health care are familiar with its principles. For further discussion of the ICF and alternative models for rehabilitation, see Fougeyrollas et al (2002) and Hammell (2004a).

THE CONCEPT AND RELEVANCE OF MEANING

The occurrence of a neurological impairment such as stroke, spinal cord injury or brain injury is not important solely because of the damage it wreaks on a physical body, but for the havoc it wreaks in a life. Morris (1991, p. 3), for instance, wrote that following her spinal cord injury: 'My terror was not about disability as such, but that I might have destroyed the structure of my life'. What rehabilitation clients want is help to manage their bodies so they can get on with their lives: the roles, relationships, valued routines and occupations that give meaning and purpose to existence and that contribute to life's quality.

Reynolds (2004, p. 111) explained: 'Medically similar illnesses may have widely different meanings and implications for individuals, depending upon their social context, personal priorities and resources'. For example, a 20-year-old man and a 70-year-old woman both have complete C6 spinal cord injuries. Although their neurological damage is very similar, their individual needs will not be met by adhering to a standard treatment protocol dictated by their neurological deficits. Rather, rehabilitation interventions will be tailor-made to address priorities informed by their interests, personal, cultural and social values, life-stage, family situation, economic supports, legal and political context (e.g. rights to access transportation, educational and employment opportunities) and the natural and constructed physical environments in which they live. A rehabilitation process that enables each client to live a meaningful life in their chosen environments will be a dynamic process; one that is as concerned with teaching the therapist about the meaning, consequences and significance of an impairment for the individual's life as it is about teaching the client about how to live well with a neurological impairment (Hammell 2004b).

CLIENT-CENTRED PRACTICE

Client-centred practice is an approach to rehabilitation that seeks to respect clients' right to autonomy (the ability to act on choices and to be in control of one's own life (French 2004). Client-centred practice has specific characteristics (Cott 2004, Hammell 2006, Law et al 1995, MacDonald et al 2001, Sumsion & Law 2006; see Box 3.3).

Therapists who aspire to client-centred practice will not tell a client that they must not get into the bath, for example, but will respect the client's expressed wish to do so, state their concerns about safety and assist the client to consider how any problems might be dealt with, should these arise (Hammell 2004b). Research has shown that physical function does not have a demonstrable effect on quality of life, and the ability and opportunity to make choices and exert control over one's life is a positive contributor to perceptions of quality of life following neurological injury (Hammell 2004c). There is also an association between perceptions of reduced control and low life satisfaction (Hammell 2004c).

Of central importance are the therapist's interpersonal qualities (Bibyk et al 1999, Blank 2004, French 2004, Johnson 1993, Marquis & Jackson 2000, Reynolds 2004), which clients view as more important than their technical or practical expertise (French 2004, Marquis & Jackson 2000; Box 3.4).

Box 3.3

Characteristics of client-centred practice
- Respect for clients' values, priorities and perspectives
- Respect for clients' autonomy and rights to choose and enact choices
- Seeks to realign and equalize power between therapist and client
- Provides client-orientated information to enable informed choices
- Enables clients to identify their priorities, needs and goals
- Facilitates client participation in the rehabilitation process
- Strives for collaboration and partnership in achieving clients' goals
- Individualizes service delivery
- Assesses the achievement of outcomes that matter to the client
- Focuses on ensuring that service provision is useful and relevant

---

Box 3.4

Examples of interpersonal qualities valued by clients
- Respect
- Acceptance
- Genuineness
- Empathy
- Openness
- Equality
- A 'caring' rather than a 'professional' manner

Research demonstrates clearly that these qualities also have an important impact on outcomes such as client self-esteem (French 2004, Marquis & Jackson 2000) and motivation (French 2004, Johnson 1993).

Applying client-centred practice to the rehabilitation process

In the assessment phase, therapists enable clients to identify their problems, prioritize their needs and catalogue their skills and resources (Law et al 1995). Client-centred assessment requires client-focused tools, such as those developed by Law et al (2005) and Stratford et al (1995), and not generic forms.

During the intervention planning phase, the therapist provides sufficient breadth and depth of information to enable clients to establish meaningful, relevant and achievable goals (Law et al 1995, MacDonald et al 2001). The client-centred therapist adopts a role, not as prescriber/dictator, but as collaborator/enabler. Intervention is the process of implementing plans; therapists maximize both their own skills and resources and those of the client in striving to achieve the client's goals (Law et al 1995).

When evaluating rehabilitation outcomes, client-centred practice emphasizes outcomes that assess the effect of interventions on issues of importance to clients' lives (Guyatt et al 1997). Research evidence demonstrates clearly the positive impact of client-centred practice on outcomes such as clients' satisfaction and symptoms (Ford et al 2003, Guadagnoli & Ward 1998), functional abilities (Maitra & Erway 2006, Neistadt 1995), commitment to therapy (Ford et al 2003, Maitra & Erway 2006) and length of stay (Guadagnoli & Ward 1998, Neistadt 1995).

SUMMARY

Evidence outlined in this chapter demonstrates that client-centred practice is an effective way of meeting clients' needs and goals. It is because human function is indivisible from the environmental context in which it occurs that therapy interventions must be informed by the meaning of impairments in the context of each individual's life, in a client-centred approach to practice that informs every phase of the rehabilitation process.

References

Abberley P 1995 Disabling ideology in health and welfare: the case of occupational therapy. Disability and Society 10(2):221–232.

Bibyk B, Day DG, Morris L et al 1999 Who's in charge here? The client's perspective on client-centred care. OT Now Sept/Oct:11–12.

Blank A 2004 Clients' experience of partnership with occupational therapists in community mental health. British Journal of Occupational Therapy 67(3):118–124.

Canadian Association of Occupational Therapists (CAOT) 2002 Enabling occupation. An occupational therapy perspective, 2nd edn, CAOT, Ottawa.

Cott CA 2004 Client-centred rehabilitation: client perspectives. Disability and Rehabilitation 26(24):1411–1422.

Cott CA, Finch E, Gasner D et al 1995 The movement continuum theory of physical therapy. Physiotherapy Canada 47(2):87–95.

Ford S, Schofield T, Hope T 2003 What are the ingredients for a successful evidence-based patient choice consultation? A qualitative study. Social Science and Medicine 56:589–602.

Fougeyrollas P, Noreau L, Boschen K 2002 Interaction of environment with individual characteristics and social participation: theoretical perspectives and applications in persons with spinal cord injury. Topics in Spinal Cord Injury Rehabilitation 7(3):1–16.

French S 2004 Enabling relationships in therapy practice. In: Swain J, Clark J, Parry K et al (eds) Enabling relationships in health and social care. Butterworth-Heinemann, Oxford, pp 95–107.

Guadagnoli E, Ward P 1998 Patient participation in decision-making. Social Science and Medicine 47(3):329–339.

Guyatt GH, Naylor CD, Juniper E, Heyland DK, Jaeschke R, Cook DJ for the Evidence-Based Medicine Working Group 1997 Users' guide to the medical literature XII. How to use articles about health-related quality of life. Journal of the American Medical Association 277(15):1232–1237.

Hammell KW 2004a Deviating from the norm: a sceptical interrogation of the ICF. British Journal of Occupational Therapy 67(9):408–411.

Hammell KW 2004b The rehabilitation process. In: Stokes M (ed) Physical management in neurological rehabilitation, 2nd ed. Elsevier, Edinburgh, pp 379–392.

Hammell KW 2004c Exploring quality of life following high spinal cord injury: a review and critique. Spinal Cord 42(9):491–502.

Hammell KW 2006 Perspectives on disability and rehabilitation. Contesting assumptions; challenging practice. Elsevier, Edinburgh.

Johnson R 1993 'Attitudes don't just hang in the air . . .': Disabled people's perceptions of physiotherapists. Physiotherapy 79(9):619–627.

Law M, Baptiste S, Mills J 1995 Client-centred practice: what does it mean and does it make a difference? Canadian Journal of Occupational Therapy 62:250–257.

Law M, Baptiste S, Carswell A et al 2005 Canadian Occupational Performance Measure, 4th edn. CAOT Publications ACE, Ottawa.

MacDonald C, Houghton P, Cox P, Bartlett D 2001 Consensus on physical therapy professional behaviours. Physiotherapy Canada, Summer:212–218, 222.

Maitra KK, Erway F 2006 Perception of client-centred practice in occupational therapists and their clients. American Journal of Occupational Therapy 60(3):298–310.

Marquis R, Jackson R 2000 Quality of life and quality of service relationships: experiences of people with disabilities. Disability and Society 15(3):411–425.

Morris J 1991 Pride against prejudice. Transforming attitudes to disability. The Women's Press, London.

Neistadt M 1995 Methods of assessing clients' priorities: a survey of adult physical dysfunction. American Journal of Occupational Therapy 49(5):428–436.

Reynolds F 2004 Two-way communication. In: Swain J, Clark J, Parry K et al (eds) Enabling relationships in health and social care. Butterworth-Heinemann, Oxford, pp 109–130.

Stratford P, Gill C, Westaway M, Binkley J 1995 Assessing disability and change on individual patients: a report of a patient-specific measure. Physiotherapy Canada 47(4):258–262.

Sumsion T, Law M 2006 A review of evidence on the conceptual elements informing client-centred practice. Canadian Journal of Occupational Therapy 73(3):153–162.

World Health Organization (WHO) 2001 International Classification of Functioning, Disability and Health. WHO, Geneva.

CHAPTER 4

Motor control

Patricia Bate

INTRODUCTION

Understanding of the processes by which the motor control system (MCS) generates movements can guide therapists in the design of rehabilitation programs. The MCS can often generate functional actions in the presence of neural damage, but final outcomes may be improved by movement re-training. Therapists aim to optimize the person's capacity for action and to minimize the effects of reduced mobility and inactivity.

This chapter outlines the major classes of theories describing how actions are generated, lists properties and principles of the MCS and illustrates these for three tasks: reaching and grasping an object, maintaining stability in standing, and locomotion. The motor roles of major neural circuits, effects of lesions, and the implications for physiotherapy, are summarized.

THEORIES OF MOTOR CONTROL

The versatility of the MCS allows it to generate actions in different ways to match various circumstances. This diversity is reflected in a multiplicity of theories of motor control, outlined in Box 4.1 (Shumway-Cook & Woollacott 2007, pp. 27–32).

PRINCIPLES OF MOTOR CONTROL

Principles and properties of movement generation which may guide rehabilitation are listed in Box 4.2.

Reaching to grasp

Visual exploration generates cues which control action. Prior to, and during reach visual information is conducted from the primary visual cortex to the posterior parietal cortex, where it is matched to motor information so that the hand can meet the target (Castiello 2005). The trajectory of the hand is determined by the relative positions of target and hand (Desmurget et al 1998). Other cues defining properties such as size of the contact surface, texture and weight, determine hand shape and grasp force.

Box 4.1

Theories of motor control
- **Reflex theories** – describe movement as a series of reactions to preceding sensory stimuli (Bate 1997).
- **Hierarchical theories** – emphasize the contributions of circuits at different levels of the CNS (Bate 1997).
- **Motor programming theories** – propose rules to simplify generation of actions; termed 'motor programmes' (MP) (Keele et al 1990).
- **Dynamic action theories** – propose actions emerging from interaction between components of the MCS without requiring instructions or commands (Turvey et al 1982).
- **Ecological theories** – emphasize detection of the information in the environment which guides actions (Gibson 1979; Kugler & Turvey 1988).
- **Systems theory** – proposes movement is organized around a behavioural goal, and emerges from interaction between the individual, the task and the environment (Shumway-Cook & Woollacott 2007, pp. 4–5).

Stability in standing

To maintain standing the MCS must align body parts, support the body in relation to gravity and other external forces, and stabilize supporting parts of the body while other parts move (Ghez 1991c). In quiet standing alignment is primarily maintained by passive mechanisms such as ligaments, joints and bony mortices. Sway is detected by sensory systems and appropriate motor commands are generated to stabilize the body's orientation; i.e. feedback mechanisms may utilize visual, vestibular, proprioceptive or tactile information (Shumway-Cook & Woollacott 2007, pp. 176–180). Stability is enhanced by anticipatory ('feedforward') mechanisms: e.g. muscle stiffness is set by descending signals at levels that will limit postural sway, and effects of the reaction forces produced by arm movements are anticipated to regulate position of the centre of mass (COM) (Patla 2003). It seems likely that stretch reflexes at the ankle, and possibly other joints, assist in controlling sway in quiet standing. Muscle stiffness or length can be set by descending signals to the alpha-gamma motor neurone pool, which controls the sensitivity of intrafusal fibres. These nuclear bag and chain receptors transduce muscle length and rate of change of length. If these values do not match those set by the descending tracts the alpha motoneurons supplying homologous extrafusal fibres are activated, and antagonist muscles inhibited, through the stretch reflex arc.

Box 4.2

Properties and principles of the motor control system

● Actions are organized to achieve functions such as eating and socializing. Actions are complex movements to which we can easily attribute a purpose (rarely involving just a single joint).
● The components of the MCS include bones, soft tissues, neural networks, physical and social aspects of the environment.
● The MCS adapts very quickly. Lack of opportunity for motor exploration and activity leads to atrophy of muscle, shortening of soft tissues, and modification of neural networks (Nudo et al 2001).
● If some components of the MCS ('degrees of freedom' – Bernstein 1967) are unavailable or damaged, actions may be configured in a different way.
● Ability to detect and discriminate environmental features such as the position and properties of an object may determine skill level (Gibson 1979).
● Actions may be organized for efficiency:
    ● to minimize energy use, effort, or torque change,
    ● to maximize smoothness of trajectory,
    ● to distribute movement among all available joints (Gielen et al 1995).
● Many neural networks participate in any action; it is inaccurate to attribute motor abilities to individual locations in the nervous system.
● Generation of actions can be simplified by activating stored rules e.g. motor programmes (Keele et al 1990).
● In repetitive actions like walking, 'Central Pattern Generators' (CPGs) behave like motor programmes (Mackay-Lyons 2002). CPGs in the spinal cord can rhythmically generate alternating ('coupled') contractions of flexor and extensor muscles; the left and right legs can also be coupled in this way (Dietz 2002).

Locomotion

In locomotion the COM is maintained above a moving base of support (BOS) which changes size and shape. To initiate gait the COM moves towards the support side before the first step (Jian et al 1993). When configured for locomotion, the MCS acts predictively to compensate for expected perturbations to balance (Patla 1998). For example, a change of direction while walking is planned during the previous step (Patla et al 1991). The MCS also counters potential perturbations that are anticipated by interpreting visual input. For example, if you see that the floor ahead is slippery you may step slowly and contact with a flat foot in order to avoid slipping. Visual information also determines velocity of locomotion (Warren & Hannon 1988). The acquisition of relevant visual information is such an integral part of locomotion function that adjustments of gait are more effective if an obstacle is observed while walking towards it than if the person observes while stationary (Thomson 1980).

Errors can be corrected through spinal circuitry. Consider the reactive control (Patla 2003) that operates if your toe catches on a stone during swing phase: e.g. the MCS organizes so that body parts return to their original trajectory. The tendons lying over the ankle are lengthened and the resulting muscle contractions increase stiffness around the ankle within 40 to 50 ms. Long latency, central feedback loops alter foot placement for the next several steps to reposition the BOS under the COM.

MAJOR CIRCUITS OF THE MOTOR CONTROL SYSTEM

Key brain structures include the cortex, the basal ganglia (BG), the diencephalon (thalamus/hypothalamus), the cerebellum, the brainstem and the spinal cord. Figure 4.1 shows major neural pathways of the motor control system. The thalamus is a major relay station receiving information from all sensory systems and other brain areas.

The three motor circuits of the BG (Kingsley 2000) appear to enable changes in motor sets (Monchi et al 2006). The circuits all include the thalamus which has excitatory effects on the cerebral cortex. Examining the excitatory and inhibitory natures of the synapses demonstrated in Figure 4.1, it can be seen that (1) lesions of the direct pathway lead to excessive inhibition of the thalamus by the BG and hence reduce the amount of movement generated (hypokinesia), (2) lesions of the indirect pathway reduce inhibition received by the thalamus leading to exaggerated movement (hyperkinesia), and (3) lesions of the dopaminergic pathway lead to over-inhibition of thalamus: movements are slow, rigid and often tremulant (Van Emmerik et al 1999).

The cerebellum also contributes to motor control through three circuits. The spinocerebellar circuit generates online corrections of evolving actions, particularly of proximal and axial body parts, supporting the body in standing. The vestibulocerebellar circuit controls posture and orientation in space and resists gravity. The cerebrocerebellar circuit seems to act like a 'feedforward controller': it stores an internal model of the body and uses this to generate predictive modifications of distal circuits (Bastian et al 2000).

Table 4.1 summarizes the motor roles of major neural circuits and the effects of lesions.

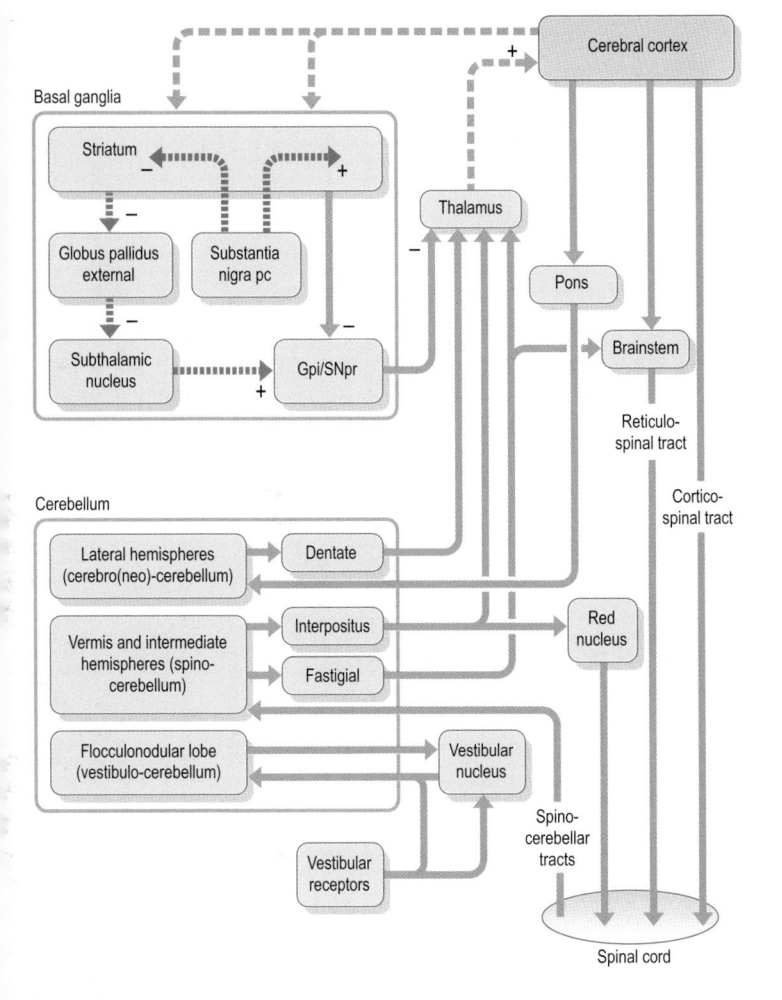

Figure 4.1
Descending tracts of the central nervous system, and circuits of the basal ganglia and cerebellum. Circuits of the basal ganglia: direct circuit – solid blue line; indirect circuit – dotted grey lines; dopaminergic circuit – dotted blue lines. (After Alexander & Crutcher 1990, Ghez 1991b.) Gpi = Globus pallidus internal segment; SNpr = Substantia nigra pars reticulata; Substantia nigra pc (SNpc) = Substantia nigra pars compacta.

Table 4.1 Major pathways of the motor control system (taken from Barker et al 2003, Ghez 1991a, Kingsley 2000, Martini 2004, Zigmond et al 1998).

Circuit or pathway	Features/roles in movement generation	Effects of lesions
• Dorsal column • Anterior spinothalamic tract • Lateral spinothalamic tract • Spinoreticular division	• Fine tactile, 2 pt discrimination, vibratory, proprioceptive info. • Crude touch and pressure, tickle, itch. • Nociception and temperature. • Arousal and emotional responses to sensory stimuli.	• Lesions of ascending sensory tracts: contralateral loss of touch, proprioception, nociception and temperature sensation.
• Somatosensory cortex (S1) • Prefrontal cortex (PFC)	• Modality mapping. • Selects appropriate motor response for context. Anticipates and stimulates actions with basal ganglia (BG).	• Impairment of contralateral sensation. • Problem with goal directed movement and storage of spatial information.
• Supplementary motor area (SMA)	• Planning and initiation of complex movement sequences and bimanual tasks. Generates the postural components of an activity. Learning new tasks.	• Apraxia (disorder of skilled movement), mirroring. Problem using internal cues for action. Bilateral lesion: akinesia.
• Premotor cortex (PMC)	• Planning of complex acts. Learning new tasks. May store/control skilled movements.	• Mild paresis. Problem using external cues for action.
• Posterior parietal cortex	• Integrates multimodal sensory information. Links perception and action. Dominant: language; non-dominant: spatial.	• Neglect of stimuli on contralateral side of body (non-dominant hemisphere). Astereognosis (loss of object recognition by touch). Apraxia (dominant hemisphere).
• Primary motor cortex (M1)	• Active prior to movement; and during delicate and precise movements by distal muscles.	• Weakness and clumsiness. Loss of independent finger movements.
• BG–cortex circuit: direct • BG–cortex circuit: indirect	• Enables actions. • Slows or stops actions.	• Hypokinesia (slow, low amplitude actions). • Hyperkinesia (superfluous, fast, jerky or writhing actions).
• BG–cortex circuit: dopaminergic	• Initiation and agility of action.	• Actions may fail to initiate or stop mid action (freezing); often tremorous.

Spinocerebellar and cuneocerebellar circuits	• Online corrections of evolving actions. Supports body in standing.	• Ipsilateral hypotonia, ataxia of limb and eye movements. Cannot correct error. Ataxic gait and stance.
Vestibulocerebellar circuit	• Controls posture and orientation in space. Resists gravity.	• Truncal ataxia; ataxic stance and gait.
Cerebrocerebellar circuit	• Predictively modifies motor signals. Maintains internal model of the body.	• Intention tremor. Failure to adapt.
Vestibulo-ocular circuit	• Stabilizes gaze during head movement.	• Loss of visual tracking, abnormal vestibulo-ocular reflex
Corticobulbarspinal tract (CBST)	• Excites distal muscles and proximal flexor muscles. Mediates dextrous hand and finger movements.	• UMN syndrome (paresis, hyperactive stretch reflexes, sensory loss).
Rubrospinal tract (RT)	• Contributes to movements of arm, hand and fingers.	• **Lesion of RT/ RST:** UMN syndrome (see lesion of CBST).
Vestibulospinal tract (VST)	• Resists gravity. Controls posture and orientation in space. Facilitates extensor muscles (lateral VST). Facilitates neck muscles (medial VST).	• **Lesion of VST/TST:** Postural instability. Weakness of antigravity actions.
Reticulospinal tract (RST)	• Postural functions. Facilitates proximal and flexor muscles (lateral RST). Facilitates proximal and extensor muscles (medial RST).	
Tectospinal tract (TST)	• Generates reflexive changes in position of head in response to bright lights, sudden movements and loud noises.	
Alpha-gamma linkage	• Inputs determine muscle resting length and stiffness, the gain of spinal feedback loops, and drive actions.	• Signs of spasticity, paresis and ataxia; exaggerated stretch reflexes, clasp knife, clonus, pendular reflexes.

UMN, upper motor neurone.

Box 4.3

Implications for physiotherapy

- Re-training may be most effective if actions are practised in functional contexts.
- Rehabilitation should include assessment and support of the patient's ability to detect and utilize information from the environment to guide action (Newell 1991).
- Rehabilitation should ensure a patient can organize actions to meet task requirements (Carr & Shepherd 2003, pp. 21–24).
- Physiotherapists can change the environment in such a way that the interaction of the patient with the environment elicits the required action. For example, the patient could practise producing an accurate wrist trajectory by reaching for a fragile vase and practise generating a smooth trajectory by carrying a full cup.
- The biomechanical environment can be changed by lengthening tight structures and strengthening weak muscles (Kugler & Turvey 1988).
- The cognitive environment can be changed by instructions and verbal feedback (Carr & Shepherd 2003, pp. 15–20).
- All the components of the MCS must be considered in designing rehabilitation. Each patient's motor disorder must be individually assessed.
- Early activity after a lesion may minimize undesirable effects of rest on the damaged motor control system (Nudo et al 2001).
- The concept of the MP allows physiotherapists to predict conditions under which rules for actions could be learned (Shumway-Cook & Woollacott 2007, pp. 11–17).
- The concept of the CPG suggests it may be possible to facilitate action of paretic limbs by eliciting repetitive, coupled actions from other limbs (Mackay-Lyons 2002).
- Rehabilitation of prehension should include training to grasp objects of various properties at various positions in space (Carr and Shepherd 2003, pp. 159–206).
- Rehabilitation of standing and gait should include training the activation of postural muscles prior to expected perturbations, and extraction of pertinent information from the visual environment (Patla 1998).
- Training strategies should include opportunity to explore (Newell 1991).

SUMMARY

Therapists aim to optimize the person's capacity for action and to minimize the effects of reduced mobility and inactivity. Understanding how actions are generated suggests strategies for rehabilitation of movement capacity in people with lesions of the central nervous system. Implications for physiotherapy are presented in Box 4.3. Physiotherapists should utilize functional contexts and address the roles of the external physical environment, biomechanical factors and patients' abilities to detect visual cues in movement generation.

References

Alexander GE, Crutcher MD 1990 Functional architecture of basal ganglia circuits: neural substrates of parallel processing. Trends in Neurosciences 13(7):266–271.

Barker RA, Barasi S, Neal MJ 2003 Neuroscience at a glance. Blackwell Publishing, Manchester.

Bate P 1997 Motor control theory: insights for physiotherapists. Physiotherapy 83(8):397–405.

Bastian AJ, Zackowski KM, Thach WT 2000 Cerebellar ataxia: torque deficiency or torque mismatch between joints. Journal of Neurophysiology 83(5):3019–3030.

Bernstein NA 1967 The coordination and regulation of movement. Pergamon Press, Oxford.

Carr J, Shepherd R 2003 Stroke rehabilitation. Butterworth-Heinemann, Oxford.

Castiello U 2005 The neuroscience of grasping. Nature Reviews Neuroscience 6:726–736.

Desmurget M, Pelisson D, Rosetti Y et al 1998 From eye to hand: planning goal-directed movements. Neuroscience and Biobehavioral Reviews 22(6):761–788.

Dietz V 2002 Do human bipeds use quadripedal coordination? Trends in Neurosciences 25(9): 462–467.

Ghez C 1991a Voluntary Movement. In: Kandel ER, Schwartz JA Jessell TM (eds) Principles of neural science, 3rd edn. Elsevier, New York, pp 610–625.

Ghez C 1991b The cerebellum. In: Kandel ER, Schwartz JA Jessell TM (eds) Principles of neural science, 3rd edn. Elsevier, New York, pp 627–646.

Ghez C 1991c Posture. In: Kandel ER, Schwartz JA Jessell TM (eds) Principles of neural science, 3rd edn. Elsevier, New York, pp 596–606.

Gibson JJ 1979 An ecological approach to visual perception. Houghton Mifflin, Boston.

Gielen CCAM, van Bolhuis BM, Theeuwen M 1995 On the control of biologically and kinematically redundant manipulators. Human Movement Science 14(4–5):487–509.

Jian Y, Winter DA, Ishac MG et al 1993 Trajectory of the body COG and COP during initiation and termination of gait. Gait & Posture 1(1):9–22.

Keele SW, Cohen A, Ivry R 1990 Motor programs: concepts and issues. Attention and Performance 13:77–110.

Kingsley R.E 2000. Concise text of neuroscience, 2nd edn. Lippincott Williams and Wilkins, Philadelphia.

Kugler PN, Turvey MT 1988 Self-organization, flowfields and information. Human Movement Science 7(2–4):97–129.

MacKay-Lyons M 2002 Central pattern generation of locomotion: a review of the evidence. Physical Therapy 82(1):69–83.

Martini FH 2004 Fundamentals of anatomy and physiology, 6th edn. Pearson Education, United Kingdom.

Monchi O, Petrides M, Strafella AP et al 2006 Functional role of the basal ganglia in the planning and execution of actions. Annals of Neurology 59(2):257–264.

Newell KN 1991 Motor skill acquisition. Annual Review of Psychology 42:213–237.

Nudo RJ, Plautz EJ, Frost SB 2001 Role of adaptive plasticity in recovery of function after damage to motor cortex. Muscle Nerve 24(8):1000–1101.

Patla AE 1998 How is human gait controlled by vision? Ecological Psychology 10(3–4):287–302.

Patla AE 2003 Strategies for dynamic stability during adaptive human locomotion. IEEE Engineering in Medicine and Biology Magazine 22(2):48–52.

Patla AE, Prentice SD, Robinson C et al 1991 Visual control of locomotion – strategies for changing direction and going over obstacles. Journal of Human Perception and Performance 17(3):603–634.

Shumway-Cook A, Woollacott M H 2007 Motor control: translating research into clinical practice. Williams and Wilkins, Baltimore.

Thomson JA 1980 How do we use visual information to control locomotion? Trends in Neuroscience 3(10):247–250.

Turvey MT, Fitch HL, Tuller B 1982 The Bernstein Perspective. In: Kelso AS (ed) Human motor behavior: an introduction. Laurence Erlbaum Associates, New Jersey, pp 239–281.

Van Emmerik REA, Wagenaar RC, Winogrodzka A et al 1999 Identification of axial rigidity during locomotion in Parkinson's disease. Archives of Physical Medicine and Rehabilitation 80(2):186–191.

Warren WH, Hannon DJ 1988 Direction of self-motion is perceived from optical flow. Nature 336:162–163.

Zigmond MJ, Bloom FE, Landis SC 1998 Fundamental neuroscience. Academic Press, San Diego.

CHAPTER 5

Neural plasticity in motor learning and motor recovery

Jeffrey A Kleim

INTRODUCTION

Virtually all adult behaviour involves the expression of an acquired motor skill and consequently a large portion of the central nervous system (CNS) is devoted to the control of skilled movement (see Chapter 4). Motor learning can be defined as permanent changes in motor behaviour as a result of practice or learning (Schmidt 2000); practice, feedback and skill acquisition are key concepts of motor learning (see Carr & Shepherd 1998 and Gilmore & Spaulding 2001 for further information). The capacity to produce skilled movements is acquired through extensive practice and persists when training ceases, suggesting that motor skills are encoded as enduring neurobiological changes (neural plasticity) within motor areas of the CNS. A wealth of empirical evidence now exists showing that the acquisition of motor skill is supported by neural plasticity within various motor regions of the CNS (Adkins et al 2006).

Improvements in motor performance after brain damage through rehabilitation can be thought of as a motor relearning process whereby lost action patterns are restored and new compensatory action patterns are acquired to re-establish motor faculties. Furthermore, motor relearning following brain damage appears to be supported by neural plasticity within residual brain regions that resembles that seen in the intact brain during normal motor learning (Nudo 2003). Understanding the basic principles that govern neural plasticity may help to guide the development of novel rehabilitation interventions or optimize existing interventions to enhance motor recovery after brain damage (Kleim & Jones 2008).

NEURAL PLASTICITY

Neural plasticity can be loosely defined as any enduring changes in neurone structure or function. Plasticity can be observed at the level of individual neurones as changes in neuronal excitability, single unit activity, dendritic arborization, spine density or synapse number (Figure 5.1). These changes are indicative of changes in neural circuitry within specific brain areas. Plasticity can also be observed across large populations of neurones as changes in regional brain activity or reorganiza-

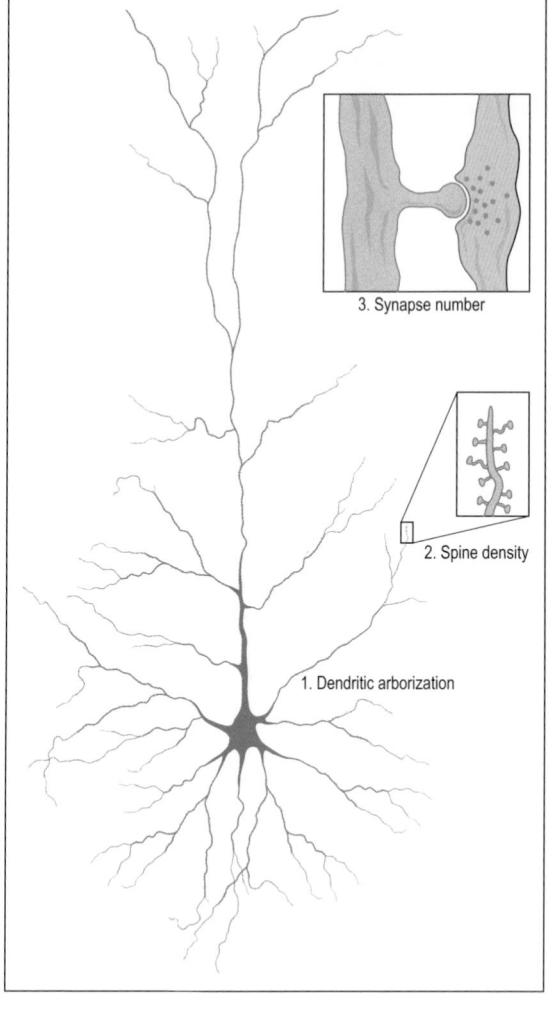

3. Synapse number

2. Spine density

1. Dendritic arborization

Figure 5.1
Examples of measures of neuronal plasticity observable at the level of individual neurones.
Plastic changes in neuronal morphology include: (1) increases in the complexity of dendritic
arborization; (2) increases in dendritic spine density; (3) increases in synapse number. All
three measures are indicative of changes in neuronal connectivity and functional change
within a given brain area.

tion of sensory or motor representations. Although neural plasticity occurs in response to a variety of different internal and external manipulations including behavioural training (Adkins et al 2006), injury (Nudo 2003), pharmacological (Meintzschel & Ziemann 2006), central (Kleim et al 2003, Teskey et al 2003) and peripheral stimulation (Wu et al 2005), here we focus on plasticity in the intact and damaged brain in association with motor training.

Evidence for neural plasticity with motor learning in the intact brain

Although numerous brain structures are involved in motor learning, there is a wealth of evidence demonstrating motor learning-dependent plasticity within the primary motor cortex (Adkins et al 2006, Monfils et al 2005). Motor skill training in both monkeys (Nudo et al 1996a) and rats (Kleim et al 2004) induces a reorganization of movement representations in the motor cortex. The cortex devotes more territory towards the control of the trained rather than untrained movements. This reorganization of movement representations is thought to occur through changes in the synaptic connections between cortical neurones (Monfils et al 2005). Indeed, areas of cortex that show motor map reorganization also show increases in synapse number (Kleim et al 2004).

Human neuroimaging and cortical stimulation studies have revealed similar results. Functional magnetic imaging studies show a progressive increase in motor cortex activity as motor learning progresses (Karni et al 1995). Transcranial magnetic stimulation (TMS) studies show a reorganization of corticospinal output associated with increased motor skill level (Pearce et al 2000; Tyc et al 2005). Together these animal and human experiments demonstrate that the acquisition and performance of motor skills are associated with neural plasticity within the motor cortex.

Evidence for neural plasticity with motor rehabilitation in the damaged brain

Motor deficits after brain damage are not solely due to the functions lost in the injured motor brain area. They are also an expression of the ability of the rest of the brain to maintain motor function without the injured area. For example, movement after stroke is associated with aberrant patterns of brain activation that reflects the brain's attempt at adapting to the lost neural tissue (Ward et al 2006). Therefore, motor recovery that occurs during rehabilitation relies on two general processes that can be achieved through several different mechanisms (Box 5.1).

Animal and human studies demonstrate that motor rehabilitation after stroke causes a restoration and reorganization of function within motor cortex (Table 5.1).

Box 5.1

Processes of recovery:
- *Pure recovery*: lost movement sequences are restored.
- *Compensation*: new movement sequences are developed to accomplish old tasks.

Mechanisms of recovery:
- Restoration of function within the motor cortex of the damaged hemisphere. Function within residual cortical tissue that was compromised after damage is restored with rehabilitation.
- Reorganization of motor function within the motor cortex of the damaged hemisphere. Rehabilitation can drive residual neural tissue to reorganize in order to compensate for lost function.
- Recruitment of motor function within the undamaged (contralesional) hemisphere. When insufficient resources are found in the damaged hemisphere, the contralateral motor cortex can be recruited.

Table 5.1 Neural plasticity following motor rehabilitation.

Rehabilitation	Plasticity	Source
Acrobatic training (rat)	Increased synapse number Increased dendritic arborization	Voorhies & Jones 2002, Chu & Jones 2000
Reach training (rat)	Increased synapse number Motor map reorganization	Kleim et al 2003, Allred & Jones 2004
Kulver board (monkey)	Motor map reorganization Axonal sprouting	Nudo et al 1996b, Dancause et al 2005
Constraint Induced Movement Therapy (Humans)	Increased MEP amplitude Motor map reorganization Changes in fMRI activity	Wittenberg et al 2003, Koski et al 2004, Forrester et al 2006, Ro et al 2006
Cortical stimulation (rat)	Increased synaptic strength Motor map reorganization	Teskey et al 2003, Kleim et al 2003

MEP, motor evoked potential; fMRI, functional magnetic resonance imaging.

PRINCIPLES OF NEURAL PLASTICITY FOR REHABILITATION

Although these studies show that plasticity occurs in association with motor rehabilitation, simply demonstrating brain plasticity does not, on its own, help therapists to provide more effective therapies (see Box 5.2).

Box 5.2

- Neuroplasticity can be considered the neural mechanism of motor recovery that is driven by physiotherapeutic intervention. Physiotherapists need to identify which interventions are most effective at restoring movement and inducing plasticity following brain damage.
- Further research is required to establish direct links between commonly applied rehabilitation interventions, neuroplastic change and functional improvement in human subjects.

5

Box 5.3

Key clinical messages
- Motor recovery after brain damage is a relearning process supported by the same or similar neural mechanisms mediating motor learning in the intact brain.
- Enduring neuroplastic changes in motor cortex accompany motor learning in the intact brain and motor relearning in the damaged brain.
- Basic science studies reveal fundamental principles of neural plasticity that can be applied to motor rehabilitation.
- Rehabilitation interventions that induce maladaptive motor compensation that rely on 'quick fix' or 'crutch dependent' strategies become instantiated in the brain and are difficult to undo, and ultimately may impede the ultimate level of recovery.
- Parameters of rehabilitation that best drive recovery with respect to the specificity, intensity, timing of training, and age of patient need to be identified.

However, by identifying the basic principles that govern experience-dependent plasticity, new insights into how therapy should be administered may be gained. Table 5.2 lists ten principles of plasticity, derived from decades of basic neuroscience research, that are likely to be especially relevant to rehabilitation after brain damage (Kleim & Jones 2008).

CONCLUSIONS: UNDERSTANDING PLASTICITY CAN ENHANCE REHABILITATION

Key messages are outlined in Box 5.3. Our task is now to use our understanding of both the principles of neural plasticity and the cellular mechanisms underlying these phenomena to enhance the efficacy of motor rehabilitation. For example,

Table 5.2 Principles of neural plasticity for rehabilitation.

Principle	Description	Source
1. Use it or lose it	• Neural circuits not actively engaged in task performance for an extended period of time begin to degrade. • Further deprivation of one sensory modality may cause its corresponding cortical area to be at least partially taken over by another modality. • Failure to engage the motor system due to learned non-use may lead to further degradation of function.	• Hubel & Weisel 1965, Merzenich et al 1984
2. Use it and improve it	• Improvements in motor performance through specific skills training tasks are accompanied by profound plasticity within motor cortex. • Combining rehabilitative training with constraint of the ipsilesional arm (constraint induced movement therapy, CIMT) in humans with unilateral strokes improves the function of the impaired limb.	• Monfils et al 2005 • Wolf et al 2006
3. Specificity matters	• Neural plasticity is driven by the acquisition and performance of motor skills, not increased motor activity associated with training. • Task related rehabilitation can induce greater functional gains.	• Adkins et al 2006 • Winstein et al 2004
4. Repetition matters	• Repetition of a newly learned (or re-learned) movement sequence is required to induce lasting neural changes. • Repetition is required to maintain and make further functional gains outside of therapy.	• Kleim et al 2004, Lang et al 2007
5. Intensity matters	• Induction of plasticity requires sufficient training intensity.	• Kleim et al 2004

6. Time matters	• Different forms of plasticity occur at different times during training. Neural plasticity is a complex cascade of molecular, cellular, structural and physiological events.	• Adkins et al 2006
	• Rehabilitation should occur early rather than late. There may be time windows in which it is particularly effective in directing the lesion-induced reactive plasticity.	• Biernaskie et al 2004, Barbay et al 2006
7. Salience matters	• The training experience must be sufficiently important (relevant) and demand attention to induce plasticity.	• Stefan et al 2004, Meintzschel & Ziemann 2006
	• Training on tasks that are relevant to the patient will facilitate functional improvements.	
8. Age matters	• Training-induced plasticity occurs more readily in younger brains; neuroplastic responses are reduced in the aged brain.	• Nieto-Sampedro & Niet-Diaz 2005
	• Good recovery can be observed in aged animals when rehabilitation is paired with adjuvant therapies known to promote plasticity.	• Markus et al 2005, Zhao et al 2005
9. Transference matters	• Plasticity in response to one experience can enhance the acquisition of behaviours similar to those acquired in the original training experience.	• Butefisch et al 2004
	• Training in one behaviour does not automatically generalize to other behaviours; behaviours must be similar.	• Sawaki et al 2006
	• Training towards restoring lost movements will facilitate further motor improvements.	
10. Interference matters	• Plasticity in response to one experience can interfere with the acquisition of other behaviours.	• Rosenkranz et al 2000, Taub et al 2003
	• Rehabilitation interventions that induce maladaptive motor compensation can interfere with restoration of lost movement capacity.	• Boyd & Winstein 2006
	• Brain injury may also change sensitivities to interference effects, e.g. providing explicit instruction on a motor sequence task improved learning in healthy controls but interfered with learning in subjects post-stroke.	

adjuvant therapies such as cortical stimulation manipulations that augment neural plasticity also enhance motor recovery (see Table 5.1).

It is important to point out that simply upregulating the capacity for plasticity will only set the stage for driving the specific changes in neural circuitry required for restoring motor function. Any effective motor rehabilitation therapy must include extensive motor training during which movement sequences are acquired and sufficiently repeated. Understanding the key elements of therapy that maximize plasticity will optimize the therapist's ability to induce meaningful changes in neural circuits that support enduring gains in motor performance.

References

Adkins DL, Boychuk J, Remple MS et al 2006 Motor training induces experience-specific patterns of plasticity across motor cortex and spinal cord. Journal of Applied Physiology 101(6):1776–1782.

Allred RP, Jones TA 2004 Unilateral ischemic sensorimotor cortical damage in female rats: forelimb behavioral effects and dendritic structural plasticity in the contralateral homotopic cortex. Experimental Neurology 190(2):433–445.

Barbay S, Plautz EJ, Friel KM et al 2006 Behavioural and neurophysiological effects of delayed training following a small ischemic infarct in primary motor cortex of squirrel monkeys. Experimental Brain Research 169(1):106–116.

Biernaskie J, Chernenko G, Corbett D 2004 Efficacy of rehabilitative experience declines with time after focal ischemic brain injury. Journal of Neuroscience 24(5):1245–1254.

Boyd L, Winstein C 2006 Explicit information interferes with implicit motor learning of both continuous and discrete movement tasks after stroke. Journal of Neurologic Physical Therapy 30(2):46–57.

Butefisch CM, Khurana V, Kopylev L et al 2004 Enhancing encoding of a motor memory in the primary motor cortex by cortical stimulation. Journal of Neurophysiology 91(5):2110–2116.

Carr JH, Shepherd R 1998 Neurological physiotherapy: optimising motor performance. Butterworth-Heinemann, London, Chapter 2.

Chu CJ, Jones TA 2000 Motor skills training enhances lesion-induced plasticity in the motor cortex of adult rats. Journal of Neuroscience 19(22):10153–10163.

Dancause N, Barbay S, Frost SB et al 2005 Extensive cortical rewiring after brain injury. Journal of Neuroscience 25(44):10167–10179.

Forrester LW, Hanley DF, Macko RF 2006 Effects of treadmill exercise on transcranial magnetic stimulation-induced excitability to quadriceps after stroke. Archives of Physical and Medical Rehabilitation 87(2):229–234.

Gilmore PE, Spaulding SJ 2001 Motor control and motor learning: implications for treatment in individuals post stroke. Physical and Occupational Therapy in Geriatrics 20(1):1–15.

Hubel DH, Wiesel TN 1965 Comparison of the effects of unilateral and bilateral eye closure on cortical unit responses in kittens. Journal of Neurophysiology 28:1029–1040.

Karni A, Meyer G, Jezzard P et al 1995 Functional MRI evidence for adult motor cortex plasticity during motor skill learning. Nature 377(6545):155–158.

Kleim JA, Jones TA 2008 Principles of experience-dependent neural plasticity: implications for rehabilitation. American Journal of Speech Hearing and Language Research 51:225–239.

Kleim JA, Bruneau R, VandenBerg P et al 2003 Motor cortex stimulation enhances motor recovery and reduces peri-infarct dysfunction following ischemic insult. Neurology Research 25(8):789–793.

Kleim JA, Hogg TM, VandenBerg PM et al 2004 Cortical synaptogenesis and motor map reorganization occur during late, but not early phase of motor skill learning. Journal of Neuroscience 24(3):628–633.

Koski L, Mernar TJ, Dobkin BH 2004 Immediate and long-term changes in corticomotor output in response to rehabilitation: correlation with functional improvements in chronic stroke. Neurorehabilitation and Neurological Repair 18(4):230–249.

Lang CE, MacDonald JR, Gnip C 2007 Counting repetitions: an observational study of outpatient therapy for people with hemiparesis post-stroke. Journal of Neurologic Physical Therapy 31:1–10.

Markus TM, Tsai SY, Bollnow MR et al 2005 Recovery and brain reorganization after stroke in adult and aged rats. Annals of Neurology 58(6):950–953.

Meintzschel F, Ziemann U 2006 Modification of practice-dependent plasticity in human motor cortex by neuromodulators. Cerebral Cortex 16(8):1106–1115.

Merzenich MM, Nelson RJ, Stryker MP et al 1984 Somatosensory cortical map changes following digit amputation in adult monkeys. Journal of Comparative Neurology 224(4):591–605.

Monfils MH, Plautz EJ, Kleim JA 2005 In search of the motor engram: motor map plasticity as a mechanism for encoding motor experience. Neuroscientist 11(5): 471–483.

Nieto-Sampedro M, Nieto-Diaz M 2005 Neural plasticity: changes with age. Journal of Neural Transmission 112(1):3–27.

Nudo RJ 2003 Adaptive plasticity in motor cortex: implications for rehabilitation after brain injury. Journal of Rehabilitation Medicine 41(7):7–10.

Nudo RJ, Milliken GW, Jenkins WM et al 1996a Use-dependent alterations of movement representations in primary motor cortex of adult squirrel monkeys. Journal of Neuroscience 16(2):785–807.

Nudo RJ, Wise BM, SiFuentes F et al 1996b Neural substrates for the effect of rehabilitative training on motor recovery after infarct. Science 272:1791–1794.

Pearce AJ, Thickbroom GW, Byrnes ML et al 2000 Functional reorganisation of the corticomotor projection to the hand in skilled racquet players. Experimental Brain Research 130(2):238–243.

Ro T, Noser E, Boake C et al 2006 Functional reorganization and recovery after constraint-induced movement therapy in subacute stroke: case reports. Neurocase 12(1):14–24.

Rosenkranz K, Nitsche MA, Tergau F et al 2000 Diminution of training-induced transient motor cortex plasticity by weak transcranial direct current stimulation in the human. Neuroscience Letters 296(1):61–63.

Sawaki L, Wu CW, Kaelin-Lang A et al 2006 Effects of somatosensory stimulation on use-dependent plasticity in chronic stroke. Stroke 37(1):246–247.

Schmidt RA, Wrisberg CA 2000 Motor learning and performance: a problem-based learning approach. Champaign IL, Human Kinetics.

Stefan K, Wycisio M, Classen J 2004 Modulation of associative human motor cortical plasticity by attention. Journal of Neurophysiology 92(1):66–72.

Taub E, Uswatte G, Morris DM 2003 Improved motor recovery after stroke and massive cortical reorganization following constraint-induced movement therapy. Physical and Medical Rehabilitation Clinics of North America 14(1):77–91.

Teskey GC, Flynn C, Goertzen CD et al 2003 Cortical stimulation improves skilled forelimb use following a focal ischemic infarct in the rat. Neurology Research 25(8):794–800.

Tyc F, Boyadjian A, Devanne H 2005 Motor cortex plasticity induced by extensive training revealed by transcranial magnetic stimulation in human. European Journal of Neuroscience 21(1):259–266.

Voorhies AC, Jones TA 2002 The behavioral and dendritic growth effects of focal sensorimotor cortical damage depend on the method of lesion induction. Behavioural Brain Research 133(2):237–246.

Ward NS, Newton JM, Swayne OB et al 2006 Motor system activation after subcortical stroke depends on corticospinal system integrity. Brain 129(3):809–819.

Winstein CJ, Rose DK, Tan SM et al 2004 A randomized controlled comparison of upper extremity rehabilitation strategies in acute stroke: a pilot study of immediate and long-term outcomes. Archives of Physical and Medical Rehabilitation 85(4): 620–628.

Wittenberg GF, Chen R, Ishii K et al 2003 Constraint-induced therapy in stroke: magnetic-stimulation motor maps and cerebral activation. Neurorehabilitation and Neural Repair 17(1):48–57.

Wolf SL, Winstein CJ, Miller JP et al 2006 Effect of contraint-induced movement therapy on upper extremity function 3 and 9 months after stroke. The EXCITE randomized clinical trial. Journal of the American Medical Association 296(17):2095–2104.

Wu CW, van Gelderen P, Hanakawa T et al 2005 Enduring representational plasticity after somatosensory stimulation. Neuroimage 27(4):872–874.

Zhao CS, Puurunen K, Schallert T et al 2005 Effect of cholinergic medication, before and after focal photothrombotic ischemic cortical injury, on histological and functional outcome in aged and young adult rats. Behavioural Brain Research 156(1):85–94.

CHAPTER 6

Common neurological conditions

Sheila Lennon and Maria Stokes

INTRODUCTION

Some of the conditions you are likely to encounter in neurological physiotherapy are shown in Box 6.1.

This chapter outlines background information on these neurological conditions, summarized from Stokes (2004). A detailed overview of medical management can be found in Warlow (2006). Aspects of physical management are dealt with elsewhere in this pocketbook: physiotherapy management (including assessment, treatment, maintenance and prevention of complications) of the most commonly encountered conditions is covered in Chapter 10; neurological investigations and common drug treatments are presented in the Appendices; the wider impact of neurological disability, including carers, is considered in Chapters 2 and 3; transfer of care and long-term management are addressed in Chapter 12. Common complications which may arise across these conditions are identified in Box 6.2.

Specific management of paediatric conditions is not included in this book but guiding principles for neurological physiotherapy that are transferable are presented in Chapter 8. Three factors to consider in childhood disorders in comparison to adult neurological conditions are that: pathology underlying disorders, such as stroke, may have different effects on the developing nervous system than on the fully mature nervous system of adults (De Sousa & Rattue 2004); an increased potential for structural deformity during growth, and the complexity of transfer of care when children become young adults and thus are discharged from paediatric services to adult neurology services. Further details for neurological paediatrics can be found in Aicardi (1998) and Belderbos (2007).

STROKE

Stroke is the third most common cause of death worldwide and a major cause of disability; age standardized incidence for people aged 55 years or more ranges from 4.2 to 6.5 per 1000 population per annum (Dewey et al 2006). The diagnosis of stroke is reliant on a comprehensive neurological examination, supported by imaging to exclude conditions that mimic stroke. Recurrence within the first year

Box 6.1

Common conditions	Less frequent conditions
Stroke	Motor neurone disease
Acquired brain injury	Polyneuropathies e.g. Guillain–Barré syndrome
Multiple sclerosis	Huntington's disease
Parkinson's disease	Peripheral nerve injuries
Spinal cord injury	Muscle disorders
	Cerebral palsy
	Spina bifida

Box 6.2

Complications
- Respiratory problems e.g. aspiration pneumonia
- Skin breakdown
- Soft-tissue shortening e.g. painful joints, joint contracture
- Deep vein thrombosis

is 5% to 10%. Stroke should be considered as a medical emergency so that appropriate treatment can be started. Three interventions which help prevent death or dependency are: (1) stroke unit care regardless of age or stroke type, and for ischaemic stroke; (2) aspirin; (3) thrombolysis with alteplase (Dewey et al 2006).

Key features of stroke are summarized in Table 6.1; physical management is outlined in Chapter 10 (subchapters 10.1 and 10.2). During stroke management, emphasis is placed on prevention of further episodes by reducing risk factors, such as lowering blood pressure and cholesterol levels, a diet rich in fresh fruit, vegetables and essential fats (fish oils), and low in salt and saturated fats, taking regular exercise and avoiding smoking.

TRAUMATIC BRAIN INJURY

Acquired brain injury (ABI) describes insults to the brain that are not congenital or perinatal usually applied to single event pathology and not to progressive degenerative disease (Campbell 2004). The most frequent causes of ABI are: trauma, infections, e.g. meningitis, cerebrovascular diseases, e.g. aneurysm, and tumours (Rabinstein & Wijdicks 2006). This chapter will focus on the management of traumatic brain injury (TBI), although the general principles can be adapted to ABI from other causes. Sporting accidents, transport accidents, assaults and falls are the primary causes of TBI. Incidence ranges from 200 to 300 new cases of TBI

Table 6.1 Key features of stroke (summarized from Baer & Durward 2004, with permission).

	Stroke
Definitions	**Stroke**: the sudden onset of a focal neurological deficit lasting more than 24 hours in which causes other than vascular have been excluded (WHO 2001). Also termed cardiovascular accident (CVA). **Hemiplegia**: the paralysis of muscles on one side of the body affecting the arm, trunk, face & leg (contralateral to the side of the lesion in the brain). **Transient ischaemic attack (TIA)**: a stroke-like syndrome in which recovery is complete within 24 hours.
Pathology	**Ischaemic stroke**: 85 % of strokes are due to occlusion of one of the major cerebral arteries as a result of atheroma or secondary to emboli (small clots) from the heart or vessels: Middle cerebral artery – MCA (hemiplegia) Posterior cerebral artery – PCA (visual/memory deficits) Anterior cerebral artery – ACA (frontal deficits/leg paresis) Vertebral or basilar arteries – brain stem stroke (dizziness/vomiting/balance/dysphagia) **Haemorrhagic stroke**: 10 % of first strokes are caused by intracerebral bleeding. **Subarachnoid haemorrhage** (SAH): 5 % are caused by bleeding into the subarachnoid space, usually from ruptured aneurysm at or near the Circle of Willis.
Symptoms	Effects of stroke are determined by the areas of brain damage, irrespective of the cause. **Left hemisphere lesion**: normally associated with severe communication problems. **Right hemisphere lesion**: normally associated with perceptual disturbances. **Common signs & symptoms are**: ● *paralysis/paresis* ● *dysphasia/aphasia*: either a receptive or expressive problem affecting the understanding and use of correct words in speech or writing ● *dysarthria*: problems of articulation in speech

(continued)

6

Table 6.1 Key features of stroke (summarized from Baer & Durward 2004, with permission)—cont'd.

Stroke	
	• *dysphagia*: problem with swallowing • *hypertonia*: increased muscle tone • *hypotonia*: reduced muscle tone • *spasticity*: velocity-dependent stretch reflex hyperactivity • *hemianopia*: visual field deficit • *orofacial paresis*: leads to problems with drooling, swallowing & feeding • *fatigue* • *urinary incontinence* • *reduced level of consciousness* • *confusion/agitation* • *unilateral neglect*: failure to respond to stimuli presented on the hemiplegic side • *psychological problems*: depression; emotional lability & personality changes.
Time course	The most rapid period of recovery occurs within the first 8–12 weeks: • 40–50%: residual disability • 30%: full recovery • 20%: death within first 4 weeks; and 30% within first year The Bamford Classification provides a simple prognostic tool for differential recovery (adapted from Dewey et al 2006, with permission): • TACI (total anterior circulation infarct): likelihood of death and dependency • PACI (posterior anterior circulation infarct): better prognosis for recovery than TACI but high risk of early recurrence • LACI (lacunar infarct): relatively good prognosis • POCI (posterior circulation infarcts – brainstem or cerebellar signs): variable prognosis Haemorrhagic strokes – haematoma and oedema may be reabsorbed in some surviving the acute episode, giving better recovery than indicated by initial prognosis.

per year; peak risk of injury occurs between 16 to 25 years, rising again around 65 years (Campbell 2004).

Physiotherapists are likely to encounter people with the more severe physical deficits; however it must be acknowledged that it is often the more hidden cognitive and behavioural deficits that are the most challenging for community re-integration (Campbell 2004). Key features are summed up in Table 6.2; physical management is outlined in Chapter 10 (subchapters 10.1 and 10.2).

Table 6.2 Key features of traumatic brain injury (summarized from Campbell 2004, with permission).

Traumatic brain injury	
Definition	**Traumatic brain injury** (TBI): insult to the brain caused by an external force which may alter level of consciousness. Injury may be **closed** (intact skull) or **penetrating** (risk of infection). Severity of injury ranges from mild concussion to very severe injury resulting in death.
Pathology	**Primary damage**: direct impact on the skull, penetration through the skull into the brain, collision between the brain and the inside of the skull; all may cause widespread shearing and tearing of brain tissue such as axons. **Secondary damage**: oedema, haematoma, and infection may result in displacement and compression of brain tissue with occlusion of major arteries.
Symptoms	**Impairments of physical function** are wide ranging e.g. abnormal tone, paresis, ataxia, dizziness, posttraumatic epilepsy. **Impairments of cognitive and perceptual abilities** include disorders of attention, memory, reasoning, dyspraxia (difficulty with purposeful actions). **Impairments of behaviour and emotional functioning** e.g. verbal aggression, sexual disinhibition. **Increased intracranial pressure** (ICP) may lead to decreased cerebral perfusion and ischaemia. Treat with caution if ICP >15–20 mmHg. **Associated injuries**: a high percentage of patients have associated injuries e.g. fractures.
Time course	Varies according to severity of injury. **Glasgow Coma Scale** (GCS) gives summated score injury severity from 3 to 15, based on eye opening, best motor response and verbal response (GCS: mild = 13–15; moderate = 9–12; severe = 3–8). **Coma** is numerically defined as GCS of 8 or less. **Post traumatic amnesia** (PTA): period from injury until return of day to day memory. More than one day of PTA is considered severe TBI.

MULTIPLE SCLEROSIS

Multiple sclerosis (MS) is the major cause of neurological disability in young adults with peak incidence between 20 and 40 years. In view of this age of onset, MS has a serious impact on employment, financial status and family life. Incidence is about 3.5 to 6.6 people per 100 000 per annum in England & Wales (NICE 2004); its variable and unpredictable course requires continual adaptation and changes in management due to new symptoms and increasing disability (Palace 2006). MS-related fatigue, defined as a subjective lack of physical and or mental energy that is perceived by the individual or carer to interfere with usual and desired activities, is one of the most disabling symptoms (Costello & Harris 2003). Physiotherapists tend to see people who are more seriously affected, but it is important to realize that many people maintain their preferred life style remaining stable in between relapses. Breaking the news of a diagnosis of MS is always a stressful event for patients and their carers. NICE (2004) recommends that an individual should be informed of the potential diagnosis of MS by a doctor with specialist knowledge about MS as soon as it is considered reasonably likely. Key features are summarized in Table 6.3 (p. 57); physical management is outlined in Chapter 10 (subchapter 10.4).

SPINAL CORD INJURY

Spinal cord injury (SCI) occurs in approximately 17.2 per million of the population in Europe (Paddison & Middleton 2004). SCI is an example of an upper motor neurone lesion leading to varied amounts of spasticity and weakness. Since the spinal cord is shorter than the vertebral column, only extending to L1 or L2 level, lower vertebral injuries normally at a cut off level of T12 will not involve damage to the cord but damage to the nerve roots, a peripheral nerve injury. Key features are summarized in Table 6.4 (p. 58); physical management is outlined in Chapter 10 (subchapter 10.3).

PARKINSONS'S DISEASE

Parkinsons's disease (PD) is the second most common cause of chronic neurological disability in the UK with an incidence of 18 per 100 000 of population per year (Jones & Playfer 2004). PD is a movement disorder that also causes disorders of cognitive function, emotional expression and autonomic function (Jones & Playfer 2004). The most common onset is in the seventh decade but 5–10% of patients present with PD at age <40 years (Fung & Morris 2006). It is important to remember that PD usually progresses slowly. Key features are summed up in Table 6.5 (p. 60); physical management is outlined in Chapter 10 (subchapter 10.5).

Table 6.3 Key features of multiple sclerosis (summarized from De Souza & Bates 2004, with permission).

	Multiple sclerosis
Definition	A chronic progressive demyelinating disease, characterized by focal disturbance of function, with a relapsing and remitting course (periods of attacks and remission), usually presenting between the ages of 20–40 years and occurring more commonly in females than males. **Types of MS** (NICE 2004): *benign* (1 or 2 relapses with full recovery); *relapsing/remitting* (with partial or complete recovery in between relapses applicable to 80% at onset); *secondary progressive* (slowly progressive deterioration with or without relapses); *primary progressive* (progressive deficit without remission applicable to 10–15% at onset). About 50% of people with relapsing/remitting disease develop secondary progressive disease during first 10 years of illness.
Pathology	**Demyelination** – immune-mediated destruction of myelin around nerve fibres, producing characteristic lesions (plaques) throughout the CNS (see Fig. Ap.1.2 on p. 279). Loss of insulation causes interruption of normal nerve conduction (travel of impulses along a nerve). **Axonal degeneration**: later stages of the disease are associated with scarring at the site of inflammatory plaques and axonal degeneration leading to residual disability.
Symptoms	Lesions are randomly distributed throughout the white matter of the nervous system resulting in widespread deficits. **Common presentations** Symptoms of **cerebellar disease** – unsteadiness; ataxia (disturbance in the coordination of movement); nystagmus (defined below); intention tremor. Symptoms of **spinal cord disease** – spastic paresis with bowel & bladder disturbance. **Early symptoms** may be vague: fatigue, lack of energy, aching limbs, sensory disturbances. Symptoms then become more specific, often with initial episode of blurred or double vision. **Other symptoms**, some of which may be exacerbated by temperature changes, include: *Sensory,* e.g. numbness and paraesthesia *Motor,* e.g. weakness, unsteadiness, slurred speech, increased tone, hyperactive tendon reflexes, extensor plantar response and absent abdominal reflexes, pyramidal distribution weakness *Visual,* e.g. acute optic neuritis (retrobulbar neuritis) with visual loss, most commonly unilateral, diplopia (double vision); nystagmus (rapid, repetitive eye movement in one direction, alternating with a slower movement in the opposite direction) *Vestibular,* e.g. vertigo (false sensation of movement) *Cognitive,* e.g. depression.
Time course	Individual variation – pattern cannot be predicted, but remember does not always lead to severe disability and loss of mobility.

Table 6.4 Key features of spinal cord injury (summarized from Paddison & Middleton 2004, with permission).

	Spinal cord injury
Definitions	**Paraplegia**: impairment or loss of motor, sensory and/or autonomic function in thoracic, lumbar or sacral segments of the spinal cord. Upper limb function is spared. **Tetraplegia**: impairment or loss of motor, sensory and/or autonomic function in cervical segments of the spinal cord. 84% of spinal cord damage results from trauma and 16% from non-traumatic causes e.g. expanding lesions such as tumours, ischaemia.
Pathology	**Primary**: loss of axons due to contusion or tearing damage of the white matter. **Secondary damage**: loss of cells in the grey matter resulting from the body's response to injury and repair leading to swelling and increased cord compression.
Symptoms	**ASIA** – Use American Spinal Injury Association (ASIA) classification to establish the level of injury that can be complete or incomplete (see Chapter 10.3). **Complete**: Paralysis and loss of sensation below the level of lesion. **Incomplete**: Variable levels of motor or sensory sparing below the lesion with neurological preservation extending through sacral segments S4/5. **Disruption to respiration**: Injuries from C1 to C3 level paralyse all muscles of respiration including the diaphragm. Paralysis of some respiratory muscles is a feature of any lesion above T6 with reduced vital capacity and ineffective cough due to loss of abdominal muscles. Cervical lesions above the C4 level of injury will require ventilation. Paralytic ileus and gastric distension can further restrict movement of the diaphragm compromising breathing. **Sympathetic disruption** occurs in cervical and upper thoracic lesions with impairment of tachycardia response, and lowering of blood pressure. Vagal overstimulation can lead to bradycardia (slowed heart rate) and autonomic dysreflexia (see below). **Disruption of postural control (balance)** in any lesion above T12. A new postural sense is developed by visual control. In lesions above T6, postural control is also achieved through muscles with high innervation and low distal attachment e.g. latissimus dorsi (Bromley 2006). **Denervated skin** is at risk from pressure damage within 20–30 minutes of injury.

Table 6.4 Key features of spinal cord injury (summarized from Paddison & Middleton 2004, with permission)—cont'd.

	Spinal cord injury
	Incontinence due to disruption of the neural control of the bladder means that the patient requires catheterization. Disruption to neural control of the bowel requires retraining to ensure bowel evacuation; constipation can be an issue.
	Pain associated with neck and back pain and other injuries, as well as from overuse at a later stage.
	Sexual dysfunction: fertility is usually maintained in women, but problematic in men. Automatic erections occur in complete lesions above the conus, but there is no sensation during intercourse (Bromley 2006).
	Autonomic dysreflexia: dysfunction of the sympathetic nervous system producing hypertension, bradycardia and headache leading to fainting which should be treated as an emergency; hypertension may rise sufficiently to induce cerebral haemorrhage.
	Osteoporosis (loss of bone mass) may lead to fractures.
	Heterotopic ossification (calcification in denervated muscle) can result in loss of range and difficulty in sitting.
	Other syndromes Symptoms are related the anatomical areas of the cord affected. *Anterior cord syndrome* – complete motor loss caudal to the lesion, and loss of pain and temperature sensation. *Brown-Sequard syndrome* – ipsilateral paralysis with contralateral loss of temperature and pain sensation. *Central cord lesion* – upper limbs affected > lower limbs; partial bowel and bladder dysfunction is common; often in older people with spondylosis (spinal degeneration). *Conus medullaris* – either upper or lower motor neurone lesions. Bladder and bowel dysfunctions with lower limb deficits. *Cauda equina lesion* – peripheral nerve damage causes flaccid paralysis. *Posterior cord lesion* – rare condition causing disturbed sensation [light touch, proprioception (causing ataxia) and vibration] with preservation of motor function.
Time course	90% of tetraplegic patients with incomplete SCI have some recovery of motor level in their upper limbs compared with 70–85% complete injuries (Ditunno et al 2000). Pinprick preservation is a good indicator of motor recovery (Poynton et al 1997) with 75% of patients regaining an ability to walk. The most rapid phase of recovery occurs within the first 2 years.

Table 6.5 Key features of Parkinson's disease (summarized from Jones & Playfer 2004, with permission).

	Parkinson's disease
Definition	A chronic progressive neurodegenerative disorder.
Pathology	**Neurodegeneration** of grey matter structures – the basal ganglia. Reduced production of the neurotransmitter dopamine by the substantia nigra resulting in rigidity and releasing the inhibition of tremor. **Decreased production of dopamine** leads to an increased inhibition to the thalamus leading to bradykinesia.
Symptoms	**Early** – *the three cardinal symptoms are*: *Bradykinesia* – slowness of movement. *Rigidity* – increased muscle tone with resistance to passive movement in all directions. Causes the face to appear mask-like. *Tremor at rest* – limbs ('pill rolling' in hands), jaw or lightly closed eyes but does not present early in 50% of cases. Also action tremor. **Later** – **Postural instability** develops with a dominance of flexor tone over extensor tone resulting in a stooped posture with a tendency to fall. A **shuffling gait** with inability to initiate movement (freezing) or to stop (festination). **Speech impairment** with voice becoming low volume and monotonous, and associated problems with swallowing leading to drooling. **Respiratory problems**: characteristic stooped posture and problems with swallowing may in turn lead to respiratory complications. **Autonomic problems** include constipation and bladder hyperreflexia. **Cognitive changes** such as depression, and psychiatric complications may occur.
Time course	Longevity has improved since dopamine replacement was introduced in 1960s, with near normal life expectancy. Symptoms still progress and some patients have severe disability.

The remaining disorders listed in Box 6.1 are less frequently encountered by physiotherapists and are presented in table format only (see Tables 6.6–6.12 on pp. 61–70). Key aspects of physical management specific to these disorders are referred to in the tables. See relevant chapters in Stokes (2004) for a more detailed overview.

Table 6.6 Key features of polyneuropathies (summarized from Nicklin 2004, with permission).

	Polyneuropathies
Definition	A group of disorders affecting peripheral nerves in one or more pathological processes, resulting in motor, sensory and/or autonomic symptoms. Broadly divided into acquired and inherited types. **Causes** include metabolic (diabetes, renal disease, alcoholism, vitamin deficiencies), inflammatory, drug- or toxin-induced disorders; can be associated with infection, malignant disease or collagen vascular disease. **Guillain–Barré syndrome** (GBS) is an acute inflammatory demyelinating neuropathy with prevalence reported as 0.5–4.0 per 100,000. Time from onset to peak disability should be less than 4 weeks.
Pathology	**Pathology** is defined according to structures involved: *Axonopathy*: interruption to axon; metabolic and hereditary. *Myelinopathy*: damage to Schwann cells producing myelin affecting nerve conduction. *Neuronopathy*: damage to cell body, recovery unlikely.
Symptoms	***Muscle weakness***: generally diffuse, symmetrical and predominantly distal. ***Sensory symptoms***: range from complete loss of sensation to mild tingling to unbearable painful dysaesthesia. ***Autonomic symptoms***: such as disturbances of blood pressure, e.g. in diabetic neuropathy. **GBS** ***Paralysis***: some patients become fully paralysed presenting with tetraplegia, facial weakness and bulbar weakness leading to dysphagia. Paralysis of respiratory muscles causes reduced vital capacity (VC), requiring elective ventilation when VC falls below 15 mm/kg. ***Autonomic dysfunction*** can lead to cardiac arrhythmias. ***Altered sensation***: predominantly a motor neuropathy but with some altered sensation, e.g. numbness and paraesthesias. ***Pain*** related to inflamed and tightened neural structures.
Time course	Variable depending on type of neuropathy. **GBS** (see Karni et al 1984) is usually associated with a complete recovery, although 10–15% of patients fail to fully recover; mortality rate of 10–15%. 3 phases: deterioration phase over 4 weeks; plateau phase (few days to months); and recovery phase (dependent on severity and rate of remyelination, and presence of axonal degeneration).

Table 6.7 Key features of peripheral nerve injuries (summarized from Jaggi et al 2004, with permission).

Peripheral nerve injuries	
Definition	Injury to a peripheral nerve may include: loss of sensation, paralysis leading to atrophy of muscle and skin, and pain. Main causes are: **Open lesions**: tidy – knife, glass; untidy – missile, burn. **Closed lesions**: compression-ischaemia from pressure neuropathy in anaesthetized patient, compartment syndrome; traction ischaemia from fracture-dislocation; thermal; irradiation; injection – regional anaesthetic block.
Pathology	Types of nerve injury are classified according to behaviour of axon after injury: **Neurapraxia**: a conduction block (intact axon and nerve fibre). Rapid recovery with removal of source of compression. **Axonotmesis**: interruption of axon and distal Wallerian degeneration (fragmentation of axoplasm with gradual myelin deterioration). High chance of spontaneous recovery. **Neurotmesis**: whole nerve trunk is cut. Wallerian degeneration. Surgical repair is necessary. **Common sites of injury**: Brachial plexus. Axillary nerve (associated with fractures of neck of the humerus). Radial nerve (associated with humeral fractures). Ulnar/median nerves at the level of the wrist or elbow. Sciatic nerve (associated with hip dislocation). Common peroneal nerve (associated with fractured neck of fibula or plaster cast compression). Posterior tibial nerve from supracondylar femoral fractures.
Symptoms & management	See MRC (1982) for motor and sensory loss with specific nerve injury. **Paralysis** leading to atrophy (wasting). **Sensory loss** with risk of damage to skin and joints. **Neuropathic pain states** (Jaggi et al 2004): 1. Causalgia (complex regional pain syndrome; CRPS type 2). Partial damage to proximal nerve trunks; intense pain, spontaneous, persistent, often burning; skin hypersensitive; disturbance of circulation and sweating.

6

Table 6.7 Key features of peripheral nerve injuries (summarized from Jaggi et al 2004, with permission)—cont'd.

	Peripheral nerve injuries
	2. Reflex sympathetic dystrophy (RSD-CRPS type 1). Also termed Sudeck's atrophy, shoulder-hand syndrome, algoneurodystrophy. Often associated with fractures or crush injuries of wrist, hand or foot. No major nerve trunk damage; inflammation, pain, limited range of movement, vasomotor instability, sweating, allodynia (exaggerated response to stimuli), trophic skin changes and discoloration, and patchy bone demineralization. 3. Post-traumatic neuralgia. 4. Neurostenalgia – due to compression, distortion or ischaemia. 5. Central pain in brachial plexus injury – severe, with two components, one constant (burning or compressing), the other intermittent, worst in hand and forearm. Usually occurs within hours of closed traction injuries. 6. Pain maintained deliberately or subconsciously. **Physical management**: Focuses on monitoring recovery (if applicable, may involve surgical transfers of muscles and tendons) and management of complications: pain control, oedema control, ROM, muscle power, and care/protection of the affected limb (skin checks, prevention/management of deformity).
Time course	Early repair of damaged nerves and prompt treatment of associated injuries to blood vessels, bones, muscle and skin. Surgical exploration to confirm diagnosis and repair of damaged nerves, which may involve grafting. Varies according to cause and severity of injury, and the delay between nerve injury and repair. Injuries to the brachial plexus are the most serious. *Neurapraxia*: recovery within 8–12 weeks. *Axonal degeneration* recovers more slowly and usually incompletely.

6

Table 6.8 Key features of motor neurone disease (summarized from O'Gorman et al 2004 with permission).

	Motor neurone disease (MND)
Definition	Progressive degeneration of upper and lower motor neurones (UMN & LMN). Annual incidence about 2 per 100,000; most patients aged 50 to 70 years. **Three main forms:** *Amyotrophic lateral sclerosis* (ALS) – 65% of MND cases, mainly affecting older men (<50 years). *Progressive bulbar palsy* – 25% of cases. *Progressive muscular atrophy* – 10 % of cases, with earlier onset than other forms (<50 years), mainly affecting males. Electrophysiological tests important for differential diagnosis (see Table Ap.1.2, p. 282).
Pathology	**Lower motor neurone lesions:** anterior horn cell degeneration. **Upper motor neurone lesions:** corticospinal tract degeneration. **Bulbar palsy:** degeneration of brain stem nuclei.

Symptoms & management	**ALS** – LMN changes include muscle weakness, fasciculation (muscle twitch) and flaccidity, with no loss of sensation. UMN changes include spasticity, weakness and exaggerated reflexes.
	Progressive bulbar palsy – dysarthria (impaired articulation) and dysphagia (impaired swallowing). LMN involvement causes atrophy and fasciculation of the tongue, and dysphagia. With UMN changes the tongue is spastic and causes dysarthria.
	Progressive muscular atrophy – LMN degeneration causing limb weakness and loss of mobility. Many patients develop a mixed picture of symptoms and signs of the three main forms of MND.
	Dysphagia develops in 75% of patients.
	Dysarthria develops in 80 % of patients.
	Pain is a common problem in up to 73% of patients.
	Dyspnoea (breathlessness) is also a frequent problem.
	Eye soreness occurs due to reduced eye blinking.
	Insomnia can be due to breathlessness, insecurity, fear, pain.
	Fatigue.
	Terminal stages – severe muscle weakness, loss of communication, and respiratory failure.
	Physical management:
	Depends on symptoms present and rate of progression. Anticipation of potential problems is essential. Consider: pain control; respiratory care; energy conservation strategies; low resistance, submaximal exercise; maintenance of joint range and muscle length; tone management; maintaining mobility; provision of adaptations and equipment in a timely fashion. Teaching carers moving and handling strategies.
Time course	Median survival of just over 2 years from symptom onset, although some patients live much longer (Chancellor & McNaughton 2006). A palliative care team approach is essential.

Table 6.9 Key features of Huntington's disease (summarized from Quarrell & Cook 2004, with permission).

	Huntington's disease
Definition	An inherited (autosomal dominant) progressive degenerative disease featuring a triad of a movement disorder, an affective disturbance and cognitive impairment.
Pathology	Defect in chromosome 4 (IT15 gene). Cell loss mainly in the basal ganglia (especially caudate and putamen nuclei); reduction of the inhibitory neurotransmitter gamma-aminobutyric acid (GABA). Cell loss also occurs in the cortex.
Symptoms & management	Onset is insidious (gradual) usually between 35 and 55 years. ***Movement***: chorea (sudden, involuntary movements) is most common; dystonia (sustained, slow contractions), bradykinesia (slow movements) and rigidity. ***Speech***: dysarthria – rate and rhythm affected, progressing to become intelligible. ***Swallowing***: dysphagia, particularly for liquids in middle to late stages. Cachexia (severe weight loss). ***Incontinence***: urinary and faecal incontinence in late stage. ***Psychiatric features***: affective disturbances – depression, aggression and apathy. ***Cognitive impairment***: deficits in executive function may contribute to behavioural problems – difficulty with concentration, forward planning and cognitive flexibility. Retain ability to comprehend. **Secondary complications**: injury, asymmetry, loss of range (contracture/deformity), pain, and chest infections. **Physical management:** Focuses on prevention of complications and maintaining independence for as long as possible. ***Early stage*** – Maintain balance and mobility. Education about maintenance of range, functional activity and postural awareness. Prescription of walking aids. Relaxation techniques. ***Middle stage*** – Maintain range, function, prevent contracture and deformity. Consider stretching and positioning to counteract misalignment of body segments and loss of rotation. Provision of adaptations, aids and equipment. Teaching carers moving and handling strategies. ***Late stage*** – Focus on optimal positioning and comfort. Specially padded adapted seating may be required. Consider wheelchair provision.
Time course	A slowly progressive disease. Duration of illness varies from 10 to 17 years.

Table 6.10 Key features of muscle disorders (adapted from Quinlivan & Thompson 2004, and Thompson & Quinlivan 2004, with permission).

	Muscle disorders
Definition	Muscle disorders are inherited or acquired, classified according to site of defect in the motor unit. Often progressive conditions leading to physical disability and, in cases, reduced life expectancy.
Pathology	Varies according to type of disorder. Different gene protein deficiencies have been identified and are diagnostic markers (see Karpati et al 2001).
Symptoms & management	These vary according to disorder. **Examples of childhood onset**: Muscular dystrophies are associated with progressive degeneration of skeletal muscle with weakness followed by progressive wasting and disability. **Duchenne muscular dystrophy** *(DMD):* X-linked recessive inherited disorder affecting boys, with gradual loss of functional muscle fibres, replaced by fat and connective tissue. Most severe form of MD. Delayed motor milestones 3–5 years. Raised creatine kinase (CK) levels in blood indicative of muscle damage. Progressive weakness and development of contractures, with loss of ambulation by early teens. Scoliosis (lateral spinal curvature) occurs in 95% of boys, requiring stabilization. Respiratory and cardiac problems are progressive and lead to premature death between 2nd and 3rd decades. **Becker MD**: milder form of X-linked dystrophy than DMD. **Spinal muscular atrophies** *(SMA):* degeneration of anterior horn cells and spinal cord, causing severe muscle weakness. **Physical management**: **DMD**: Key milestones in disease progression require sensitive management e.g. diagnosis, loss of ambulation, final illness and bereavement. Consider: passive movements, stretching, positioning, splinting; use of standing frame; respiratory care; provision of adaptations and equipment e.g. wheelchairs. A palliative care team approach is essential. **Becker BD**: Consider prevention of contracture, prolonging ambulation, standing frame and provision of adaptations and equipment. **Examples of adult onset**: **Post-polio syndrome** *(PPS):* new set of symptoms 30 years after acute polio – fatigue, weakness, muscle or joint pain, functional loss. **Myasthenia gravis**: defect at the neuromuscular junction causing muscle fatigue and weakness.

(continued)

Table 6.10 Key features of muscle disorders (adapted from Quinlivan & Thompson 2004, and Thompson & Quinlivan 2004, with permission)—cont'd.

	Muscle disorders
	Fascioscapulohumeral muscular dystrophy *(FSH)*: facial weakness characterized by inability to whistle. Onset by 30 years, with variable symptoms ranging from minimal facial weakness with slow progression to marked progression with lower limb weakness and severe disability early in life.
	Myotonic dystrophy *(DM1)*: congenital form present at birth; juvenile and classic forms in 2nd–3rd decades, with ptosis (drooping eyelids) frontal balding, myotonia (slow to relax muscle contraction, e.g. to release grip) and muscle weakness; symptoms vary in severity between patients; high anaesthetic risk and malignant hyperthermia reaction can occur with certain combinations of anaesthesia.
	Limb girdle muscular dystrophies: weakness of muscles in shoulder and pelvic girdles, with or without contractures; cardiac and respiratory involvement, with loss of ambulation 10–20 years after onset in 2nd–3rd decades.
	Glycogen storage diseases: abnormal glycogen metabolism e.g. McArdle's disease, a glycogen storage disorder caused by deficiency of the enzyme myophosphorylase, results in muscle pain and fatigue during anaerobic exercise.
	Inflammatory myopathies: three groups – dermatomyositis (facial rash, muscle pain, proximal weakness); polymyositis (proximal weakness), and inclusion body myositis (facial weakness, distal weakness, does not respond to steroids).
	Endocrine myopathies: muscle pain (myalgia) and weakness due to endocrine disorders, such as hypothyroidism (underactive thyroid).
	Physical management: Minimize complications to maximize abilities and maintain optimal level of function. Consider: maintenance of muscle strength, retarding contracture progression, promoting or prolonging ambulation, maintenance of activities, management of scoliosis, and respiratory complications.
Time course	Severity varies with type of muscle disorder. DMD is the most severe form of MD.

**Table 6.11 Key features of the cerebral palsies (summarized from Pountney &
Green 2004, with permission).**

	The cerebral palsies
Definition	**Cerebral palsy** (CP) is an umbrella term for a range of causative factors producing a disorder of posture and movement, as a result of damage to the developing nervous system before or during birth, or in early infancy.
Pathology	Causes are still speculative but brain damage can result from hypoxia, vascular accidents, infections and toxicitiy. 10% of cases due to birth asphyxia. 50% of cases are pre-term infants. Associated with low birth weight.
Symptoms & management	Condition is classified according to its type, distribution and severity. Type is categorized according to the impairment: spastic, dyskinetic, ataxic and hypotonic. **Motor impairments** of weakness and spasticity, with bone and joint deformities, spinal curvatures, and pain. *Hemiplegia* – one side of the body primarily involved. *Diplegia* – lower half of the body involved. *Quadriplegia* – entire body involved. **Cognitive impairment** is common. **Associated complications** include: epilepsy, disorders of the sensory system e.g. visual impairment, musculoskeletal deformity, growth delay (below normal growth curves for height and weight), sleep disturbance and reduced life expectancy. The neurological lesion will slow the development of movement patterns often resulting in adoption of asymmetrical postures and limited ranges of movement. Underdevelopment of affected body parts may occur. Muscle and bone will develop differently resulting in muscle imbalances, and deformities of joints and bones. Different distributions and types of CP result in different patterns of deformity. **Physical management** e.g. specialized handling, strength training, positioning, orthotics to prevent deformities, but, in cases, multilevel orthopaedic surgery, e.g. tendon release, bony surgery, is used to balance muscle length and correct deformity. Botulinum toxin may be used to reduce increased tone in selected muscles, to establish new motor patterns and reduce contractures. The effects last for several months.
Time course	Varies according to severity. Lifestyle and opportunities have improved and many adults live independent, supported, lives.

6

Table 6.12 Key features of spina bifida (summarized from Pountney & McCarthy 2004, with permission).

Spina bifida	
Definition	A neural tube defect (NTD) in which the neural tube fails to fuse somewhere along its length in the spine.
Pathology	Types of spinal lesion: *Meningocele* – no neural tissue outside the vertebral canal. *Myelomeningocele* – neural tissue and nerve roots may be outside the vertebral canal. *Rachischisis* – neural tissue lies open on the surface of the vertebral canal, as a flattened plaque.
Symptoms & management	**Spinal level** of the lesion determines the symptoms and functional abnormality e.g. muscles involved (weakness, spasticity), abnormal skin sensation, and involvement of bladder or bowel function. Spinal curvature may be congenital or occur during development. **Hydrocephalus**: excess cerebrospinal fluid (CSF) circulates in and around the brain due to obstruction in its flow caused by the NTD in 80% of cases. Some problems are caused by structural neurological abnormalities during brain development: learning difficulties are common; visual disruption e.g. reduced visual acuity, blindness. **Physical management** aims to promote sensorimotor development within the limits of the neurological constraints, and to achieve as much functional independence as possible through: ● development of physical skills; ● achievement of independent mobility, either walking or in a wheelchair; ● prevention of deformity. Most common deformities are: talipes equinovarus (club foot) and congenital dislocation of the hip (CDH). Growth spurt in adolescence may accelerate progression of spinal deformity.
Time course	Varies according to severity. Many adults live independently.

References

Aicardi J 1998 Diseases of the nervous system in childhood, 2nd edn. Mac Keith Press, Oxford.

Baer G, Durward B 2004 Stroke. In: Stokes M (ed) Physical management in neurological rehabilitation, 2nd edn. Elsevier, London, pp 75–101.

Belderbos R 2007 Oxford specialist handbook in paediatric neurology. Oxford University Press, Oxford.

Bromley I 2006 Tetraplegia and paraplegia, 6th edn. London, Churchill Livingstone.

Campbell M 2004 Acquired brain injury: trauma and pathology. In: Stokes M (ed) Physical management in neurological rehabilitation, 2nd edn. Elsevier, London, pp 103–124.

Chancellor AM, McNaughton HK 2006 Motor neurone disease, disorders of the spine and spinal cord. In: Warlow C (ed) The Lancet handbook of treatment in neurology. Elsevier, London, pp 89–126.

Costello K, Harris C 2003 Differential diagnosis and management of fatigue in multiple sclerosis: considerations for the nurse. Journal of Neuroscience Nursing 35: 139–148.

De Sousa C, Rattue H 2004 General introduction to paediatric neurology. In: Stokes M (ed) Physical management in neurological rehabilitation, 2nd edn. Elsevier, London, pp 283–296.

De Souza L, Bates D 2004 Multiple sclerosis. In: Stokes M (ed) Physical management in neurological rehabilitation, 2nd edn. Elsevier, London, pp 177–201.

Dewey HM, Chambers BR, Donnan GA Stroke 2006 In: Warlow C (ed) The Lancet handbook of treatment in neurology. Elsevier, London, pp 89–126.

Ditunno JF, Ditunno PL, Graziani V et al 2000 Walking index for spinal cord injury (WISCI): an international multi centre validity and reliability study. Spinal Cord 38(4):234–243. Revision: (WISCI II) Spinal Cord 2001 39:654–656.

Fung VCS, Morris J 2006 Parkinson's disease and other movement disorders. In: Warlow C (ed) The Lancet handbook of treatment in neurology. Elsevier, London, pp 127–159.

Jaggi A, Birch R, Dean L et al 2004 Peripheral nerve injuries. In: Stokes M (ed) Physical management in neurological rehabilitation, 2nd edn. Elsevier, London, pp 153–175.

Jones D, Playfer J 2004 Parkinson's disease. In: Stokes M (ed) Physical management in neurological rehabilitation. Elsevier, London, pp 203–219.

Karni Y, Archdeacon L, Mills K R, Wiles C M 1984 Clinical assessment & physiotherapy in Guillain Barre syndrome. Physiotherapy 70:288–292.

Karpati G, Hilton-Jones D, Griggs RC 2001 Disorders of voluntary muscle, 7th edn. Cambridge University Press.

Medical Research Council (MRC) of the United Kingdom 1982 Aids to the examination of the peripheral nervous system. Eastbourne, Baillière-Tindall.

National Institute for Clinical Excellence (NICE) 2004 Multiple Sclerosis: national clinical guidelines for diagnosis and management in primary and secondary care. Royal College of Physicians, London.

Nicklin J 2004 Disorders of nerve II: polyneuropathies. In: Stokes M (ed) Physical management in neurological rehabilitation. Elsevier, London, pp 253–268.

O'Gorman B, Oliver D, Nottle C, Prisley S 2004 Disorders of nerve 1: Motor neurone disease. In: Stokes M (ed) Physical management in neurological rehabilitation. Elsevier, London, pp 233–251.

Paddison S, Middleton F 2004 Spinal cord injury. In: Stokes M (ed) Physical management in neurological rehabilitation. Elsevier, London, pp 125–152.

Palace J 2006 Multiple sclerosis and other inflammatory CNS disorders. In: Warlow C (ed) The Lancet handbook of treatment in neurology. Elsevier, London, pp 201–222.

Pountney T, Green E 2004 The cerebral palsies and motor learning. In: Stokes M (ed) Physical management in neurological rehabilitation. Elsevier, London, pp 313–332.

Pountney T, McCarthy G 2004 Neural tube defects: spina bifida and hydrocephalus. In: Stokes M (ed) Physical management in neurological rehabilitation. Elsevier, London, pp 333–346.

Poynton AR, O'Farrel DA, Shannon F et al 1997 Sparing of sensation to pinprick predicts motor recovery of a motor segment after injury to the spinal cord. Journal of Bone and Joint Surgery Br 79:952–954.

Quarrell O, Cook B 2004 Huntington's disease. In: Stokes M (ed) Physical management in neurological rehabilitation, 2nd edn. Elsevier, London, pp 221–232.

Quinlivan R, Thompson N 2004 Disorders of muscle and post-polio syndrome. In: Stokes M (ed) Physical management in neurological rehabilitation, 2nd edn. Elsevier, London, pp 269–280.

Rabinstein AA, Wijdicks EF 2006 Surgery for intracerebral hematoma: the search for the elusive right candidate. Reviews in Neurological Diseases 3(4):163–172.

Stokes M (ed) 2004 Physical management in neurological rehabilitation. Elsevier, London.

Thompson N, Quinlivan R 2004 Muscle disorders of childhood onset. In: Stokes M (ed) Physical management in neurological rehabilitation, 2nd edn. Elsevier, London, pp 347–363.

Warlow C 2006 The Lancet handbook of treatment in neurology. Elsevier, London.

World Health Organization 2001 International classification of functioning, disability and health. Geneva: Switzerland. Accessed 2007 from: www.who.int/icf.

CHAPTER 7

Common motor impairments and their impact on activity

Louise Ada and Colleen G Canning

INTRODUCTION

Neurological conditions can involve upper motor neurone lesions (UMNL), e.g. stroke, or lower motor neurone lesions (LMNL), e.g. Guillain–Barré syndrome, or both, e.g. motor neurone disease. The pathology produces primary impairments – defined as an abnormality of a physiological, psychological or anatomical structure or function. The classification of impairments as negative or positive is a useful framework for investigating the underlying causes of activity limitation (Carr & Shepherd 2003, pp. 210–221; Box 7.1). Furthermore, since neurological conditions usually result in impairments that take time to resolve, common secondary impairments (such as contracture, shoulder subluxation, and swelling) arise as adaptations to the primary impairments.

Maintaining balance on any base of support is a complex functional motor goal, and its loss is neither an impairment nor an activity limitation. In neurological conditions, it is usually the result of various impairments e.g. if a person is weak and cannot select appropriate movements with appropriate timing after suffering a stroke, then they may have difficulty balancing their body mass over a small base of support such as a foot, which in turn will result in difficulty with activities such as standing and walking. The only situation, in which loss of balance may be thought of as a primary impairment, is when balance is affected due to a lesion of the vestibular system. This chapter examines the more common motor impairments that arise from neurological conditions and offers some general suggestions for training interventions; other chapters (see Chapters 13–16) cover non-motor impairments. See Chapter 6 for an overview of common conditions. See Chapter 9 for assessment of impairments and activity limitations. See Chapter 10 for specific treatment suggestions for different types of patient.

PRIMARY MOTOR IMPAIRMENTS

Weakness

Weakness is a reduction in ability to produce normal levels of voluntary force, typically measured as maximum isometric force. Weakness is the only motor

Box 7.1

Primary negative impairments:
- **represent a loss of function** previously present
- common impairments are: weakness, loss of dexterity/ataxia, and bradykinesia/akinesia

Primary positive impairments:
- **are additional** such as abnormal postures, increased reflexes, and abnormal tone
- common impairments are: spasticity, hypertonia, hypotonia, rigidity, tremor, and dyskinesia

---

Box 7.2

In UMNL there is:
- disruption to descending input
- decreased number of motor units activated
- decreased motor unit discharge rate
- disrupted motor unit recruitment

In LMNL there is:
- disruption to nerve
- loss of cross sectional area
- disuse atrophy

---

impairment that is commonly present in all UMNL and LMNL. However, the mechanism is different between the two types of lesion (see Box 7.2).

Weakness is a major contributor to persistent activity limitations (Canning et al 2004; Morris et al 2004). See characteristics in Box 7.3 and evidence in Table 7.1.

In UMNL the evidence suggests that strength training does not increase spasticity (Ada et al 2006a and b, Bourbonnais et al 2002, Bütefisch et al 1995, Engardt et al 1995, Sharp & Brouwer 1997). In LMNL there is also some evidence that strength training does not result in overwork weakness (prolonged reduction in the absolute strength and endurance of a muscle due to excessive activity) (Aitkens et al 1993, Drory et al 2001, Kilmer et al 1994, McCartney et al 1988, Milner-Brown & Miller 1988, Ruhland & Shields 1997). See Box 7.4.

Loss of dexterity and ataxia

We consider loss of dexterity to be synonymous with incoordination, loss of selective movement or lack of motor control. Dexterity is 'the ability to solve any motor task. . . . precisely, quickly, rationally and deftly' (Bernstein 1991) where flexibility with respect to the changing environment is an important feature.

Table 7.1 Some evidence for strength training.

Studies	Subjects	Intervention	Outcome
Systematic reviews (SR)			
Morris et al (2004)	Stroke	Progressive resistance exercise (PRE)	→ strength ? activity
Ada et al (2006a)	Stroke	PRE, electrical stimulation (ES), biofeedback, activity-triggered ES	→ strength → activity
Glanz et al (1996)	Stroke	ES	→ strength
Schleenbaker & Mainous (1993)	Stroke	Biofeedback	→ activity
Moreland & Thomson (1994)	Stroke	Biofeedback for upper limb	No diff
Moreland et al (1998)	Stroke	Biofeedback for lower limb	→ strength No diff activity
Controlled trials			
Ruhland & Shields (1997)	Chronic peripheral neuropathy	Progressive resisted exercise	→ strength
McCartney et al (1988)	Neuromuscular (NM) diseases	Progressive resisted exercise	→ strength
Aitkens et al (1993)	NM diseases	Progressive resisted exercise	No difference strength
Dibble et al (2006)	Parkinson's disease	Progressive resisted eccentric exercise	→ strength → activity
Kilmer et al (1994)	NM diseases	Progressive resisted exercise	→ concentric strength ← eccentric strength

Box 7.3

Weakness in UMNL may include the following characteristics

- weakness makes an independent contribution to activity limitations above that of dexterity (Canning et al 2004)
- there is selective weakness in shortened range (Ada et al 2003)
- there is ↑ time to peak torque (Canning et al 1999)
- there is greater ↓ in torque with increasing speed of concentric contraction (Ponichtera-Mulcare 1993)
- there is ↓ ability to sustain a contraction (Schwid et al 1999)
- there is ↓ number of functional motor units over time (McComas et al 1973)

Box 7.4

Strength training for UMNL should:
- be started early
- include varied types of contractions e.g. at short muscle lengths, at fast speeds, sustained contractions
- include mental practice if physical effort is not possible

For both UMNL & LMNL

When muscles <u>do not have</u> antigravity strength:
- encourage a contraction by using gravity modification/elimination, suspension, electrical stimulation (ES), electromyographic (EMG) biofeedback, and activity-triggered ES

When muscles <u>do have</u> antigravity strength:
- apply resistance to produce near maximum contractions according to the guidelines set out by the American College of Sports Medicine (ACSM 2002)

Ataxia is a specific type of incoordination (usually arising from lesions to the cerebellum) which is often summarized as 'errors in rate, range, direction and force of movement'. Loss of dexterity is commonly present in UMNL (see Box 7.5); it is not usually a problem in LMNL, where loss of strength is consistently the major motor impairment.

Dexterity training should include task-specific training (see evidence in Table 7.2; and training strategies in Box 7.6).

Table 7.2 Some evidence for task-related training.

Studies	Subjects	Intervention	Outcome
Systematic reviews			
Van Peppen et al (2004)	Stroke	CIMT, TT, auditory cues during walking	→ activity
Moseley et al (2003)	Stroke	TT with BWS in dependent walkers TT with BWS in independent walkers	No diff activity → activity
Pollock et al (2004)	Stroke	Orthopaedic vs neurophysiologic vs motor learning approaches	No diff activity
Barclay-Goddard et al (2004)	Stroke	Visual and/or auditory feedback	No diff activity
RCTs not included in SR			
Dean & Shepherd (1997)	Chronic stroke	Task-related training (sitting)	→ activity
Engardt et al (1993)	Stroke	Feedback during sit to stand	→ activity
Kautz et al (2005)	Stroke	Task practice of pedalling	→ activity
Winstein et al (2004)	Acute stroke	Task training	→ activity
Michaelsen & Levin (2004)	Chronic stroke	Reaching with trunk restraint	→ dexterity
Duncan et al (2003)	Stroke	Task-specific training	→ activity
Dean et al (2000)	Stroke	Lower limb (LL) group circuit training	→ activity
Salbach et al (2004)	Stroke	LL individual circuit training	→ activity
Mudie et al (2002)	Acute Stroke	BPM feedback vs task specific reach vs Bobath	No diff in symmetry
Jones et al (1996)	MS ataxia	Proximal stabilization, balance and weighting	→ activity No diff in dexterity
Ellis et al (2005)	PD	Strengthening, balance and fitness	→ activity
Protas et al (2005)	PD	TT	→ activity

BPM, Balance Performance Monitor; CIMT, constraint-induced movement therapy; MS, multiple sclerosis; PD, Parkinson's disease; RCTs, randomized controlled trials; TT, treadmill training with body weight support.

7

Box 7.5

> **Impaired dexterity involves the loss of:**
> - skilful coordination of voluntary muscle activity to meet environmental demands
> - fractionation e.g. loss of independent use of individual fingers required for tasks such as typing, manipulating objects
> - spatial and/or temporal accuracy of movements
>
> **Loss of dexterity may include the following characteristics:**
> - jerky movement trajectories (Levin 1996)
> - dysmetria (disorder of movement termination) – hypermetric movement (overshooting) or hypometric movement (undershooting) (Bastian et al 1996)
> - rebound phenomenon (lack of check/restraint)
> - dysdiadochokinesia (difficulty in performing rapidly alternating movements)
> - dyssynergia (inability to coordinate timing of muscle contractions)
> - intention tremor (rhythmical, involuntary oscillation during voluntary movements)

Box 7.6

> **Task-specific training includes:**
> - part practice (such as outlined in Carr & Shepherd 2003)
> - modified practice (such as raising the height of the bed to practise standing up)
> - whole task practice (when antigravity strength is present), emphasizing speed and accuracy
> - whole task plus concurrent additional task(s) (i.e. dual or triple task) practice when whole task performance is nearing normal level

Bradykinesia and akinesia

Bradykinesia and akinesia are defined as reduced velocity and amplitude of movements, respectively (Berardelli et al 2001); see Box 7.7 and Box 7.8. However, these two terms are commonly used synonymously to describe both reduced velocity and amplitude of movement. Akinesia refers to difficulty in movement initiation and episodes of freezing (or motor blocks) occurring during the execution of a movement (Morris 2000). Bradykinesia and akinesia are seen in lesions of the

Box 7.7

Bradykinesia
- occurs bilaterally, but may be asymmetrical in severity
- occurs at single joint level (Hallett & Khoshbin 1980)
- is more pronounced in complex movements performed sequentially or simultaneously (Agostino et al 1998)
- presents as reduced speed and stride length in walking, with a compensatory increase in cadence for any given speed (Morris et al 1994)
- presents as reduced speed, amplitude and coordination of activities such as reaching and manipulation, standing up and sitting down, transfers, turning in bed and getting into/out of bed

Box 7.8

Akinesia:
- Slowness to commence activities
- Freezing (motor blocks) during activities (Kamsma et al 1995)
- Freezing during walking greatly increasing the risk of falling (Gray & Hildebrand 2000)
- Progressive shortening of steps and hastening of gait (festination) characteristically occurs prior to freezing (Iansek et al 2006)
- Typically occurs on initiation of and during walking, during turning and when performing simultaneous tasks (Nieuwboer et al 2001)

basal ganglia such as Parkinson's disease; both are worse when more than one task is being performed simultaneously, such as walking and talking (Bloem et al 2001).

Evidence for training to overcome bradykinesia and/or akinesia is presented in Table 7.3; see Box 7.9 for training suggestions and also refer to Chapter 10 (sub-chapter 10.5).

Impairments of tone

'Tone is the resistance of the limb to passive stretch . . . It is determined by the physical inertia of the limb as well as the passive mechanical properties of the soft tissues because in a normal, relaxed muscle, there is no reflex response to the stretch' (Burke, 1988). The most common impairments of tone are presented in Box 7.10.

Box 7.9

Training should include:

In the early stages of Parkinson's disease, when no activity limitations are evident:

● Exercise therapy (including dexterity, lower limb strength and fitness training) to maintain optimal mobility

● Walking over longer distances, using cueing can emphasize walking with long strides as well as fitness

In the middle stages of Parkinson's disease:

● Cognitive movement strategies (e.g. breaking the task down into components, preparing for threats to balance in advance)

● Cueing strategies (visual, auditory, tactile or combined) are used in the context of everyday tasks (Morris et al 1997)

● Maintaining muscle strength (especially of the lower limbs) and fitness

Table 7.3 Some evidence for training to overcome bradykinesia and/or akinesia.

Studies	Subjects	Intervention	Outcome
Systematic reviews			
Smidt et al (2005)	Various	Exercise therapy	↑ activity
Lim et al (2005)	PD	Rhythmical cueing	↑ activity (gait speed)
Randomized controlled trials not included in systematic reviews			
Nieuwboer et al (2007)	PD	Rhythmical cueing	↑ activity ↓ akinesia
Keus et al (2006)	PD	Cueing and cognitive movement strategies	↑ activity
Morris et al (2006)	PD	Movement strategies vs exercises	↓ impairment ↑ activity

There is debate about hypotonia; the small amount of available evidence suggests that clinical perception of hypotonia is most likely to be the result of the complete relaxation felt when passively moving paralysed or severely weak limbs (Burke 1988, Van der Meché & van Gijn 1986).

Spasticity is often used interchangeably with hypertonus; this is incorrect and confusing. Hypertonia (measured by resistance to stretch) needs to be distinguished from spasticity (best measured by electromyographic (EMG) activity

Box 7.10

Hypotonia
- the resistance to passive movement is less than normal

Hypertonia
- an increase in stiffness with resistance to stretch in one direction
- the result of **neural** impairments e.g. spasticity and/or **musculoskeletal** impairments e.g. contracture

Spasticity
- '. . . a motor disorder characterized by a velocity-dependent increase in tonic stretch reflexes with exaggerated tendon jerks resulting from hyperexcitability of the stretch reflex as one component of the UMN syndrome' (Lance 1980)
- Clasp knife phenomenon – as resistance builds up, there is a 'catch', and as movement slows, there is a 'give' as resistance melts away.
- Clonus – repetitive contractions of the muscle in response to a maintained stretch

Rigidity
- is bidirectional
- does not involve hyperexcitable stretch reflexes, and is not velocity-dependent (Kandel et al 2000)

response to stretch), and contracture (Ada et al 2006b, O'Dwyer & Ada 1996, O'Dwyer et al 1996). Spasticity may have a fast and a slow course in UMNL (Chapman & Wiesendanger 1982). The slow time course implies that spasticity is an adaptation to injury (probably mediated by the same sort of changes to synaptic connections that mediate recovery of activity) and that this adaptation can be influenced by external events, i.e. intervention. The evidence suggests that spasticity is a separate entity to the difficulty or inability to contract muscles (Neilson & McCaughey 1982, Sahrmann & Norton 1977, Tang & Rymer 1981). It would appear that the major contribution to movement disability after stroke is the result of the negative impairments, e.g. weakness, rather than the positive impairments, e.g. spasticity.

Evidence for reducing spasticity is presented in Table 7.4. However, even where hyperreflexia is considered to be a major problem, a reduction in hyperreflexia is not necessarily followed by an improvement in motor activity. Where spasticity is mild, intervention should focus on improving activity. Where spasticity is severe, intervention should focus on making the patient more comfortable (see Box 7.11).

Table 7.4 Some evidence for reducing spasticity.

Studies	Subjects	Intervention	Outcome
Systematic reviews			
Mortensen & Eng (2003)	Stroke or TBI	Casting	Moderate recommendation for casting
Randomized controlled trials not included in systematic reviews			
Verplancke et al (2005)	TBI	BTA + casting vs placebo + casting	↓ contracture with casting alone
Gracies et al (2000)	Stroke	Dynamic lycra splinting for 3 hrs	↓ spasticity short-term
Agerionoti et al (1990)	Stroke	Vibration	↓ spasticity short-term

BTA, botulinum toxin A; TBI, traumatic brain injury.

Box 7.11

When spasticity is mild to moderate, intervention could include:
- dexterity training that focuses on eliminating unnecessary activity
- eccentric training of muscles that commonly develop spasticity
- maintenance of muscle length

When spasticity is moderate to severe, intervention to reduce severe contracture could include:
- casting
- centrally acting drugs e.g. baclofen, diazepam or peripherally acting drugs e.g. botulinum toxin

Tremor

Tremor is a rhythmical, involuntary oscillation of a body part (see Box 7.12); tremor commonly results from cerebellar and basal ganglia lesions. When severe, intention, action and postural tremors can impact heavily on activity (Bain et al 1993).

Interventions to decrease tremor are presented in Box 7.13.

Dyskinesia

The most common presentations of dyskinesia are tremor, chorea and dystonia (Box 7.14). Dyskinesia is an umbrella term for involuntary movements of whatever

Box 7.12 Types of tremor (Deuschl et al 1998)

- Resting – occurs with no voluntary activation and limb supported
- Action or kinetic – occurs with voluntary activation (includes postural, isometric and intention)
- Intention – occurs during target-directed voluntary movements (terminal tremor, most marked near target)
- Postural – occurs when voluntarily maintaining a position against gravity
- Isometric – occurs during isometric contraction

Box 7.13

Interventions to temporarily control tremor (Parkinson's disease; Morris et al 1997):
- Performing a purposeful movement with the affected limb
- Applying gentle pressure through the affected limb

Medical and surgical interventions to decrease tremor (Parkinson's disease):
- drugs – e.g. levodopa, dopamine agonists (Sethi 2003)
- for drug-resistant tremor, thalamotomy of the ventral intermediate nucleus (VIM) or thalamic stimulation (Liu et al 2000)

Intervention to temporarily reduce intention tremor (cerebellar lesions):
- use of weights (Langton Hewer et al 1972; Morgan et al 1975)
- adaptive equipment and strategies (McGruder et al 2003)

Medical and surgical interventions to decrease tremor (cerebellar lesions):
- drugs – e.g. ondansetron (Rice et al 1997)
- surgery – e.g. thalamotomy of the ventral intermediate nucleus (Liu et al 2000)
- thalamic stimulation (Montgomery et al 1999)

cause. The relationship to activity limitations is variable. Dyskinesia may be primary (e.g. cervical dystonia, occupational dystonia such as writer's cramp), or secondary due to long-term treatment with anti-psychotic drugs which block dopamine transmission and may make dopamine receptors hyperreceptive in the management of Parkinson's disease.

Interventions are unlikely to prevent or permanently reduce dyskinesias (see Box 7.15). If severe disabling dyskinesia persists with optimal medication and

Box 7.14

Types of dyskinesia
- tremor – repetitive rhythmic movement consistent in time and space (see above)
- chorea – rapid, irregular, purposeless movement of any part of the body
- dystonia – sustained muscle contractions, frequently causing twisting and repetitive movements or abnormal postures
- myoclonus – brief shock-like jerks of a limb or body part, encephalopathy, drug treatment
- ballism – violent flailing movements

Box 7.15

Interventions for dyskinesia
- prolonged stretch and weight bearing in normal alignment for dystonia of the calf muscles (Schenkman et al 1989)
- voluntary activation which involves fixing the distal segment, e.g. clasping the hands behind back while walking, squeezing movements in sitting, supporting arms in sitting and pushing down through arms for chorea (Morris et al 1997)
- relaxation for anxiety reduction (Morris et al 1997)

physiotherapy, then surgical options such as pallidotomy and deep brain stimulation of globus pallidus internus and subthalamic nucleus are considered (Piper et al 2005).

SECONDARY MUSCULOSKELETAL IMPAIRMENTS

The most common secondary musculoskeletal impairments are:
- length-associated changes such as shortening and stiffness, e.g. contracture
- use-associated changes such as subluxation and swelling.

Although the implication is that secondary impairments should be preventable; the fact that their incidence is still so high means that they are not very easy to prevent. There are neural, musculoskeletal and environmental contributors such as:
- paralysis → immobility
- paralysis → gravity dependence of limbs
- trauma.

Contracture

Contracture is a clinical term meaning a decrease in passive range of motion (ROM) at a joint. It may be the result of loss of length in muscle(s) or periarticular connective tissues (cartilage, capsule, and ligament) with increased stiffness in these structures. All neurological conditions which involve muscle weakness and spasticity are prone to developing contracture. The most detrimental effect on activity when muscles shorten and stiffen tend to be in those muscles where the full range is needed in everyday tasks, e.g. gastrocnemius for standing and walking. Evidence for interventions to decrease contracture is presented in Table 7.5; see Box 7.16 for intervention.

Table 7.5 Some evidence for intervention to decrease contracture.

Studies	Subjects	Intervention	Outcome
Systematic reviews			
Lannin & Herbert (2003)	Stroke	Hand splinting	Insufficient evidence
Mortensen & Eng (2003)	Stroke or TBI	Casting	Moderate recommendation for casting
Randomized controlled trials not included in systematic reviews			
Verplancke et al (2005)	TBI	BTA + casting vs placebo + casting	↓ contracture with casting alone
Moseley (1997)	TBI	Casting vs control	↑ ROM
Ada et al (2005)	Acute stroke	Positioning vs nothing	↓ loss of ROM
Ben et al (2005)	SCI	Standing stretch vs nothing	Small ↑ ROM
Harvey et al (2003)	SCI	Stretch vs nothing	No diff
Harvey et al (2000)	SCI	Stretch vs nothing	No diff
Lannin et al (2003)	Stroke	Hand splinting + stretch vs stretch	No diff
Turton & Britton (2005)	Stroke	Positioning vs nothing	No diff
De Jong et al (2006)	Acute stroke	Positioning vs nothing	↓ loss of range of motion

BTA, botulinum toxin A; ROM, range of motion; SCI, spinal cord injury; TBI, traumatic brain injury.

Box **7.16** Intervention for contracture

● Muscles at risk of shortening that will have a detrimental impact on activity should be positioned in lengthened positions for long periods daily; i.e. for at least 20–30 min at maximum range.

Subluxation of the shoulder

Subluxation is a partial dislocation of the head of the humerus in the glenoid fossa; it is more associated with weakness than pain (Joynt 1992). Subluxation of the humerus affects up to 34% of people early after stroke (Roy et al 1994) and also affects C4/5 level tetraplegics who have some scapulothoracic muscles (such as rhomboids and upper trapezius) but not others (such as serratus anterior) innervated. There is very little evidence to suggest that once the shoulder is subluxed that it can return to normal. Furthermore, the shoulder cannot move normally when it is subluxed. Interventions to prevent subluxation are included in Box 7.17.

Box 7.17

Interventions for subluxation:
● almost continuous electrical stimulation (ES) to post deltoid and supraspinatus (Ada & Foongchomcheay 2002)
● a firm tray when seated and a triangular sling temporarily fitted when standing (Ada et al 2005)

Swelling of the extremities

A small amount of swelling in the hand can cause changes in sensation, while swelling in the lower limb can contribute to deep vein thrombosis (DVT) formation. Any neurological condition, acute, chronic or degenerative, that is severe enough to effectively immobilize the person in an upright but seated position with both the upper and lower limbs dependent, will exhibit swelling of the extremities. The main causes of swelling are dependency of the limbs as a result of early resumption of upright position, and lack of muscle pump due to severe weakness. See Box 7.18 for intervention.

Box 7.18

Intervention to prevent swelling:
● electrical stimulation (ES) to the forearm muscles and the ankle muscles since ES is also effective in increasing strength (Faghri 1997)

KEY CLINICAL MESSAGES
- Neurological conditions can involve both UMNL or LMNL.
- Classifying impairments after brain damage as primary or secondary, and negative or positive is a useful framework for investigating movement disability.
- Neurological conditions usually result in impairments that take time to resolve; common secondary impairments (such as contracture, shoulder subluxation, and swelling) arise as adaptations to the primary impairments.
- Weakness is a major contributor to persistent activity limitations.
- Loss of dexterity can be considered to be synonymous with incoordination, loss of selective movement or lack of motor control; dexterity training should include task-specific training.
- Evidence suggests that spasticity is a separate entity to the difficulty or inability to contract muscles. The major contribution to movement disability after stroke is the result of the negative impairments e.g. weakness rather than the positive impairments e.g. spasticity. Even where hyperreflexia is considered to be a major problem, a reduction in hyperreflexia is not necessarily followed by an improvement in motor activity.

References

Ada L, Foongchomcheay A 2002 Efficacy of electrical stimulation in preventing or reducing subluxation of the shoulder after stroke: a meta-analysis. Australian Journal of Physiotherapy 48:257–267.

Ada L, Canning CG, Low SL 2003 Stroke patients have selective weakness in shortened range. Brain 126:724–731.

Ada L, Goddard E, McCully J, Stavrinos T, Bampton J 2005 Thirty minutes of positioning reduces the development of shoulder external rotation contracture after stroke: a randomized controlled trial. Archives of Physical Medicine and Rehabilitation 86:230–234.

Ada L, Dorsch S, Canning CG 2006a Strengthening interventions increase strength and improve activity after stroke: a systematic review. Australian Journal of Physiotherapy 52:241–248.

Ada L, O'Dwyer N, O'Neill E 2006b Relation between spasticity, weakness and contracture of the elbow flexors and upper limb activity after stroke: an observational study. Disability & Rehabilitation 28:891–897.

Ageranioti SA 1990 Effects of vibration on hypertonia and hyperreflexia in the wrist joint of patients with spastic hemiparesis. Physiotherapy Canada 42:24–33.

Agostino R, Berardelli A, Curra A, Accornero N, Manfredi M 1998 Clinical impairment of sequential finger movements in Parkinson's disease. Movement Disorders 13:418–421.

Aitkens SG, McCrory MA, Kilmer DD, Bernauer EM 1993 Moderate resistance exercise program: its effect in slowly progressive neuromuscular disease. Archives of Physical Medicine and Rehabilitation 74:711–715.

American College of Sports Medicine 2002 Progression models in resistance training for healthy adults. Position Stand. Medicine and Science in Sports and Exercise 34:364–380.

Bain PG, Findley LJ, Atchison P et al 1993 Assessing tremor severity. Journal of Neurology, Neurosurgery and Psychiatry 56:868–873.

Barclay-Goddard R, Stevenson T et al 2004 Force platform feedback for standing balance training after stroke. Cochrane Database of Systematic Reviews (4):CD004129. UI:15495079.

Bastian AJ, Martin TA, Keating JG, Thach WT 1996 Cerebellar ataxia: abnormal control of interaction torques across multiple joints. Journal of Neurophysics 76:492–509.

Ben M, Harvey L, Denis S et al 2005 Does 12 weeks of regular standing prevent loss of ankle mobility and bone mineral density in people with recent spinal cord injuries? Australian Journal of Physiotherapy 51:251–256.

Berardelli A, Rothwell JC, Thompson PD, Hallett M 2001 Pathophysiology of bradykinesia in Parkinson's disease. Brain 124:2131–2146.

Bernstein NA 1994 On dexterity and its development. Moscow: Physical Culture and Sport Press (in Russian) 1991, cited in Latash LP, Latash MK. A new book by Bernstein: 'On dexterity and its development'. Journal of Motor Behavior 26:56–62.

Bloem BR, Valkenburg VV, Slabbekoorn M, van Dijk JG 2001 The multiple tasks test. Strategies in Parkinson's disease. Experimental Brain Research 137:478–486.

Bourbonnais D, Bilodeau S, Lepage Y et al 2002 Effect of force-feedback treatments in patients with chronic motor deficits after stroke. American Journal of Physical Medicine and Rehabilitation 81:890–897.

Burke D 1988 Spasticity as an adaptation to pyramidal tract injury. Advances in Neurology 47:401–423.

Bütefisch C, Hummelsheim H, Denzler P, Mauritz K-H 1995 Repetitive training of isolated movements improves the outcome of motor rehabilitation of the centrally paretic hand. Journal of Neurological Sciences 130:59–68.

Canning CG, Ada L, O'Dwyer N 1999 Slowness to develop force contributes to weakness after stroke. Archives of Physical Medicine and Rehabilitation 80:66–70.

Canning CG, Ada L, Adams R, O'Dwyer NJ 2004 Loss of strength contributes more to physical disability after stroke than loss of dexterity. Clinical Rehabilitation 18:300–308.

Carr JH, Shepherd RB 2003 Stroke Rehabilitation. Butterworth-Heinemann, Oxford.

Chapman CE, Wiesendanger M 1982 Recovery of activity following unilateral lesions of the bulbar pyramid in the monkey. Electroencephalography and Clinical Neurophysiology 53:374–387.

De Jong LD, Nieuwboer A, Aufdemkampe G 2006 Contracture preventive positioning of the hemiplegic arm in subacute stroke patients: a pilot randomized controlled trial. Clinical Rehabilitation 20:656–667.

Dean CM, Shepherd RB 1997 Task-related training improves performance of seated reaching tasks after stroke. A randomized controlled trial. Stroke 28:722–728.

Dean CM, Richards CL, Malouin F 2000 Task-related circuit training improves performance of locomotor tasks in chronic stroke: a randomized, controlled pilot trial. Archives of Physical Medicine and Rehabilitation 81:409–417.

Deuschl G, Bain P, Brin M and an *ad hoc* Scientific Committee 1998 Consensus statement of the movement disorder society on tremor. Movement Disorders 13:2–23.

Dibble LE, Hale TF, Marcus RL et al 2006 High-intensity resistance training amplifies muscle hypertrophy and activityal gains in persons with Parkinson's disease. Movement Disorders 21:1444–1452.

Drory VE, Goltsman E, Reznik JG, Mosek A, Korczyn AD 2001 The value of muscle exercise in patients with amyotrophic lateral sclerosis. Journal of the Neurological Sciences 191:133–137.

Duncan P, Studenski S, Richards L et al 2003 Randomized clinical trial of therapeutic exercise in subacute stroke. Stroke 34:2173–2180.

Ellis T, de Goede CJ, Feldman RG, Wolters EC, Kwakkel G, Wagenaar RC 2005 Efficacy of a physical therapy program in patients with Parkinson's disease: a randomized controlled trial. Archives of Physical Medicine and Rehabilitation 86:626–632.

Engardt M, Ribbe T, Olsson E 1993 Vertical ground reaction force feedback to enhance stroke patients' symmetrical body-weight distribution while rising/sitting down. Scandinavian Journal of Rehabilitation Medicine 25:41–48.

Engardt M, Knutsson E, Jonsson M, Sternhag M 1995 Dynamic muscle strength training in stroke patients: effects on knee extension torque, electromyographic activity and motor activity. Archives of Physical Medicine and Rehabilitation 76:419–425.

Faghri PD, Rodgers MM 1997 The effects of activity and neuromuscular stimulation-augmented physical therapy program in the recovery of hemiplegic arm in stroke patients. Clinical Kinesiology 51:9–15.

Glanz M, Klawansky S, Stason W et al 1996 Activity and electrostimulation in post stroke rehabilitation: a meta-analysis of the randomized controlled trials. Archives of Physical Medicine and Rehabilitation 77:549–553.

Gracies JM, Marosszeky JE, Renton R et al 2000 Short-term effects of dynamic Lycra splints on upper limb in hemiplegic patients. Archives of Physical Medicine and Rehabilitation 81:1547–1555.

Gray P, Hildebrand K 2000 Fall risk factors in Parkinson's disease. Journal of Neuroscience Nursing 32:222–234.

Hallett M, Khoshbin S 1980 A physiological mechanism of bradykinesia. Brain 103:301–314.

Harvey LA, Batty J, Crosbie J, Poulter S, Herbert RD 2000 A randomized trial assessing the effects of 4 weeks of daily stretching on ankle mobility in patients with spinal cord injuries. Archives of Physical Medicine and Rehabilitation 81:1340–1347.

Harvey LA, Byak AJ, Ostrovskaya M et al 2003 Randomised trial of the effects of four weeks of daily stretch on extensibility of hamstring muscles in people with spinal cord injuries. Australian Journal of Physiotherapy 49:176–181.

Iansek R, Huxham F, McGinley J 2006 The sequence effect and gait festination in Parkinson disease: contributors to freezing of gait? Movement Disorders 21:1419–1424.

Jones L, Lewis Y, Harrison J, Wiles CM 1996 The effectiveness of occupational therapy and physiotherapy in multiple sclerosis patients with ataxia of the upper limb and trunk. Clinical Rehabilitation 10:277–282.

Joynt RL 1992 The source of shoulder pain in hemiplegia. Archives of Physical Medicine and Rehabilitation 73:409–413.

Kamsma Y, Brouwer W, Lakke J 1995 Training of compensational strategies for impaired gross motor skills in Parkinson's disease. Physiotherapy Theory and Practice 11:209–229.

Kandel ER, Schwartz JH, Jessell TM 2000 Principles of neural science. New York, McGraw-Hill.

Kautz SA, Duncan PW, Perera S et al 2005 Coordination of hemiparetic locomotion after stroke rehabilitation. Neurorehabilitation and Neural Repair 19:250–258.

Keus SH, Bloem BR, van Hilten JJ et al 2006 Effectiveness of physiotherapy in Parkinson's disease: the feasibility of a randomised controlled trial. Parkinsonism and Related Disorders 13:115–121.

Kilmer DD, McCrory MA, Wright NC et al 1994 The effect of a high resistance exercise program in slowly progressive neuromuscular disease. Archives of Physical Medicine and Rehabilitation 75:560–563.

Lance JW 1980 Symposium synopsis. In: Feldman RG et al (eds) Spasticity: disordered motor control. Miami, Symposia Specialists, pp 485–494.

Langton Hewer R, Cooper R, Morgan MH 1972 An investigation into the value of treating intention tremor by weighting the affected limb. Brain 95:579–590.

Lannin NA, Herbert RD 2003 Is hand splinting effective for adults following stroke? A systematic review and methodologic critique of published research. Clinical Rehabilitation 17:807–816.

Lannin NA, Horsley SA, Herbert R et al 2003 Splinting the hand in the functional position after brain impairment: a randomized, controlled trial. Archives of Physical Medicine and Rehabilitation 84:297–302.

Levin MF 1996 Interjoint coordination during pointing movements is disrupted in spastic hemiparesis. Brain 119:281–293.

Lim I, van Wegen E, de Goede C et al 2005 Effects of external rhythmical cueing on gait in patients with Parkinson's disease: a systematic review. Clinical Rehabilitation 19:695–713.

Liu X, Aziz TZ, Miall RC et al 2000 Frequency analysis of involuntary movements during wrist tracking; a way to identify MS patients with tremor who benefit from thalamotomy. Stereotactic and Functional Neurosurgery 74:53–62.

McCartney N, Moroz D, Garner S, McComas AL 1988 The effects of strength training in patients with selected neuromuscular disorders. Medicine and Science in Sports and Exercise 24:362–368.

McComes AJ, Sica RE, Upton AR, Aguilera N 1973 Changes in motorneurones of hemiparetic patients. Journal of Neurology, Neurosurgery and Psychiatry 36:183–193.

McGruder J, Cors D, Tiernan AM, Tomlin G 2003 Weighted wrist cuffs for tremor reduction during eating in adults with static brain lesions. American Journal of Occupational Therapy 57:507–516.

Michaelsen SM, Levin MF 2004 Short-term effects of practice with trunk restraint on reaching movements in patients with chronic stroke: a controlled trial. Stroke 35:1914–1919.

Milner-Brown HS, Miller RG 1988 Muscle strengthening through high-resistance weight training in patients with neuromuscular disorders. Archives of Physical Medicine and Rehabilitation 69:14–19.

Montgomery EB, Baker KB, Kinkel RP, Barnett G 1999 Chronic thalamic stimulation for the tremor of multiple sclerosis. Neurology 53:625–628.

Moreland J, Thomson MA 1994 Efficacy of electromyographic biofeedback compared with conventional physical therapy for upper-extremity activity in patients following stroke: a research overview and meta-analysis. Physical Therapy 74:534–543.

Moreland JD, Thomson MA, Fuoco AR 1998 Electromyographic biofeedback to improve lower extremity activity after stroke: a meta-analysis. Archives of Physical Medicine and Rehabilitation 79:134–140.

Morgan MH, Hewer RL, Cooper R 1975 Application of an objective method of assessing intention tremor – further study on the use of weights to reduce intention tremor. Journal of Neurology Neurosurgery and Psychiatry 38:259–264.

Morris M 2000 Movement disorders in people with Parkinson's disease: a model for physical therapy. Physical Therapy 80:578–597.

Morris ME, Iansek R 2006 Effects of strategy training compared to exercises for gait rehabilitation in Parkinson disease: a randomized controlled trial. Movement Disorders 21:S515.

Morris ME, Iansek R, Matyas TA, Summers JJ 1994 The pathogenesis of gait hypokinesia in Parkinson's disease. Brain 117:1169–1181.

Morris M, Bruce M, Smithson F 1997 Physiotherapy strategies for people with Parkinson's disease. In: Morris M, Iansek R (eds) Parkinson's disease: a team approach. Melbourne, Kingston Centre Southern Health Care Network, pp 27–64.

Morris SL, Dodd KJ, Morris ME 2004 Outcomes of progressive resistance strength training following stroke: a systematic review. Clinical Rehabilitation 18:27–39.

Mortenson PA, Eng JJ 2003 The use of casts in the management of joint mobility and hypertonia following brain injury in adults: a systematic review. Physical Therapy 83:648–658.

Moseley AM 1997 The effect of casting combined with stretching on passive ankle dorsiflexion in adults with traumatic head injuries. Physical Therapy 77:240–247.

Moseley AM, Stark A, Cameron ID, Pollock A 2003 Treadmill training and body weight support for walking after stroke. Stroke 34:3006.

Mudie MH, Winzeler-Mercay U, Radwan S, Lee L 2002 Training symmetry of weight distribution after stroke: a randomized controlled pilot study comparing task-related reach, Bobath and feedback training approaches. Clinical Rehabilitation 16:582–592.

Neilson PD, McCaughey J 1982 Self-regulation of spasm and spasticity in cerebral palsy. Journal of Neurology, Neurosurgery and Psychiatry 45:320–330.

Nieuwboer A, Dom R, De Weerdt W et al 2001 Abnormalities of the spatiotemporal characteristics of gait at the onset of freezing in Parkinson's disease. Movement Disorders 16:1066–1075.

Nieuwboer A, Kwakkel G, Rochester L 2007 Cueing training in the home improves gait-related mobility in Parkinson's disease: The RESCUE trial. Journal of Neurology, Neurosurgery and Psychiatry 78:134–140.

O'Dwyer NJ, Ada L 1996 Reflex hyperexcitability and muscle contracture in relation to spastic hypertonia. Current Opinion in Neurology 9:451–455.

O'Dwyer NJ, Ada L, Neilson PD 1996 Spasticity and muscle contracture following stroke. Brain 119:1737–1749.

Piper M, Abrams GM, Marks WJ 2005 Deep brain stimulation for the treatment of Parkinson's disease: overview and impact on gait and mobility. NeuroRehabilitation 20:223–232.

Pollock A, Baer G, Pomeroy V, Langhorne P 2003 Physiotherapy treatment approaches for the recovery of postural control and lower limb activity following stroke. Cochrane Database Systematic Review (2):CD001920.

Ponichtera-Mulcare JA 1993 Exercise and multiple sclerosis. Medicine and Science in Sports & Exercise 25:451–465.

Protas EJ, Mitchell K, Williams A et al 2005 Gait and step training to reduce falls in Parkinson's disease. NeuroRehabilitation 20:183–190.

Rice GPA, Lesaux J, Vandervoort P et al 1997 Ondansetron, a 5-HT3 antagonist, improves cerebellar tremor. Journal of Neurology, Neurosurgery and Psychiatry 62:282–284.

Roy CW, Sands MR, Hill LD 1994 Shoulder pain in acutely admitted hemiplegics. Clinical Rehabilitation 8:334–340.

Ruhland JL, Shields RK 1997 The effects of a home exercise program on impairment and health-related quality of life in persons with chronic peripheral neuropathies. Physical Therapy 77:1026–1039.

Sahrmann SA, Norton BJ 1977 The relationship of voluntary movement to spasticity in the upper motor neuron syndrome. Annals of Neurology 2:460–465.

Salbach NM, Mayo NE, Wood-Dauphinee S et al 2004 A task-orientated intervention enhances walking distance and speed in the first year post stroke: a randomized controlled trial. Clinical Rehabilitation 18:509–519.

Schenkman M, Donovan J, Tsubota J et al 1989 Management of individuals with Parkinson's disease: rationale and case studies. Physical Therapy 69:944–955.

Schleenbaker RE, Mainous AG 1993 Electromyographic biofeedback for neuromuscular reeducation in the hemiplegic stroke patient: a meta-analysis. Archives of Physical Medicine and Rehabilitation 74:1301–1304.

Schwid SR, Thornton CA, Pandya S 1999 Quantitative assessment of motor fatigue and strength in MS. Neurology 53:743–750.

Sethi KD 2003 Tremor. Current Opinion in Neurology 16:481–485.

Sharp SA, Brouwer BJ 1997 Isokinetic strength training of the hemiparetic knee: effects on activity and spasticity. Archives of Physical Medicine and Rehabilitation 78:1231–1236.

Smidt N, de Vet HC, Bouter LM et al 2005 Effectiveness of exercise therapy: a best-evidence summary of systematic reviews. Australian Journal of Physiotherapy 51: 71–85.

Tang A, Rymer WZ 1981 Abnormal force – EMG relations in paretic limbs of hemiparetic human subjects. Neurology, Neurosurgery and Psychiatry 44:690–698.

Turton AJ, Britton E 2005 A pilot randomized controlled trial of a daily muscle stretch regime to prevent contractures in the arm after stroke. Clinical Rehabilitation 19:600–612.

Van der Meché FGA, van Gijn J 1986 Hypotonia: an erroneous clinical concept? Brain 109:1169–1178.

Van Peppen RP, Kwakkel G, Wood-Dauphinee S et al 2004 The impact of physical therapy on activity and outcomes after stroke: what's the evidence? Clinical Rehabilitation 18:833–862.

Verplancke D, Snape S, Salisbury CF et al 2005 A randomized controlled trial of botulinum toxin on lower limb spasticity following acute acquired severe brain injury. Clinical Rehabilitation 19:117–125.

Winstein CJ, Rose DK, Tan SM et al 2004 A randomized controlled comparison of upper-extremity rehabilitation strategies in acute stroke: a pilot study of immediate and long-term outcomes. Archives of Physical Medicine and Rehabilitation 85: 620–628.

CLINICAL DECISION MAKING

CHAPTER 8

Guiding principles for neurological physiotherapy

Sheila Lennon and Clare Bassile

INTRODUCTION

This chapter discusses the role and aims of neurological physiotherapy, explaining the factors that influence physiotherapy management priorities across settings. Physiotherapists in neurology base their assumptions about intervention on different philosophical perspectives, which determine how patients are assessed and treated (Lennon 2004). Therapists need to incorporate a wide range of strategies that are supported by the current evidence base into their treatment programmes regardless of their philosophical origin (Pollock et al 2007). Despite subscribing to different philosophical perspectives and working in radically different health care systems and cultures, the authors of this chapter have identified guiding principles underlying current physiotherapy practice for adults with clinical problems arising from damage to the nervous system within a core conceptual framework which is applicable to all physiotherapists working in neurological rehabilitation. Specific information about assessment and intervention for different types of patients is presented in Chapters 9 and 10.

ROLE OF PHYSIOTHERAPY

The role of the physiotherapist working in neurology is to help the patient experience and relearn optimal movement and functional activity. Physiotherapists are not only interested in which activities patients have difficulty in performing with or without assistance, but also in how the patient moves (the quality of movement) to execute these activities. Movement re-education and the practice of functional activity are two essential components of neurological physiotherapy (see Figure 8.1); the degree of overlap between these components varies according to therapist preference and patient and carer's needs. However, physiotherapy is not just about assessing and re-educating movement and function, a significant proportion of therapy time is devoted to educating, advising, and supporting patients and their families as well as liaising with other members of the health care team.

Figure 8.1
Essential components of neurological physiotherapy.

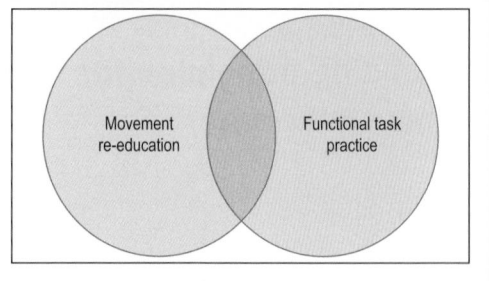

Figure 8.2
RAMP – aims of neurological physiotherapy (adapted from Lennon 2004, with permission).

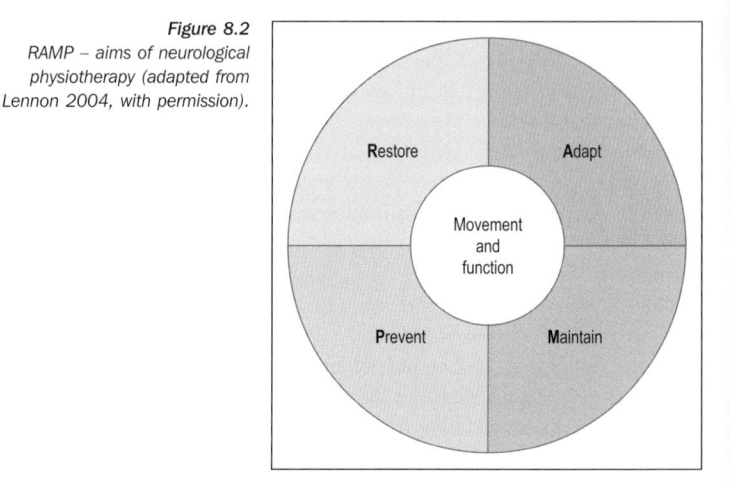

AIMS OF NEUROLOGICAL PHYSIOTHERAPY

Rehabilitation aims to achieve the best possible functional outcome and quality of life for each individual (Duncan et al 2005). Physiotherapists within the package of rehabilitation use the process of clinical reasoning combined with current evidence and the patient and carer's perspective to assess, develop and evaluate an appropriate plan of care for each patient (Chapter 9; APTA 2003). Therapists use a common assessment process across neurological conditions supplemented by standardized measures with published reliability and validity (Chapter 11). Final elements within the assessment form, the treatment strategies and outcome tools selected, will vary according to the aims of intervention and other management priorities (see Chapter 10 for physiotherapy interventions at different stages of care). The aims of neurological physiotherapy can be summed up using the acronym RAMP (Figure 8.2).

Physiotherapy ideally aims to restore movement and function in people with neurological pathology, but this may not always be possible. Maintenance of function is just as important as recovery, and should be viewed as a positive achievement. A wealth of literature in the domain of progressive neurological conditions such as multiple sclerosis (Motyl et al 2005, MS Society 2004, NICE 2003) and Parkinson's disease (De Goede et al 2001, Keus et al 2007) has demonstrated that functional ability can be maintained despite deteriorating impairments. There is also some evidence to suggest that disease progression may be modulated with physiotherapy (Heesen et al 2006).

Adaptation (compensation) is another important issue in neurological physiotherapy. Compensation refers to the use of alternative movement strategies to complete a task (Shumway-Cook & Woollacott 2007, pp. 21–45). It can be viewed as both a negative and a positive contributor to movement dysfunction following brain damage. Therapists focus on promoting compensatory strategies that are necessary for function and discouraging those that may be detrimental to the patient; e.g. promoting musculoskeletal damage like genu recurvatum (Edwards 2002, p. 2). The initiation of compensatory strategies into intervention may depend on the health care system as much as on philosophical perspective.

Different philosophical approaches treat restoration of function with varying degrees of actual functional task practice; e.g. practising a movement pattern is impairment focused not function focused. Current evidence suggests that the practice of motor skills needs to be both task and context specific (Kwakkel et al 2004, Van Peppen et al 2004), however when the patient has impairments that make it difficult to practise the ultimate task directly, therapists may also need to address impairments (Lennon 2004) either before or during a modified version of functional task practice. It is important to remember that for the patient to regain a functional arm and hand, you must practise reach and grasp activities (Winstein et al 2004). The key message is that interventions should always focus on the function and goals of the individual, and not simply be aimed at improving impairments without carry over into functional activity (Edwards 2002, p. 100). Thus assessing the effects of an intervention should always encompass the use of measures at both the impairment and activity levels of the International Classification of Functioning, Disability and Health (ICF) (WHO 2001).

FACTORS INFLUENCING MANAGEMENT PRIORITIES

The aims stated in Figure 8.2 have differential priorities at various stages in patient management and the timing at which each aim is incorporated into the plan depends upon a number of factors (Box 8.1).

Box 8.1

Factors in determining management priorities
- type of pathology (static vs progressive)
- type of setting (acute vs sub acute vs rehab vs home vs outpatient dept)
- prognosis
- patient and family needs and preferences

Box 8.2

Common secondary complications
- contractures
- pneumonia
- deep vein thrombosis
- pulmonary emboli
- pressure sores
- disuse atrophy
- autonomic nervous system deregulation e.g. fluctuations in heart rate or blood pressure

---

Type of pathology

Neurological lesions can generally be viewed as static (e.g. spinal cord injury, stroke), or progressive (e.g. multiple sclerosis – MS). Recovery is usually emphasized in a lesion like stroke, but progressive diseases usually require compensation especially if disease progression is rapid, i.e. motor neurone disease. However, there are always exceptions to this rule so understanding the nature of the pathology is essential to determine which aims [recovery vs adaptation (compensation)] should be emphasized by the physiotherapist. For example, in the complete spinal cord injured patient compensation needs to be emphasized, as recovery is not an option.

Type of setting

During the acute care stay the emphasis may be on identifying which patients are most likely to benefit from rehabilitation, and selecting the most appropriate type of setting for onward referral. Physiotherapy in this setting normally includes prevention of secondary complications from immobility (Box 8.2) along with a programme that includes interventions to reduce neurological deficits (impairments) and retraining of mobility skills (activities).

Interventions aimed at recovery of function need to be emphasized over compensation if the patient has the potential to change and is being considered for rehabilitation. If the patient is being discharged home quickly, then the priority may be interventions which teach compensations for a safe discharge (Rundek et al 2000).

Service delivery issues will also affect the aims of physiotherapy management. For example in the United States of America, given the prospective payment system of reimbursement, functional goals in the home setting usually emphasize compensation to adapt to residual disabilities rather than to reduce neurological deficits.

Predictors of recovery (prognosis)

Therapists take into account several factors when discussing within the health care team which setting the patient should be transferred to (Box 8.3).

As predictors of recovery vary according to the neurological condition, therapists also need to consider the usual patterns of recovery (time windows) for each condition, and the type of pathology when making the decision to aim for adaptation rather than recovery in their interventions. For example, for patients following stroke outcome appears largely defined within the first few weeks post stroke with the biggest functional gains occurring within 3 to 6 months (Kwakkel et al 2004); however, when the literature is scrutinized in more depth, the prognosis for recovery is multifactorial, and the time windows vary depending on whether you are working for regaining functional hand use or improving the patient's ability to walk. Using an example from the stroke population, some finger flexion or extension, and wrist extension appear to be key movements associated with upper

Box 8.3

Factors affecting recovery
- mental status
- medical stability
- importance of presenting complications e.g. raised intracranial pressure vs chest infection
- movement available
- affect (motivation and cooperation in therapy)
- functional ability
- tolerance of activity
- home context e.g. the patient lives alone or has family to care for
- presence of co-morbidities e.g. severe arthritis, previous level of mobility

extremity recovery (Fritz et al 2005). The variation in time window is large, with the Copenhagen cohort study reporting 12.5 weeks (Nakayama et al 1995) and the EXCITE study reporting up to 9 months after stroke (Wolf et al 2006); thus it is suggested that patients after stroke showing some signs of recovery of wrist and finger movement should receive interventions specifically to encourage hand movements for at least up to 9 months post stroke. Another example from patients with incomplete spinal cord injury suggests a time window for rehabilitation focusing on recovery of up to 8 weeks post injury to determine whether they will recover ambulation. If by 8 weeks the patient moves from an ASIA B to an ASIA C impairment level, then ambulation recovery usually occurs (Dobkin et al 2006).

Although it is difficult to predict outcome reliably in terms of recovery of motor deficits, for patients with stable pathology, a good rule of thumb is to push for recovery over compensation in patients deemed appropriate for in-patient rehabilitation in the early stages (e.g. within the first 3–4 weeks) depending on the patient's response to intervention, and proposed location of transfer of care, then start building in compensatory strategies. This gives the patient an opportunity to recover optimal movement and function rather than to use compensatory strategies which may hinder movement recovery because the patient is learning how <u>not</u> to use a limb (see Chapter 5 on training principles for neuroplastic change).

Patient and family preferences

Collaborative communication and involvement of patients and caregivers in deciding on treatment priorities, and setting their own rehabilitation goals, leads to improvements in self care and satisfaction with services (see Chapters 2 and 3). Negotiating with patients and carers when devising the treatment plan will help the therapist to decide whether to aim for recovery or compensation in conjunction with maintenance and prevention.

GUIDING PRINCIPLES FOR NEUROLOGICAL PHYSIOTHERAPY

The next section provides an overview of guiding principles for neurological physiotherapy some of which are also generic to all members of the rehabilitation team (Figure 8.3).

These principles which represent a conceptual framework to guide assessment and treatment in neurological physiotherapy are outlined in Table 8.1.

Appropriate components within therapy sessions

A comprehensive physiotherapy programme may include a wide range of components such as postural control training, movement re-education (trunk/pelvis/limbs), aerobic training, strengthening exercises, flexibility exercises, and

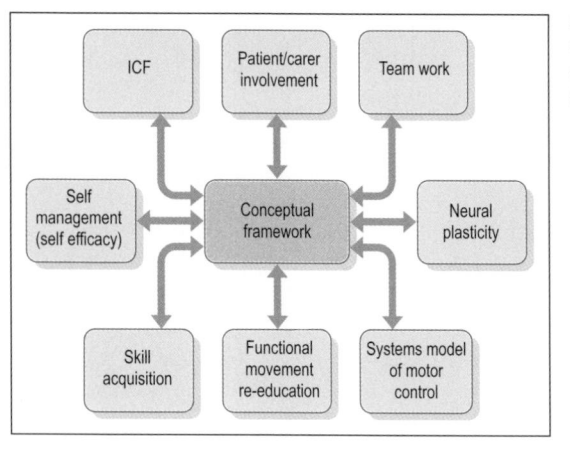

Figure 8.3
Guiding principles for neurological physiotherapy.

functional task practice (e.g. reach and grasp, bed mobility, transfer and ambulation activities).

Guidelines of critical features for training actions and functional tasks have been published in expert text books (Carr & Shepherd 2003, Edwards 2002). The choice and emphasis of the components will vary depending on the results of each patient's assessment (Chapters 9 & 10). Therapy programmes should be structured so patients can perform them independently or with as little set-up as possible from other individuals as staffing and visits from family/friends cannot be counted on consistently (Bear-Lehman et al 2001, Bernhardt et al 2004).

Structuring the therapy session

Therapists can be viewed as teachers of motor skill acquisition; therefore knowledge from motor learning and skill acquisition needs to be applied in patient intervention [see for an example Malouin & Richards (2005) recommendations for gait re-education after stroke].

The therapist always starts by asking what is the activity (action level e.g. goal) that needs to be worked on and what is the best position to start with. Box 8.4 sums up a simple way to remember the different elements that need to be addressed when answering these two questions. These elements are not hierarchical; they all interact together. Always consider starting by practising the chosen activity. If that would be too difficult then prioritize practising movements, or simplify the activity or practise part of the task.

Table 8.1 Guiding principles for neurological physiotherapy.

The ICF	• Neurological physiotherapy targets both impairments and activity within the ICF (WHO 2001). • Link the patient's impairments to activity limitations to direct a targeted approach to the re-education of movement, function and participation (Chapter 10).
Patient and carer involvement	• Enable patients and carers to be actively involved in deciding on treatment priorities, and collaborative goal setting (Chapters 2 and 3).
Interdisciplinary team work	• Adopt an interdisciplinary approach across services to coordinate care, prevent duplication, minimize secondary complications, re-inforce a 24 hour management approach and to improve outcomes of intervention (Duncan et al 2005).
Neural plasticity	• Training and experience changes the form and function of the nervous system: neural plasticity is the underlying rationale for rehabilitation (Chapter 5).
A systems model of motor control	• Adopt a systems model of motor control, which analyses the interaction between the individual, the task and the environment. Consider the neurophysiological, the biomechanical, and the behavioural constraints that influence the patient's everyday function (Chapter 4).
Functional movement re-education	• Consider both movement re-education and functional task practice. • Compare the patient's movements and functional mobility to parameters derived from both the healthy population and where possible from the impaired population to devise appropriate management plans. • Retrain optimal movement, actions and everyday activities (Carr & Shepherd 2003, pp. 8–24; Edwards 2002, p. 36).
Skill acquisition	When a patient practises a particular task, the therapist should (see Table 8.2 for more information): • Identify the critical task or movement components for successful performance (Carr & Shepherd 2003, pp. 15–18). • Decide how these components should be manipulated during training and determine the order/schedule for the practice session. • Use the variables that affect learning in an effective manner to promote skill acquisition e.g. feedback.
Self management (self efficacy)	• Encourage patients to develop core self-management skills such as problem solving; planning, setting targets and reflecting on individual successes will assist with strengthening their belief in their ability to succeed (self-efficacy – Chapter 12).

Box 8.4

- **Initial position**: Consider alignment and symmetry for more efficient muscle activation.
- **Loading**: Observe how the centre of mass (CoM) is moving within the chosen activity and individual's position. Consider how the patient is able to actively move their CoM with respect to their base of support (BOS) to target postural control (balance).
- **Movement**: Select the best movement to start with, try minimizing gravity and friction. Consider degrees of freedom (single joint and multijoint movement patterns) and putting movements into actions for task performance.
- **Functional task practice**: Consider the components of the task and the environmental set up to determine how best to modify the task for success.

Variables of practice

Practice for the purpose of skill acquisition is essential; in general the more time that is spent learning a skill the more performance is improved e.g. practice makes perfect; however a critical issue for physiotherapy is how much practice is required to improve functional skills (Kwakkel 2006). When looking at the variables that affect practice and learning, therapists often manipulate multiple variables simultaneously without thought to how these variables might interact. Some tips for structuring therapy using these variables are outlined in Table 8.2; these variables have mainly been researched in the motor learning literature related to psychology and sports exercise science.

ISSUES FOR DEBATE

Three current contentious issues are discussed briefly in this section: abnormal tone, associated reactions and therapeutic handling.

Abnormal tone

Should physiotherapists treat hypertonus or hypotonus (see Chapter 7)? The bottom line is if abnormal tone is exacerbating patient problems, hindering function and leading to complications; it should be treated (NCGS 2004). Although many therapists believe they are changing abnormal tone at a neural level, Mayston (2002) suggests that therapists change abnormal tone at a non-neural level by influencing muscle length and range. This enables improved alignment for more efficient muscle activation, thus allowing patients to experience more effective movement.

Table 8.2 Key variables for neurological physiotherapy.

Key variables	Issues to consider
Practice	● Amount (intensity or dose – Kwakkel 2006). ● Frequency (number of repetitions). ● Duration (number of minutes per session). ● Variety (alter regulatory features – Gentile 2000) e.g. transfers from different height chairs and different surface types. ● Type of practice (for example blocked practice (e.g. 5 reps at each seat height) vs random practice (e.g. different seat heights each time); Gilmore & Spaulding 2001). Choosing the practice schedule depends on a number of patient centred issues such as experience, age, memory, and task. However, there is insufficient data on which sequence works best for which patient (Gilmore & Spaulding 2001).
Specificity of training	● Functional task practice must be both task and context specific; therefore whenever possible practise the task (Kwakkel et al 2004, Van Peppen et al 2004). ● Consider critical requirements for each task (Carr & Shepherd 2003), as well as the impairments being targetted (Edwards 2002).
Transfer of training (generalizability)	● Impairment-focused training such as strength, range, symmetry, postural sway may improve the parameters being trained but these changes do not generalize to the activity or participation level (Kwakkel et al 2004, Van Peppen et al 2004). ● Consider two types of transfer of training (Winstein 1991): a) part task training: break the task down into simple steps, then put the steps back together again by practising the whole task. b) adaptive training: simplify the task by controlling a particularly difficult part e.g. using a body weight support system that gradually adds the body weight into gait. ● Task-related practice: some transferability will occur to a task which incorporates the components of transferring the centre of mass from the trunk to the lower extremities (e.g. practice of reaching greater than arm's length in sitting transfers to the sit to stand transitional activity – Dean & Shepherd 1997).

8

Table 8.2 Key variables for neurological physiotherapy—cont'd.

Key variables	Issues to consider
Feedback	• Type of feedback (info about behaviour or about movement). • Frequency (how often? All or some of the time? Never 100% of the time – Winstein 1994). • Timing (when to deliver the info – before, during or after). • Delivery mode (visual, verbal, manual). • Consider using extrinsic feedback or feedback with an external focus. Do not give feedback on every trial (van Vliet & Wulf 2006).
Modelling	• Demonstrate what you want the patient to do. • Consider delivery mode e.g. live vs videotaped vs written instruction (Laguna 2000, Reo & Mercer 2004, Williams & Hodges 2004, pp. 145–174). • Consider who is modelling (patient, therapist, another patient similar level/slightly ahead, expert).
Mental practice	• Defined as the act of repeating imagined movements several times with the intention of improving motor performance (Jackson et al 2001). An adjunct to physical practice, it is not better than physical practice (Braun et al 2006). • Consider when to use it; e.g. when patient needs additional personnel to set up environment for independent practice, during rest periods, or when patients are not safe to practise independently.

Associated reactions

Do we view associated movements during the execution of a motor task as abnormal or just part of the learning process? This depends on the therapist's philosophical perspective. Proponents of motor learning would explain that associated movements are part of early skill acquisition which should diminish as the patient's ability to perform the task improves. However, proponents of the Bobath Concept believe these associated reactions are a sign that the activity that the patient is practising requires too much effort, and would voice concerns that these stereotypical patterns will become ingrained and prevent further recovery. Whatever the preferred explanation, therapists would agree that associated reactions exist (Edwards 2002, pp. 93–99). They tend to manifest themselves when patients perform tasks that are effortful and new. Therapists should be alert to the flexibility of the patterns demonstrated by the performer and the triggers for these reactions should be identified. Therapy intervention will vary according to treatment philosophy.

Therapeutic handling

Do therapists spend too much time and effort on movement re-education using therapeutic handling; i.e. 'hands on' therapy in comparison to functional task practice? Lennon (2004) suggests a pragmatic approach, both 'hands on' and 'hands off' therapy may be required; it is not always possible to directly practise functional tasks; for example, the patient may not have any signs of motor activity in the lower limb in order to practise the task of walking. In this case the patients will require either hands-on assistance from therapists or support from assistive technologies, e.g. a partial body weight system in order to practise the task of walking. With regard to return of upper limb recovery, most large randomized controlled trials agree that patients need to have a minimum level of residual movement to demonstrate functional improvement (Van Peppen et al 2004). This means that therapists will need to use both impairment- and function-focused strategies depending on the patient.

Therapists must remember that therapeutic handling is only one of many strategies, which can help elicit return of movement. Therapeutic handling is a form of manual feedback. The motor learning literature corroborates that certain types of feedback should be used at different points in skill acquisition (Gilmore & Spaulding 2001). For example, manual guidance should mainly be used at the early cognitive stage of motor learning, whereas physical and verbal guidance may actually interfere with motor learning in the later associative (refining the skill) and autonomous (automaticity of the skill) stages of skill acquisition (Shumway-Cook & Woollacott 2007, pp. 32–39, Winstein 1991). In addition, using therapeutic handling most of the time is like giving patients feedback 100% of the time; this has been shown to actually hinder skill acquisition and creates a dependence on guidance (Winstein et al 1994). Therapists also need to consider that allowing patients to make errors can be a valuable training strategy.

KEY CLINICAL MESSAGES

- Eight principles have been identified to guide physiotherapy practice: the ICF, patient/carer involvement, interdisciplinary team work; neural plasticity, a systems model of motor control, functional movement re-education, skill acquisition and self-management (self efficacy).
- Movement re-education and functional task practice are the two core elements of functional movement re-education.
- Therapists may need to use a combination of impairment- and function-focused strategies. Whenever possible a task-oriented training approach should be adopted [tasks to improve ambulation may be either task related (e.g. sit to stand practice) or task specific (e.g. walking practice)] to promote motor learning and skill acquisition.

- Good quality evidence to support many interventions applied in neurological practice is lacking, however when good quality evidence to support clinical interventions is available we need to use that evidence.
- Neurological physiotherapy is a complex intervention. Best practice remains to be defined in terms of which interventions should be used for which patients in which dose and at what time post brain damage (Pomeroy & Tallis 2003).

References

[APTA] American Physical Therapy Association 2003 Guide to physical therapy practice. APTA, Alexandria, Va.

Bear-Lehman J, Bassile CC, Gillen G 2001 A comparison of time use on an acute rehabilitation unit: subjects with and without a stroke. Physical and Occupational Therapy in Geriatrics 20(1):17–27.

Bernhardt J, Dewey H, Thrift A, Donnan G 2004 Inactive and alone: physical activity within the first 14 days of acute stroke care. Stroke 35(4):1005–1009.

Braun SM, Beurskens AJ, Borm PJ et al 2006 The effects of mental practice in stroke rehabilitation. Archives of Physical Medicine and Rehabilitation 87:842–852.

Carr JH, Shepherd RB 2003 Stroke rehabilitation: guidelines for exercise and training to optimise motor skills. Butterworth Heinemann, London.

Dean C, Shepherd RB 1997 Task-related training improves performance of seated reaching tasks after stroke. A randomized controlled trial. Stroke 28:722–728.

De Goede C, Keus S, Kwakkel G et al 2001 The effects of physical therapy in PD: a research synthesis. Archives of Physical Medicine and Rehabilitation 82:509–515.

Dobkin BH, Apple D, Barbeau H et al 2006 Weight supported treadmill vs. overground training for walking after acute incomplete spinal cord injury. Neurology 66: 484–493.

Duncan PW, Zorowitz R, Bates B et al 2005 Management of adult stroke rehabilitation care. Stroke 36:3100-e143.

Edwards S 2002 An analysis of normal movement as the basis for the development of treatment techniques. In: Edwards S (ed) Neurological physiotherapy. Churchill Livingstone, London.

Fritz SL, Light KE, Patterson TS, Behrman AL et al 2005 Active finger extension predicts outcomes after constraint-induced movement therapy for individuals with hemiparesis after stroke. Stroke 36:1172–1177.

Gentile AM 2000 Skill acquisition: action, movement and neuromotor processes. In: Carr J, Shepherd R (eds) Movement science foundations for physical therapy in rehabilitation, 2nd edn. Aspen Publishers, Maryland.

Gilmore PE, Spaulding SJ 2001 Motor control and motor learning: implications for treatment in individuals post stroke. Physical and Occupational Therapy in Geriatrics 20 (1):1–15.

8

Heesen C, Romberg A, Gold S, Schulz KH 2006 Physical exercise in multiple sclerosis: supportive care or a putative disease-modifying treatment. Expert Reviews in Neurotherapeutics 6(3):347–355.

Jackson PL, Lafleur MF, Richards C et al 2001 Potential role of mental practice using motor imagery in neurologic rehabilitation. Archives of Physical Medicine and Rehabilitation 82:1133–1141.

Keus S, Bloem B, Hendriks E et al 2006 Evidence-based analysis of physical therapy in Parkinson's disease with recommendations for practice and research. Movement Disorders 22 (4):451–460.

Kwakkel G 2006 Impact of intensity of practice after stroke: issues for consideration. Disability and Rehabilitation 28:823–830.

Kwakkel G, Kollen B, Lindeman E 2004 Understanding the pattern of functional recovery after stroke. Restorative Neurology & Neuroscience 22:281–299.

Laguna PL 2000 The effect of model observation versus physical practice during motor skill acquisition and performance. Journal of Human Movement Studies 39: 171–191.

Lennon S 2004 The theoretical basis of neurological physiotherapy. In: Stokes M (ed) Physical management in neurological rehabilitation. Elsevier Mosby, London, pp 367–378.

Malouin F, Richards CL 2005 Assessment and training of locomotion after stroke: evolving concepts. In: Refshauge K, Ada L, Ellis E (eds) Science-based rehabilitation theories into practice. Elsevier, Oxford, pp 185–222.

Mayston M 2002 Problem solving in neurological physiotherapy – setting the scene. In: Edwards S (ed) Neurological physiotherapy. Churchill Livingstone, London, pp 3–19.

Motyl RW, McAuley E, Snook EM 2005 Physical activity and multiple sclerosis: a meta-analysis. Multiple Sclerosis 11:459–463.

MS Society 2004 Translating the NICE MS guideline into practice: a physiotherapy guidance document. London. MS Society, Chartered Society of Physiotherapy and Association of Physiotherapists in Neurology.

Nakayama H, Jorgensen HS, Raaschou HO, Olsen TS 1995 Recovery of upper extremity functiton in stroke patients: the Copenhagen stroke study. Archives of Physical Medicine and Rehabilitation 75:394–398.

National Institute for Clinical Excellence (NICE) 2003 Multiple sclerosis: management of multiple sclerosis in primary and secondary care. Clinical Guideline 8. London, National Institute for Clinical Excellence.

National Clinical Guidelines for Stroke (NCGS) 2004 Royal College of Physicians (RCP), London.

Pollock A, Baer G, Pomeroy V, Langhorne P 2007 Physiotherapy treatment approaches for the recovery of postural control and lower limb function following stroke. Cochrane Database of Systematic Reviews, Issue 1: CD001920.

Pomeroy VM, Tallis RC 2003 Avoiding the menace of evidence-tinged neuro-rehabilitation. Physiotherapy 89(10):595–601.

Reo JA, Mercer VS 2004 Effects of live, videotaped or written instruction on learning an upper-extremity exercise program. Physical Therapy 84 (7):622–633.

Rundek T, Mast H, Hartmann A et al 2000 Predictors of resource use after acute hospitalization: the Northern Manhattan Stroke Study. Neurology 55(8):1180–1187.

Shumway-Cook A, Woollacott MH 2007 Motor control: translating research into clinical practice. Lippincott Williams & Wilkins, Baltimore.

Van Peppen RPS, Kwakkel G, Wood-Dauphinee S et al 2004 The impact of physical therapy on functional outcomes after stroke: what's the evidence? Clinical Rehabilitation 18:833–862.

Van Vliet P, Wulf G 2006 Extrinsic feedback for motor learning after stroke: what is the evidence? Disability & Rehabilitation 28:831–840.

Williams M, Hodges NJ 2004 Skill acquisition in sport: research, theory and practice. Routledge, London.

Winstein CJ 1991 Designing practice for motor learning: clinical implications. In: Lister MJ (ed) Contemporary management of motor control problems: proceedings of the II STEP Conference. Foundation for Physical Therapy, Alexandria, Virginia.

Winstein CJ, Pohl PS Lewthwaite R 1994 Effects of physical guidance and knowledge of results on motor learning: support for the guidance hypothesis. Research Quarterly for Exercise and Sport 64(4):316–323.

Winstein CJ, Rose DK, Tan SM et al 2004 A randomized controlled comparison of upper-extremity rehabilitation strategies in acute stroke: a pilot study of immediate and long-term outcomes. Archives of Physical Medicine and Rehabilitation 85: 620–628.

Wolf SL, Winstein CJ, Miller JP, Taub E et al 2006 Effect of constraint-induced movement therapy on upper extremity function 3 to 9 months after stroke: the EXCITE randomized clinical trial. Journal of the American Medical Association 296:2095–2104.

World Health Organization 2001 International classification of functioning, disability and health. Geneva: Switzerland.

8

CHAPTER 9

Neurological assessment: the basis of clinical decision making

Susan Ryerson

INTRODUCTION

Assessment in neurological physiotherapy is a process of collecting information about disordered movement patterns, underlying impairments, activity restrictions, and societal participation of people with neurological pathology for the purpose of intervention planning. The purpose of assessment is to help the therapist determine the best intervention (Bernhardt & Hill 2005, p. 16); assessment includes both subjective information (from the medical chart and interview) and objective information (observation, and examination). This chapter presents an overview of the components of assessment that lead to goal setting and intervention planning. A patient case scenario is used to illustrate how assessment fits into the process of clinical decision making. Further key information to guide treatment of impairments, activity limitations and participation restrictions is provided in Chapter 10.

SUBJECTIVE ASSESSMENT

During this section, the therapist gathers general information from the medical record, the various members of the multidisciplinary team (MDT) and the patient and/or family. The medical chart screening provides data about past and present medical histories and helps the therapist determine if the patient is medically stable and ready for therapeutic intervention. The interview with the patient and/or family gives the therapist a sense of the patient's previous level of functioning and personal needs. This is a time when the therapist establishes rapport and trust and may gain insight into the patient's goals and concerns. The interview also allows the therapist to note the patient's spontaneous posture, movements, mental status, and orientation and may identify areas for immediate objective assessment. Suggested questions for specific types of patients are covered in Chapter 10.

OBJECTIVE ASSESSMENT

The objective assessment consists of observation and examination; it begins with the observation of activity level and voluntary movement control. Observational

Box 9.1

REMEMBER:
- It may take a few treatment sessions to fully assess the patient.
- Always consider if you need to seek the help of an assistant before attempting to stand, walk or transfer a patient for the first time.
- DO NOT be afraid to do the tests in a different order or to omit tests that are inappropriate for the patient's ability.
- It is essential to undress the patient or you will not be able to observe the salient points.
- Since functional activities require linked trunk and extremity movement, collect information about movement in the trunk as well as in the upper and lower limbs (Ryerson & Levit 1997).
- Always start by analysing how the patient moves independently before you use handling to assist the patient.
- Compare the patients' activity and motor deficits to parameters derived from normal movement performance. Normal movement patterns are characterized by appropriate alignment, postural control to move the body against gravity, adequate muscle strength and patterns of voluntary, selective movement that allow appropriate sequencing to accomplish a task with efficiency (Edwards 2002, Shumway-Cook & Woollacott 2007, Bernhardt & Hill 2005).
- Activities initially performed with compensatory patterns may need to be re-evaluated at a later date to determine if the compensatory adjustments could be minimized or eliminated.

assessment allows the therapist to evaluate how the patient uses movement during a task and how their mental, cognitive, communicative and behavioural abilities affect task performance. There are a few simple points to remember before the therapist starts the objective assessment (see Box 9.1).

During examination, the therapist should refrain from physically assisting the patient, but may offer verbal cues or demonstration to determine potential for improved performance. The therapist asks the patient to perform specific movements of the trunk/limbs or a task, e.g. the therapist can assess trunk movements both in sitting and during a sitting activity such as putting on a shirt or donning socks and shoes.

As the patient moves, the therapist analyses the resulting movement patterns in terms of key questions (Box 9.2). Following the assessment of independent voluntary movement, physiotherapists use therapeutic handling techniques to gather

Box 9.2 Key clinical questions.

- What is the starting position of the body (alignment) and base of support? Are there asymmetries in weight distribution and postural deviations?
- How does the patient perform the movement or task? Which body parts move first, how is the rest of the sequence completed?
- What is the patient's ability to balance and maintain the end point posture (note final limb position including limb posturing)?
- What range does the patient move through?
- Are the movements and/or task performed quickly or slowly? Smoothly? Effortlessly?

additional information about the nature of impairment and/or the relationship between an impairment and activity performance.

UNDERSTANDING THE COMPONENTS OF ASSESSMENT

To gain a meaningful picture of the problems contributing to decreased activity and societal participation, this section will review how the major components within a neurological assessment are analysed (see Table 9.1): *functional activity level, intact motor abilities, postural and movement deficits, response to handling, and underlying impairments.* See also Chapter 7 on common motor impairments and their impact on activity.

Although it is essential to assess range, weakness, and functional performance similar to any other type of assessment, there are several impairments that are unique and important in neurological assessment (see Chapter 7; see Table 9.2). It is these relevant impairments linked to the appropriate activity limitations that become the focus of goal setting and rehabilitation intervention strategies to improve motor performance. However it is important to remember that interventions should always aim to improve activity and participation; they should focus on the function and goals of the individual, and should never be simply aimed at the improvement of impairments.

An example of a neurological assessment form is presented in Table 9.3 (see pp. 119–120).

CLINICAL DECISION MAKING: PUTTING IT ALL TOGETHER

Clinical decision-making is the overall process of gathering and analysing this assessment information, forming a hypothesis, and prioritizing goals for intervention in collaboration with the patient and their care givers (Bernhardt & Hill 2005,

Table 9.1 Key components of assessment.

Functional activity level	● Activities the patient is able to perform independently with or without compensatory patterns.
Intact motor abilities	● Movement and activity patterns that are already performed in an optimal manner. These movement patterns reflect the patient's strengths and can be used to build on for further independence.
Postural and movement deficits (Bernhardt & Hill 2005)	● Postural deviations and movement problems that affect activity performance. ● Postural control is assessed *statically* – determining the ability to stay upright over the base of support and withstand the force of gravity, and *dynamically* – assessing the ability of the body to remain upright during movement of the limbs outside the base of support and the ability of the body to respond to external environmental perturbations.
Response to handling (Ryerson & Levit 1997)	● Therapeutic handling is used to determine if the result of manual assistance produces new movement or allows a previously impossible activity to be performed. ● Handling may be used to correct alignment, to limit degrees of freedom of a joint, to block unwanted movement, or to stabilize a weak joint or body segment. ● Manual assistance also provides the therapist with an assessment of active tone. Normally, during assisted movement, the limb or trunk follows lightly and stays positioned when the touch is released. When tone is decreased, the limbs feel heavy when passively moved and 'fall' into the pull of gravity. Resistance to passive movement occurs with increasing tone, especially when the limb is moved quickly.
Underlying impairments (see Chapter 7)	● Impairments can be either primary (impairments that arise from the neurological system) or secondary (impairments that arise from other body systems in response to the insult to the neurological system).

Table 9.2 Common impairments in patients with neurological pathology.

PRIMARY IMPAIRMENTS **Altered volitional movement** ● Neurological weakness [loss of central ability to produce and sustain force (Canning et al 2004)]. ● Impaired selective movement deficits [initiation, cessation, timing, sequencing; co-contraction (Zachowski et al 2004)]. ● Loss of trunk-limb linked movement.	● Deficiencies in sustaining contraction, recruitment ordering and firing rates (Ada et al 1996, Dickstein et al 2000, Tanaka et al 1998). ● Activation of an inappropriate muscle sequence or substitution of stronger proximal muscles for weaker distal muscles. ● Excessive co-contraction: both the correct muscles and additional inappropriate muscles are simultaneously contracting (Dewald et al 1995, Dewald & Beer 2001). This inability to stop/quiet muscle firing may lead to permanent changes in the resting posture of the extremity and eventually contribute to muscle shortening (Kamper & Rymer 2001).
Altered sensation ● Touch, temperature, proprioception, visual, somatosensory, vestibular, hypersensitivity, pain.	● Altered sensation affects the ability to feel and correctly interpret information, to learn new movement patterns, and to plan and execute movements automatically (Horak et al 1984, Palmer et al 1996).
Altered postural control ● The inability to orient body segments and to orient the body to the environment or, the inability to keep the body within the base of support (Shumway-Cook & Woollacott 2007).	● With loss of postural control, patients may display compensatory behaviours such as using the unaffected arm for support, excessive weight shifting to the stronger side, and an avoidance of movements that compromise stability. ● Loss of postural control may be present because of trunk and/or limb weakness, altered alignment, aberrant afferent sensory information, and/or impaired central integration of sensory and motor patterns (Shumway-Cook & Woollacott 2007, Dickstein 2004).
Altered tone ● *Spasticity* ● *Clinical hypertonicity*	● An increased velocity-dependent resistance to stretch and includes a clasped-knife phenomena and hyperactive tendon responses (Lance 1980). ● An increase in tone that occurs during voluntary movement resulting for example from insufficient trunk control for a task, or compensatory training patterns. It may be fluctuating or persistent.

(*continued*)

Table 9.2 Common impairments in patients with neurological pathology—cont'd.

SECONDARY IMPAIRMENTS ● *Musculoskeletal system*	● Altered joint alignment (weakness and/or patterns of disordered motor control result in destabilizing pulls on the trunk and extremities that alter the relationship between body segments). ● Muscle shortening. ● Joint and/or muscle pain (e.g. from poor joint mechanics during movement, or excessive stretch on a tendon when a limb is weak and unsupported).
● *Integumentary system*	● Oedema (especially hand and foot – develops as a consequence of weakness, loss of movement, and hospitalization factors such as intravenous infiltrates and dependent limb positioning).
● *Cardiovascular system*	● Decreased endurance (Kelly et al 2003, Macko et al 2001). This decrease in exercise endurance is attributed to co-morbidities such as cardiovascular disease or metabolic disease such as diabetes and the effect of general aging. Additionally, decreased endurance may result from inactivity due to muscle weakness and loss of postural control.

Freeman 2002, Shumway-Cook & Woollacott 2007). The therapist then devises a treatment plan by identifying the impairments and functional activities which will be the initial focus of treatment, implements the plan, and conducts periodic reassessments to evaluate the efficacy of treatment in order to decide when to discharge the patient (see Box 9.3).

A patient case scenario is used to illustrate how the assessment process leads to goal setting and intervention planning (see Table 9.4, p. 121, and Table 9.5, p. 123). The therapist in this case has hypothesized that the loss of sitting balance/inability to transfer/move from sitting to standing are due to:

1. Weakness and loss of control in trunk.
2. Loss of voluntary/selective movement in the leg – insufficient hip/knee extension and inability to depress the leg into the supporting surface.
3. Ankle/foot weakness and loss of ankle joint range of motion.
4. Impaired lower leg proprioception.

Table 9.3 Sample physiotherapy assessment form.

Name:	D.O.B:
Hospital number:	Age:
Address:	Tel No:
Physician name & address:	
Date of hospital admission:	Date of assessment:
Diagnosis:	Date of Onset:
Therapist's name:	Signature:

HISTORY OF THE PRESENT COMPLAINT (HPC)
RELEVANT PAST MEDICAL HISTORY (PMH)
SOCIAL HISTORY (SH)
(e.g. work, hobbies, family and home conditions, social services and stairs – bedroom and bathroom, smoker).
MOBILITY STATUS
PREVIOUS MOBILITY

PATIENTS EXPRESSED GOALS/EXPECTATIONS
GENERAL OBSERVATIONS

MENTAL STATE	**COMMUNICATION**
OROFACIAL FUNCTION	**CHEST STATUS**

VISION	HEARING	SWALLOWING/FEEDING

SENSATION/PERCEPTION

TONE
(grading/associated reactions (ARs') response to handling-specify position of assessment)

SELECTIVE MOVEMENT/ROM/STRENGTH
(can they perform the movement independently, or do they need assistance? If assistance is needed, how much and to what part of body? Describe resting posture and tone)
head/trunk/pelvis
upper limbs
lower limbs

BALANCE
Static (the ability to stay upright over the base of support)
Dynamic (the ability of the body to stay upright during movement of the limbs outside the base of support and to respond to external environmental perturbations).

(*continued*)

Table 9.3 Sample physiotherapy assessment form—cont'd.

GAIT
(Note level of assistance required; any gait deviations and use of walking aids) **Stance phase** (consider weight transfer onto affected leg; extension of affected hip on weight bearing; heel strike at initial contact; knee control in mid-stance) **Swing phase** (consider standing on unaffected leg, swing through of affected leg with hip flexion, knee extension and dorsiflexion)

FUNCTIONAL MOBILITY
(determine general activity level e.g. bed bound, wheelchair dependent, ambulant; can they perform the movement independently, or do they need assistance? If assistance is needed, how much and to what part of body?) **In/out of bed:** **Lying to sitting:** **Sitting to standing:** **Stairs/curbs:** **Transfers:**

Problem List	Treatment Plan
Patient agreed short-term goals	**Patient agreed long-term goals**

Box 9.3 Clinical decision-making process.

- Assessment data collection (components that are recorded on the assessment form).
- Recognizing relevant impairments that relate to the specific activity restrictions (problem list).
- Formulating a hypothesis.
- Goal setting in collaboration with patient/family and team members.
- Establishing a treatment plan.
- Delivering the interventions.
- Reassessment (patient response: outcomes-goal achievement-problem resolution or modification).
- Transfer of care or discharge.

Table 9.4 Sample assessment for a patient post CVA.

History of present complaint:	68-year-old male; diagnosis of R middle cerebral artery infarct with left hemiplegia. Onset: 5 days ago.
Past medical history:	Diabetes mellitus, high blood pressure.
Social history:	Retired teacher, lives with wife, three grown children who live nearby. Plays golf weekly.
Previous mobility:	Active, independent with no limitations.
Expressed goals:	Return home, regain mobility and participate in recreational activities.
General observations:	● Sitting in bedside chair leaning to R side, tries to correct trunk position during interview, no spontaneous movements L arm or leg. ● Appears alert and oriented, expressive speech intact, dysarthria noted, L lower facial paralysis. ● No reports of pain or swallowing difficulties.
Activity level: **Wheelchair bound** **Bed mobility**	● Able to roll onto L side; uses R arm and head/upper trunk to initiate roll. Complaints of L shoulder pain when lying on L side for more than 2 minutes. ● Cannot scoot up or down in bed; can bridge with assistance to maintain flexed leg position. ● Able to roll onto R side with verbal cues (hold L arm, reach across body as roll, lift head) and minimal assistance to L leg (when L leg placed in flexed position on bed, patient can activate leg muscles to assist movement to side lying. ● Reports L arm feels heavy when he lifts it.
Transfers: to/from plinth	● Requires minimal support to R upper trunk and verbal cues from therapist to initially move trunk forward, requires moderate assistance when lifting buttocks from chair, rotates body during transfer with only verbal cues. ● L foot slides forward during transfers.
Sitting: on plinth	● Sits on plinth with R arm support and can initiate forward flexion/extension movements; cannot sit without arm support. ● Trunk leans to R, appears to have more weight on R buttock. Has difficulty keeping L foot flat on floor. ● Inferior shoulder subluxation present. Holds L arm in lap.

(*continued*)

Table 9.4 Sample assessment for a patient post CVA—cont'd.

Sit to stand:	● Needs verbal reminders to scoot forward, and to lean trunk forward. ● Physical assistance needed to position foot. ● Unable to keep weight over L foot during stand. ● Requires moderate assistance when lifting buttock from chair. Takes 6–8 sec to rise to stand with assistance. ● Cannot control L knee in standing; knee buckles. ● Arm postures in 20 degrees elbow flexion during attempt to stand, no posturing during sitting.
Gait/Stairs:	**Unable to assess**
Selective movement Trunk	**Sitting** ● When therapist supports pelvis/hips, patient can initiate forward flexion movements with upper trunk through $\frac{1}{2}$ range; trunk lean to R noted during movement. Ribcage/spine rotate slightly to L. ● Falls to L when reaching R arm beyond arm's length. Can lift up R leg in flexion pattern through $\frac{1}{3}$ range, further attempts result in loss of sitting balance to L. ● Cannot extend entire spine; tends to rest in forward flexion; holds L hand in lap. ● Side bending to R is accompanied by trunk rotation L. Side bending to L possible when therapist provides stability to L hip/pelvis. **Standing: unable to assess**
L Upper limb	**Sitting** ● Forward reach characterized by shoulder elevation, shoulder abduction (20 degrees), elbow flexion (30 degrees). No movement of wrist/fingers noted. Arm movement is slow and jerky. Arm feels heavy, but shoulder follows movement; cannot hold positions when handling withdrawn. ● With minimal assistance, patient able to flex shoulder to 60 and activate elbow extensors for a brief period. ● When arms supported on table, patient able to supinate forearm through $\frac{1}{2}$ range, active pronation not possible. ● When forearm stabilized, wrist extension present through $\frac{1}{2}$ range. ● No finger flexion/extension possible. Soft oedema noted on volar and dorsal aspect of hand. ● 1 cm inferior shoulder subluxation at rest. **Standing: unable to assess**

9

Table 9.4 Sample assessment for a patient post CVA—cont'd.

L Lower extremity	**Sitting**
	● Lifts leg in flexor pattern through $\frac{1}{2}$ range. Ankle dorsiflexion with supination noted during lift of leg. Able to extend knee 45 degrees with ankle plantarflexion. Unable to isolate active knee or ankle flexor movements.
	● Ankle joint ROM: dorsiflexion -5 degrees. Plantar flexion WNL.
	Supine
	● Active hip and knee synergistic flexor and extensor movements through full range.
	● Unable to place or maintain foot on bed in bridging position. With both legs flexed and L foot stabilized on bed by therapist, able to rotate both hips L/R, abduct/adduct L hip, and 'bridge'.
Sensation	● Light touch: intact upper and lower limb.
	● Proprioception: intact shoulder/elbow, hip/knee; impaired wrist/hand, ankle/foot.
	● Stereognosis: not assessed.
Activity restrictions	**Relevant impairments**
1. Unable to balance and perform washing and dressing activities in sitting.	1. Weakness in leg, especially hip.
	2. Weakness in trunk (loss of trunk-limb linked patterns).
	3. Decreased ankle range and altered proprioception in L ankle/foot.
2. Unable to transfer from chair/bed/plinth.	4. Inability to maintain sufficient weight between legs during extension phase of transfer/stand.
3. Unable to move from sitting to standing independently.	5. Loss of upper body stability.

CVA, cardiovascular accident; L, left; R, right; ROM, range of movement; WNL, with no limitations.

Table 9.5

Short-term goals (one week)	Long-term goals (three to four weeks)
1. Independence in bed mobility; rolling to either side, side lying to sitting.	1. Independence in washing and dressing in standing.
2. Independence in daily washing and upper body dressing in sitting.	2. Independent sit to stand.
3. Transfer from bed/chair/bed with contact guarding.	3. Assisted ambulation: walking aid and standby support.
4. Sit to stand with minimal assistance/verbal cues.	

Box 9.4

SOAP notes

S–Subjective: info provided by the patient and the team.
O–Objective: examination findings.
A–Assessment: analysis concerning impairments and activity limitations.
P–Plan for the therapy session.

Box 9.5 The assessment process.

Subjective assessment
● Review chart and talk with care team.
● Interview patient/family.

Objective assessment
● Observe functional abilities and document with objective measurement tools as appropriate.
● Identify impairments contributing to loss of function and movement:
  a. Observe how patient moves limbs and trunk when unassisted by therapist.
  b. Use handling to assess movement of limbs and trunk, tone, ROM, muscle strength, balance, sensation.
  c. Document with objective measurement tools as appropriate.

Problem list
● Hypothesis linking activity restrictions and relevant impairments.

Goal setting
● Patient-centred, short-term and long-term goals with time frames for achievement.

Treatment plan
● Interventions selected based on the clinical reasoning strategy.

Re-assessment/evaluation

Transfer of care/discharge

The interventions aimed at impairment level and/or activity level are selected on the basis of the therapist's clinical reasoning strategy, and re-assessed on a regular basis to evaluate the effectiveness of therapy intervention, and the need for modification to the treatment plan. Therapists often record their decision making on a daily basis using SOAP notes (Kettenbach 2003; see Box 9.4).

SUMMARY

Assessment is the cornerstone of clinical decision making (see Box 9.5).

References

Ada L, O'Dwyer N, Green J 1996 The nature of the loss of strength and dexterity in the upper limb following stroke. Human Movement Science 15:671–687.

Bernhardt J, Hill K 2005 We only treat what it occurs to us to assess: the importance of knowledge-based assessment. In: Refshauge K, Ada L, Ellis E (eds) Science based rehabilitation: theories into practice. Elsevier, Edinburgh, pp 15–48.

Canning C, Ada L, Adams R 2004 Loss of strength contributes more to disability after stroke than loss of dexterity. Clinical Rehabilitation 18:300–308.

Dewald JP, Beer RF 2001 Abnormal joint torque patterns in the paretic upper limb of subjects with hemiparesis. Muscle & Nerve 24:273–283.

Dewald J, Pope P, Given J, Buchanan T 1995 Abnormal muscle coactivation patterns during isometric torque generation at the elbow and shoulder in hemiparetic subjects. Brain 118:495–510.

Dickstein R, Sheffi S, Ben Haim Z, Shabtai E, Markovici E 2000 Activation of flexor and extensor trunk muscles in hemiplegia. American Journal of Physical Medicine & Rehabilitation 79:228–234.

Dickstein R, Sheffi S, Markovici E 2004 Anticipatory postural adjustment in selected trunk muscles in post stroke hemiparetic patients. Archives of Physical Medicine and Rehabilitation 85:261–267.

Edwards S 2002 An analysis of normal movement as the basis for the development of treatment techniques. In: Edwards S (ed) Neurological physiotherapy: a problem solving approach, 2nd edn. Churchill Livingstone, Edinburgh, pp 35–67.

Freeman JA 2002 Assessment, outcome measurement, and goal setting in physiotherapy practice. In: Edwards S (ed) Neurological physiotherapy: a problem solving approach, 2nd edn. Churchill Livingstone, Edinburgh, pp 21–34.

Horak F, Anderson M, Esselman P, Lynch K 1984 The effect of movement velocity, mass displaced and task certainty on associated postural adjustments made by normal and hemiplegic individuals. Journal of Neurology, Neurosurgery and Psychiatry 47:1020–1028.

Kamper D, Rymer WZ 2001 Impairment of voluntary control of finger motion following stroke: role of inappropriate muscle coactivation. Muscle & Nerve 24:673–681.

Kelly J, Kilbreath S, Davis G 2003 Cardiorespiratory fitness and walking ability in subactue stroke patients. Archives of Physical Medicine and Rehabilitation 84:1780–1785.

Kettenbach G 2003 Writing SOAP notes. FA Davis, Philadelphia.

Lance J 1980 Symposium synopsis. In: Feldman R et al (eds) Spasticity: disordered motor control. Chicago, Year Book Medical Publishers, pp 485–494.

Macko R, Smith G, Dobrovolny C et al 2001 Treadmill training improves fitness reserve in chronic stroke patients. Archives of Physical Medicine and Rehabilitation 82:879–884.

Palmer E, Downes L, Ashby P 1996 Associated postural adjustments are impaired by a lesion of the cortex. Neurology 46:471–475.

Ryerson SJ, Levit KK 1997 Functional movement reeducation: a contemporary model for stroke rehabilitation. Churchill Livingstone, New York.

Shumway-Cook A, Woollacott MM 2007 Motor control: translating research into clinical practice, 3rd edn. Lippincott Williams & Wilkins, Baltimore.

Tanaka M, Hachisuka K, Ogata H 1998 Muscle strength of trunk flexion-extension in post-stroke hemiplegic patients. American Journal of Physical Medicine & Rehabilitation 77:288–290.

Zachowski K, Dromerick A, Sahrmann SA, Thach W, Bastian A 2004 How do strength, sensation, spasticity and joint individuation relate to the reaching deficits of people with chronic hemiparesis? Brain 127:1035–1046.

CHAPTER 10

Treatment: minimizing impairments, activity limitations and participation restrictions

INTRODUCTION

This chapter focuses on the physiotherapy management of the types of patient commonly encountered in clinical practice with examples related to specific pathologies:

10.1: The acute patient before and during stabilization: stroke, traumatic brain injury (TBI) and Guillain–Barré syndrome (GBS)

10.2: The stable acute patient with potential for recovery: stroke, TBI and GBS

10.3: The acute patient with limited potential for recovery: complete spinal cord injury

10.4: The patient with degenerative disease: multiple sclerosis

10.5: The patient with degenerative disease: Parkinson's disease

Please see Chapter 6 for an overview of neurological conditions, Chapter 8 for overall guiding principles, Chapter 9 for principles of neurological assessment and Chapter 13 on respiratory management.

10.1 The acute patient before and during stabilization: stroke, TBI and GBS

Cherry Kilbride and Elizabeth Cassidy

Physiotherapy intervention for the acute patient is addressed in three interconnected stages: pre-physiotherapy assessment (stage 1), physiotherapy assessment (stage 2) and physiotherapy intervention (stage 3).

STAGE 1: PRE-PHYSIOTHERAPY ASSESSMENT

The pre-physiotherapy assessment prompts you to find out if the patient is stable enough for physiotherapy. Acute patients may be unstable in the early stages;

physiotherapy must be applied with careful monitoring of vital signs. Acute patients may be sedated, paralysed and intubated with impaired levels of consciousness (LOC) (Carter & Edwards 2002). Before starting the initial physiotherapy assessment a comprehensive appraisal of the patient's stability must be undertaken.

Table 10.1.1 identifies important information to gather from patient records to inform physiotherapy assessment including potential risk factors which may influence what you do. This data will help indicate the need to modify planned interventions e.g. to keep change of positions to a minimum, treat little but often or to advise only. At this stage, you are primarily liaising with doctors about planned medical and surgical management and nursing staff for timely information on the patient's condition. (See Box 10.1.1.)

Box 10.1.1

- Never talk over the patient; always introduce yourself and explain what you are doing. Assume the patient can hear and understand what you are saying.
- Modify the environment by reducing adverse factors like excessive noise e.g. radios and TVs which can adversely affect irritability levels and subsequent patient response to assessment.

STAGE 2: PHYSIOTHERAPY ASSESSMENT

Building on information collected during the pre-assessment stage, data gathered in this phase assists identification of impairments, activity limitations and participation restrictions requiring physiotherapy intervention (read this section in conjunction with Chapter 9 on assessment).

Table 10.1.2 (p. 130) identifies key physiotherapy information to guide assessment of impairments, activity limitations and participation restrictions. (See also Boxes 10.1.2 and 10.1.3 on p. 135.)

STAGE 3: PHYSIOTHERAPY INTERVENTION

Neurological physiotherapists provide stimulus via movement to engage patient response; do *not* wait for the patient to wake up or move before starting treatment (Thornton & Kilbride 2004). Core physiotherapy interventions and special considerations for intervention and team work are presented in Table 10.1.3 (p. 132).

Text continued on p. 135

Table 10.1.1 Essential information for assessment of stability.

	Stroke	TBI	GBS
Database (information from records)	• Cause of stroke e.g. haemorrhage or infarct (Lindsay & Bone 2004) • Planned medical/surgical management e.g. carotid angiography • Risk of rebleed or extension of stroke • Change in neurological status over last 24 hours • Cardiovascular stability: BP, HR, RR, ECG • Scans • GCS (Teasdale & Jennett 1974) – LOC • Chest X-ray (aspiration) • Temperature • ABGs • Glucose levels (target range 4–7 mmol/L hyperglycemia post stroke associated with poorer outcome (Gray et al 2004) • FBC (e.g. levels of Hb and WBC).	• Neurosurgical management: e.g. craniotomy, bone flap, drains, ventilation mode (may be elective), drug management (Lindsay & Bone 2004) • Positions to avoid e.g. neck flexion, rotation, dependent head position 2004) • Associated injuries • GCS – LOC • ICP (raised > 15 mm HG indicates moderate risk of intervention) • Level of sedation, paralysing agents • Cardiovascular stability: BP, HR, ECG, RR • EEG • Scans and X-rays • ABGs • Seizures • Temperature • FBC	• FVC (<15 mL/kg may indicate need for elective ventilation, Ng et al 1995) • Autonomic dysfunction (unexpected cardiac arrhythmias, arrest; McLeod 1992) • Impaired sensation-stocking and glove (Lindsay & Bone 2004) • X-rays (chest) • Temperature • ABGs • BP, HR, RR • FBC • Pain (Pentland & Donald 1994) • EMG
Subjective (obtained from the MDT)	• Nursing staff: neurological status, tissue viability, early mobilization, sitting out • Doctors: planned medical interventions • SLT: swallow	• Neurosurgeons, doctors, anaesthetists: stability for treatment, planned management • Nurses: patient's response to nursing, medical, surgical interventions, irritability e.g. change in vital signs, sleep/wake cycles, pain (Tyrer & Livesley 2003)	• Doctors: rate of change over last 24 hours: e.g. has patient reached nadir (Asbury & Cornblath 1990), planned medical interventions e.g. immunoglobulin transfusion (plasmapheresis) • Anaesthetist: respiratory status • Nurses: pain, tissue viability

ABGs, arterial blood gases; BP, blood pressure; ECG, electrocardiogram; EEG, electroencephalograph; EMG, electromyogram; FBC, full blood count; FVC, forced vital capacity; GBS, Guillain–Barré syndrome; GCS, Glasgow Coma Scale; Hb, haemoglobin; HR, heart rate; LOC, level of consciousness; ICP, intracranial pressure; MDT, multidisciplinary team; RR, respiratory rate; SLT, speech & language therapist; TBI, traumatic brain injury; WBC, white blood cells.

Table 10.1.2 Physiotherapy assessment in the medical stabilization phase.

	Stroke	TBI	GBS
Further database information	• Swallow • Hydration • Nutrition • Co-morbidities • Drug management	• Swallow • Hydration • Nutrition • Associated injuries • Antispasmodic drugs	• Communication strategies if ventilated • Swallow • Nutrition • Psychological affect • Drug management
Subjective information	Cross refer to Chapter 9	Cross refer to Chapter 9	Cross refer to Chapter 9
Objective examination **Core impairments**	• Hemiplegia • Weakness • Loss or reduced movement • Fatigue • Loss of dexterity • Altered sensation • Proprioceptive loss • Altered tone (often low) • Cognitive/perceptual impairments e.g. contraversive pushing syndrome (Karnath et al 2000), visuospatial neglect, midline awareness, orientation to time, place, person and situation, memory problems • Visual field impairment	• Quadraparesis, non-symmetrical • Altered tone, often develops rapidly and globally (Campbell 2004) • Rigidity • Decorticate (UL-flexed; LL-extended), decerebrate (UL & LL-extended; Britton 2004) • Cognitive/perceptual impairments e.g. midline awareness, initiation, planning, problem solving, memory, dyspraxia (disorder of skilled movement), orientation to time, person, place and situation (Cicerone et al 2005) • Visual impairment • Sensory inattention • Proprioceptive alteration • Cranial nerve involvement	• Quadraparesis, symmetrical • Altered sensation, note main patterns (Nicklin 2004) • Loss or reduced movement • Weakness • Fatigue • Pain • Cranial nerve involvement • Respiratory effort, accessory muscle use, ability to cough

Potential secondary complications	• Pain: HSP (Jackson et al 2003); complex regional pain syndrome type II (Weber et al 2001); thalamic pain (Lyndsey & Bone 2004) • Swollen hand • Emerging habitual postures, leading to soft tissue adaptation • Decreased ROM: lateral rotation and abduction of shoulder, wrist/finger extension, loss of hand cupping (passive or active), tendo achilles, hip flexors, hamstrings • Cardiovascular deconditioning (Kilbreath & Davis 2005)	• Decreased ROM: jaw, lateral rotation, abduction of the shoulder, hip flexors, hamstrings, tendo achilles, toe flexors (Carter & Edwards 2002) • Emerging habitual postures in response to prolonged ITU stay, limited experience of movement e.g. stiff rib cage, lumbar spine, +/- peripheral and central causes of hypertonia • Emerging behaviours; primary or secondary to pathology • Risk of heterotopic ossification (Knight et al 2002)	• Decreased ROM: tendo achilles, hamstrings, stiff lumbar spine, hips; restricted movement in flexion and extension particularly small joints • Emerging habitual postures from pain, limited experience of movement • Neural pain
Activity limitations	Bed mobility, Transfers, ADL, Mobility		
Common measurement tools (see Wade 1992)	MAS, Rivermead, Barthel index, FIM/FAM	GCS, WHIM (Shiel et al 2000)	Oxford scale (MRC 1982), myometer, VAS

ADL, activities of daily living; FAM, Functional Assessment Measure; FIM, Functional Independence Measure; GCS, Glasgow Coma Scale; HSP, hemiplegic shoulder pain; LL, lower limb; MAS, Motor Assessment Scale; ROM, range of movement; UL, upper limb; VAS, visual analogue scale; WHIM, Wessex Head Injury Matrix.

Table 10.1.3 Key physiotherapy interventions for the acute patient.

	Stroke	TBI	GBS
Key interventions	**Maintain range of movement to prevent/minimize soft tissue adaptation** ● Active/active assisted/passive movements; joints, muscles most at risk e.g. glenohumeral, ankle, knee, muscles crossing two joints ● Avoid vigorous or forced movements, vary speed, direction ● Positioning to help maintain ROM ● Mobilization of rib cage, pelvis and jaw (Carter & Edwards 2002)		
	Splinting and casting ● Low tone and weakness contribute to poor joint/limb alignment ● Emerging positive features of UMN syndrome influence development of habitual postures ● Splinting if positioning ineffective (Edwards & Charlton 2002)	**Splinting and casting** ● Proactive plastering to prevent loss of ROM at the ankle ● POPs (fibreglass casts) should be extended to fully support the toes (Edwards & Charlton 2002)	**Resting splints** ● To maintain range of movement and protect joints especially hands and feet which may be last to recover ● NB: remove splints for full passive movements
	Positioning ● Maintain optimal alignment of body parts (Sharman 2002) ● Vary postures during day and night, using rolls, pillows, wedges, supine, side lying, sitting out (Thornton & Kilbride 2004) ● Positioning for optimal oxygen saturation (Tyson & Nightingale 2004) ● Positioning/seating to enhance perceptual awareness, communication, swallow and social interaction (Pope 2002)		

Special considerations			
Weight bearing/movement re-education • When patient stable commence programmes of sitting and standing for antigravity activity, maintenance of length (Carr & Shepherd 1998) • Initially sit out for 15–20 minutes, adapted ward chair/specialist seating e.g. tilt in space to achieve optimum postures to maintain length, protect vulnerable joints e.g. glenohumeral, respiration, communication, social interaction (Pope 2002) • A standing programme starting with the tilt table (if no/only minimal movement present – Chang 2004) or other standing devices should be introduced to the patient's routine. Progressive mobilization against gravity: short periods may only be tolerated initially e.g. 5 minutes (Carter & Edwards 2002) • Ventilation does not preclude standing or sitting; monitor saturation levels and vital signs (Carter & Edwards 2002) • Monitor BP, HR particularly if autonomic disturbances			
	Sensory re-education • Consider a graded stimulation programme for patients with limited sensory stimulation e.g. prolonged ITU stay (Campbell 2004)		
Special considerations	• Direct intervention for low level of arousal • Early signs of perceptual/cognitive deficits e.g. contraversive pushing syndrome. Don't over bombard: alter one variable at a time, one step instructions, allow time for processing of information, plan short and frequent assessments • Fatigue management (Staub & Bogousslavsky 2001) • Depression management (Anderson et al 2004)	• Direct intervention for low level of arousal • Agitation • Weaning and reduction in sedation may change physical presentation e.g. emergence of high tone • Early signs of behavioural and perceptual/cognitive impairments. Alter one variable at a time, one step instructions, allow time for processing of information, plan short and frequent assessments • Fatigue management (Borgaro et al 2005)	• Pain management with consistent team approach. Large amplitude mid-range movement may have pain relieving properties (Freeman 1992)

10

(continued)

Table 10.1.3 Key physiotherapy interventions for the acute patient—cont'd.

	Stroke	TBI	GBS
Team work	Nurses: positioning, handling to prevent HSP, moving and handling, therapeutic handling for movement re-education within ADL. Family and friends: support/education. OT: movement within ADL, transfers, home visits. SLT: swallowing management, communication strategies. Orthoptist: visual dysfunction.	Doctors: medication e.g. antispasmodics, botulinum toxin. Nurses: casts/splints, handling at risk joints, positioning, moving and handling, therapeutic handling for movement re-education within ADL. Family and friends: support/education e.g. levels of stimulation. OT: specialist seating, movement within ADL, transfers, home visits. Dietician, SLT: nutritional management, communication strategies. Orthoptist: visual dysfunction.	Nursing staff: positioning, handling at risk joints, moving and handling, therapeutic handling for movement re-education within ADL. OT: resting splints, seating, transfers, home visits. Family and friends: support/education. Doctors: pain management team.

ADL, activities of daily living; BP, blood pressure; HR, heart rate; ITU, intensive care unit; OT, occupational therapist; ROM, range of movement; SLT, speech and language therapist; UMN, upper motor neurone.

Box 10.1.2

> **When assessing, remember:**
> - *WATCH* for responses from the patient to your intervention.
> - *WAIT* to find out whether vital signs fluctuate or stabilize.
> - *STOP* if you are unsure or if the patient becomes unstable.
> - *ALERT* nursing and medical staff.
> - *RECORD* your intervention inpatient health records.

Box 10.1.3

> **Key clinical questions: stop, look, think and consider:**
> - Do I need to move the patient or can I start my assessment in situ?
>   A change of posture may adversely affect patient stability and can
>   be unnecessarily fatiguing.
> - What can the patient do by themselves? Encourage active participation
>   whenever possible.
> - If the patient can move, how are they doing it? Is it effortful, easy,
>   smooth or uncoordinated?
> - Is there resistance to movement, do the muscles feel stiff or floppy?
> - If the patient is unable to move independently, does changing the
>   patient's position wake them up and help them move?

Following assessment, physiotherapists establish a problem list. At this stage patient-centred goals are set in conjunction with the patient and carers using the SMART framework (Cott & Finch 1990) in order to develop an appropriate treatment plan. Intervention should always be goal-directed (see Box 10.1.4).

Box 10.1.4

> **The SMART framework (goals are specific, measurable, achievable, realistic and timed):**
> - Mrs Smith will retain a minimum of plantargrade at both ankles over the
>   next 4 weeks.
> - Mrs Smith will be able to sit out in a wheelchair for an hour twice a day
>   in 2 weeks.
> - Mrs Smith will be able to stand on a tilt table with chest, hip and knee
>   straps for 15 minutes at 80° in two weeks.

10.2 The stable acute patient with potential for recovery: stroke, TBI and GBS

Cherry Kilbride and Elizabeth Cassidy

Once the patient is medically stable, intensive rehabilitation begins. Physiotherapists help patients to experience and relearn movement, and to regain optimal functional activity. Therapists are especially interested in how the patient moves (quality of movement) to perform functional activities.

ASSESSMENT

Before starting the initial assessment a comprehensive appraisal of the patient's status using information from relevant sources must be undertaken. Physiotherapy assessment focuses on key presenting impairments and how they impact on regaining function; assessment informs the identification of physiotherapy problems for intervention (read this section in conjunction with Chapter 9). This information helps direct future goals and treatment. Key assessment information for the recovering patient; common impairments and activity limitations are indicated in Table 10.2.1. (See also Box 10.2.1.)

Box 10.2.1

Key clinical questions: stop, look, think and consider:
- What can the patient do for themselves?
- What can the patient do with assistance?
- What can the patient do if their position is changed?
- Why does the patient move that way?
- What is impacting or interfering with movement most? e.g. Does the patient have pain?

Table 10.2.1 Physiotherapy assessment in the recovering patient.

	Stroke	TBI	GBS
Database information	See Tables 10.1.1 & 10.1.2		
Subjective	Cross refer Chapter 9		
Objective examination Key impairments	• Emerging positive features of UMN syndrome e.g. spastic dystonia, positive support response, associated reaction, spasticity (Edwards 2002) • Enduring negative features of UMN syndrome e.g. weakness, loss or reduction of voluntary movement, fatigue, loss of dexterity • Altered sensation • Proprioceptive loss • Cognitive and perceptual impairments e.g. pushing, decreased midline awareness, orientation, memory	• Emerging positive features of UMN syndrome e.g. spastic dystonia, positive support response, flexor withdrawal response, spasticity, extensor thrust (Edwards 2002) • Enduring negative features of UMN syndrome e.g. quadraparesis (non-symmetrical) or hemiplegia, weakness, reduction of movement, fatigue, loss of dexterity • Other emerging motor impairments e.g. ataxia, rigidity, titubation (rhythmic nodding of the head – Lyndsey & Bone 2004) • Altered sensation • Proprioceptive loss • Cognitive and perceptual impairments: altered midline/spatial awareness, initiation, planning, problem solving, memory, orientation	• LMN signs e.g. weakness, quadraparesis (symmetrical), distal > proximal, fatigue, loss, reduction of movement • Altered sensation • Proprioceptive loss • Pain

(continued)

10

Table 10.2.1 Physiotherapy assessment in the recovering patient—cont'd.

	Stroke	TBI	GBS
Potential secondary complications	• Pain: HSP (Jönsson et al 2006); complex regional pain syndrome type II (Weber et al 2001); thalamic pain (Lyndsey & Bone 2004) • Length changes e.g. tendo achilles, wrist, finger extension • Hypertonia (neural/non-neural contributions) • Emerging habitual postures • Biomechanical, peripheral alignment of limbs and trunk in relation to each other (Sharman 2002; Thornton & Kilbride 2004) • Disuse atrophy • Cardiovascular deconditioning (Kilbreath & Davis 2005) • Learned non-use (Taub et al 1993)	• Length changes, contractures, risk/ presence of HO • Emerging habitual postures • Hypertonia (neural/non-neural contributions) • Biomechanical and peripheral alignment of limbs and trunk in relation to each other (Thornton & Kilbride 2004) • Disuse atrophy • Cardiovascular deconditioning (Kilbreath & Davis 2005)	• Length changes, contractures • Joint stiffness flexion and extension (Sonyal et al 1992) • Disuse atrophy • Cardiovascular deconditioning (Kilbreath & Davis 2005) • Biomechanical and peripheral alignment of limbs and trunk in relation to each other (Thornton & Kilbride 2004)
Activity limitations	• Bed mobility (rolling over; sitting up; moving around in bed) • Split level transfers i.e. transfers involving different heights • Sit to stand, stepping, on/off floor • ADL • Mobility (indoors/outdoors) • Stairs		
Commonly used measurement tools (Wade 1992)	MAS, Rivermead, FIM/FAM, VAS, BBS, Get Up and Go	MAS, Rivermead, FIM/FAM, VAS	FIM/FAM, Oxford scale (MRC 1982), myometry, VAS

ADL, activities of daily living; BBS, Berg Balance Score; FAM, Functional Assessment Measure; FIM, Functional Independence Measure; HO, heterotopic ossification; HSP, hemiplegic shoulder pain; MAS, Motor Assessment Scale; ROM, range of movement; UMN, upper motor neurone; VAS, visual analogue

GOAL SETTING

Patients' views are central to informing the goal-setting process; think of the key activities they want to achieve. SMART examples are given in Box 10.2.2. Consider the following factors:

● Perceptual and cognitive impairment
● Behaviour
● Emotional and psychological issues
● Is there a mismatch between potential for participation and what they do? If so, may need to liaise with the multidisciplinary team to develop other rehabilitation strategies.

Box 10.2.2

SMART goals

● Mrs Smith will be able to stand with feet flat on the floor with minimal assistance of one person for 5 minutes in 2 weeks.
● Mrs Smith will be able to sit out in a high-backed arm chair for all meals and evening visits in 2 weeks.
● Mrs Smith will be able to transfer independently from bed to chair in 3 weeks.

INTERVENTION

Although recovering patients present with multiple impairments which impact on their ability to participate in functional activities, treatment should focus on the function and goals of the individual, and should never be simply aimed at the improvement of impairments. The treatment strategies that the physiotherapist starts with essentially depends on the patient's starting level of motor activity (see Table 10.2.2).

KEY CLINICAL MESSAGES

● Acute patients may be unstable in the early stages; physiotherapy applied inappropriately can make patients worse. However early mobilization with careful monitoring of vital signs is key.
● Neurological physiotherapists provide stimulus via movement to engage patient response; do *not* wait for the patient to wake up or move before starting treatment.
● Physiotherapy assessment focuses on key presenting impairments and how they impact on regaining function.
● Treatment should focus on the function and goals of the individual, and should never be simply aimed at the improvement of impairments.

Table 10.2.2 Key physiotherapy interventions for the recovering patient.

Key interventions	Stroke	TBI	GBS
(a) For people with no activity to minimal activity: elicit motor activity, early strength training	• Modify exercise so that small muscle activity results in movement; eliminate gravity, focus on strongest mid-range activity, reduce friction (Ada & Canning 2005) • Therapeutic handling; active, self-assisted, passive movements (Thornton & Kilbride 2004) • Activation of extensor activity, weight bearing, through standing (supported/active assisted) (Markham 1987) and sitting (Carr & Shepherd 1998); treadmill training with body weight support (Hesse et al 2003, Tuckey & Greenwood 2004). • Consider adjuncts e.g. selective electrical stimulation (Gabr et al 2005) biofeedback (Ada & Canning 2005), mental practice (Sharma et al 2006), hydrotherapy (Taylor et al 1993), orthotics (Edwards & Charlton 2002)		
For people with some activity: focus on modified task practice and strength training	• Strength training through full range and inner range, increase speed, add resistance (Ada & Canning, 2005) • Task-specific training (part or modified) (Ada & Canning 2005, Carr & Shepherd 2003, Shumway-Cook & Woollacott 2007) • Consider adjuncts: FES for foot drop (Burridge et al 1997), ankle foot orthoses (Olney 2005), treadmill training (Hesse et al 2003; Tuckey & Greenwood 2004) • Consider rehabilitation environment and conditions for practice (Carr & Shepherd 2003, Malouin & Richards 2005, Shumway-Cook & Woollacott 2007)		
For people with more activity: focus on advanced strength training, full task practice, cardiorespiratory fitness and endurance	• Resisted exercise (body weight, free weights, theraband) (Ada & Canning 2005) • Whole task training (Ada & Canning 2005, Carr & Shepherd 2003, lying to sitting (Shumway-Cook & Woollacott 2007), sit to stand, gait re-education (Malouin & Richards 2005), reach and grasp (Carr & Shepherd 2003, Duff et al 2007) • Consider rehabilitation environment and cognitive loading to develop adaptability of task performance to different environmental demands and conditions (Ada & Canning 2005) • Conduct, risk assessment for cardiorespiratory training (Kilbreath & Davis 2005), consider walking, stepping, static cycle/cycle ergonometer, treadmill (Kilbreath & Davis 2005), FES to facilitate gait speed (Burridge et al 1997)		

(b) Prevent/address soft-tissue length changes	• Weight bearing via active means wherever possible; active standing, sit to stand, strengthening (Carr & Shepherd 2003) • Splinting/casting (Edwards & Charlton 2002), stretching (Harvey et al 2002) • Strengthening (Ada & Canning 2005)
(c) Adjuncts	• Botulinum toxin (RCP 2002), other antispasmodics • Hydrotherapy (Taylor et al 1993) • Re-education of sensation through provision of meaningful sensory inputs, normally task orientated, training attention to and interpretation of sensation (Yekutiel & Guttman 1993) • CIMT: mild to moderate impairment of upper limb and learned non use (Wolf et al 2006) • HSP minimize risk of trauma, provide limb support, maintain ROM, consider integrated care pathway (Jackson et al 2003) • Consider cognitive/perceptual impairments (Cicerone et al 2005)
Special considerations	• Splinting and casting: to gain ROM especially at the ankle, knee, elbow modifications e.g. drop out splints, hinged POPs (Edwards & Charlton 2002) and CPMs may optimize ROM (Macfarlane & Thornton 1997) • Specialist seating; often required e.g. tilt in space, electric wheelchair (Pope 2002) • Ataxia: training programme concentrating on specific impairments affecting task performance (Carr & Shepherd 1998) • Vestibular rehabilitation (Meldrum & McConn Walsh 2004) • Cognitive/perceptual impairments can compound behavioural problems or be issues in themselves (Campbell 2004) • Graded time at home: patients may begin to spend short periods of time at home in preparation for discharge • Progression from resting to dynamic splints to assist aspects of ADL; custom-made back slabs to support free standing (Edwards & Charlton 2002) • Gait re-education i.e. use of parallel bars, walking aids • Graded time at home: patients may begin to spend short periods of time at home in preparation for discharge

(continued)

Table 10.2.2 Key physiotherapy interventions for the recovering patient—cont'd.

Key interventions	Stroke	TBI	GBS
Team work	Nurses: promote/integrate functional goals into ward activity. Family and friends: support/ education for discharge planning, ongoing treatment goals. OT, social worker/discharge coordinator: facilitate transfer to community setting. Physiotherapists: in the community for next stage of rehabilitation.	Doctors: review of medication. Nurses: promote/integrate functional goals into ward activity. Family and friends: support/education. Clinical psychologist: assessment/advice on enduring cognitive/perceptual impairments. OT, social worker and discharge coordinator: facilitate transfer to the community setting. Physiotherapists: in the community for next stage of rehabilitation.	Nurses: promote/integrate functional goals into ward activity. OT: resting splints. Family and friends: support and education. Doctors/pain management team: pain control.

CIMT, constraint induced movement therapy; CPM, continuous passive movement; FES, functional electrical stimulation; HSP, hemiplegic shoulder pain; OT, occupational therapy; PoP, plaster of paris; RCP, Royal College of Physicians; ROM, range of movement.

References for subchapters 10.1 and 10.2

Ada L, Canning, C 2005 Changing the way we view the contribution of motor impairments to physical disability after stroke. In: Refshauge K, Ada L, Ellis E (eds) Science Based Rehabilitation: theories into practice. Elsevier, Edinburgh, pp 87–106.

Anderson CS, Hackett ML, House AO 2004 Interventions for preventing depression after stroke. Cochrane Database of Systematic Reviews. Issue 2 Art. No: CD003689. DOI: 10–1002/14651858.CD003689.pub2.

Asbury AK, Cornblath DR 1990 Assessment of current diagnostic criteria for Guillain-Barré syndrome. Annals of Neurology 27(suppl):21–24.

Borgaro S, Baker J, Wethe J et al 2005 Subjective reports of fatigue during early recovery from TBI. Journal of Head Trauma and Rehabilitation: focus on clinical research and practice part 2, 20(5):416–425.

Britton T 2004 Abnormalities of muscle tone and movement. In: Stokes M (ed) Physical management in neurological rehabilitation, 2nd edn. Elsevier, Edinburgh pp 47–56.

Burridge J, Taylor P, Hagan S et al 1997 The effects of common peroneal stimulation on the effort and speed of walking: a randomised controlled trial with chronic hemiplegic patients. Clinical Rehabilitation 11:201–210.

Campbell M 2004 Acquired brain injury: trauma and pathology. In: Stokes M (ed) Physical management in neurological rehabilitation, 2nd edn. Elsevier, Edinburgh pp 103–124.

Carr J, Shepherd R 1998 Neurological rehabilitation optimising motor performance, Butterworth-Heinemann, Oxford.

Carr J, Shepherd R 2003 Stroke rehabilitation: guidelines for exercise and training. Butterworth Heinemann, London.

Carter P, Edwards S 2002 General principles of treatment. In: Edwards S (ed) Neurological physiotherapy: a problem solving approach, 2nd edn. Churchill Livingstone, Edinburgh, pp 121–153.

Chang A 2004 Standing with assistance of a tilt table in intensive care: a survey of Australian physiotherapy practice. Australian Journal of Physiotherapy 50:51–54.

Cicerone KD, Dahlberg C, Malec JF et al 2005 Evidence based cognitive rehabilitation: updated review of the literature from 1998 through 2002. Archives of Physical Medicine and Rehabilitation 86(8):1681–1692.

Cott C, Finch E 1990 Goal setting in physical therapy practice. Physiotherapy Canada 43:19–22.

Duff S, Shumway-Cook A, Woollacott M 2007 Clinical management of the patient with reach, grasp and manipulation disorders. In: Shumway-Cook A, Woollacott M (eds) Motor control: translating research into clinical practice, 3rd edn. Lippincott Williams & Wilkins, Philadelphia, pp 518–556.

Edwards S 2002 Abnormal tone and movement as a result of neurological impairment: considerations for treatment. In: Edwards S (ed) Neurological physiotherapy: a problem solving approach, 2nd edn. Churchill Livingstone, Edinburgh, pp 89–120.

Edwards S, Charlton P 2002 Splinting and the use of orthoses in the management of patients with neurological disorders. In: Edwards S (ed) Neurological physiotherapy:

10

a problem solving approach, 2nd edn. Churchill Livingstone, Edinburgh, pp 219–253.

Freeman J 1992 Clinical notes of physiotherapy management of the patient with Guillain-Barré syndrome. Synapse, April.

Gabr U, Levine P, Page S 2003 Home based electromyography-triggered stimulation in chronic stroke. Clinical Rehabilitation 19:737–745.

Gray CS, Hildreth AJ, Alberti GKMM et al 2004 Poststroke hyperglycemia: natural history and immediate management. Stroke 35:122–127.

Harvey L, Herbert R, Crosbie J 2002 Does stretching induce lasting increases in joint ROM? A systematic review. Physiotherapy Research International 7(1):1–13.

Hesse S, Werner C, von Frankenberg S et al 2003 Treadmill training with partial body weight support after stroke. Physical Medicine Rehabilitation Clinics of North America 14(suppl 1):S111–S123.

Jackson D, Turner-Stokes L, Williams H et al 2003 Use of an integrated care pathway: a third round audit of the management of shoulder pain in neurological conditions. Journal of Rehabilitation Medicine 3(5):265–270.

Jonsson A-C, Lingren I, Hallstrom B et al 2006 Prevalence and intensity of pain after stroke: a population based study focussing on patients' perspectives. Journal of Neurology, Neurosurgery and Psychiatry 75:590–595.

Karnath HO, Ferber S, Dichgans J 2000 The origin of contraversive pushing: evidence of a second graviceptive system in humans. Neurology 55:1298–1304.

Kilbreath S, Davis G 2005 Cardiorespiratory fitness after stroke In: Refshauge K, Ada L, Ellis E (eds) Science based rehabilitation: theories into practice. Elsevier, Edinburgh, pp 131–158.

Knight L, Thornton H, Turner-Stokes L 2002 Management of neurogenic heterotopic ossification: three case histories to illustrate the role of physiotherapy. Physiotherapy 89(8):471–477.

Lindsay KW, Bone I 2004 Neurology and neurosurgery illustrated, 4th edn. Edinburgh, Churchill Livingstone.

MacFarlane A, Thornton H 1997 Solving the problem of contractures – throw out the recipe book? Physiotherapy Research International 2:1–6.

Malouin F, Richards C 2005 Assessment and training of locomotion after stroke: evolving concepts. In: Refshauge K, Ada L, Ellis E (eds) Science based rehabilitation: theories into practice. Elsevier, Edinburgh, pp 185–222.

Markham CH 1987 Vestibular control of muscular tone and posture. Journal of Canadian Science and Neurology 14:493–496.

McLeod JG 1992 Autonomic dysfunction in peripheral nerve disease. In: Bannister R, Mathias C (eds) Autonomic failure, 3rd edn. Oxford Medical Publications, Oxford, pp 659–681.

Medical Research Council (MRC) of the United Kingdom 1982 Aids to the examination of the peripheral nervous system. Bailliere-Tindall, Eastbourne.

Meldrum D, McConn Walsh R 2004 Vestibular and balance rehabilitation. In: Stokes M (ed) Physical management in neurological rehabilitation, 2nd edn. Elsevier, Edinburgh, pp 413–430.

Ng KPP, Howard RS, Fish DR et al 1995 Management and outcome of severe Guillain Barré syndrome. Quarterly Journal of Medicine 88:243–250.

Nicklin J 2004 Disorders of nerve II: Polyneuropathies. In: Stokes M (ed) Physical management in neurological rehabilitation, 2nd edn. Elsevier, Edinburgh, pp 253–267.

Olney S 2005 Training gait after stroke: a biomechanical perspective. In: Refshauge K, Ada L, Ellis E (eds) Science based rehabilitation: theories into practice. Elsevier, Edinburgh, pp 159–184.

Pentland B, Donald SM 1994 Pain in Guillain-Barré syndrome: a clinical review. Pain 59:159–164.

Pope P 2002 Posture management and special seating. In: Edwards S (ed) Neurological physiotherapy: a problem solving approach, 2nd edn. Churchill Livingstone, Edinburgh, pp 189–217.

Royal College of Physicians (RCP) 2002 Guidelines for the use of botulinum toxin (BTX) in the management of spasticity in adults. Royal College of Physicians, London.

Sharma N, Pomeroy V, Baron JC 2006 Motor imagery: a backdoor to the motor system after stroke? Stroke 37:1941–1952.

Sharman S 2002 Diagnosis and treatment of movement impairment syndromes. Mosby, St Louis.

Shiel A, Wilson B, McLellan L et al 2000 The Wessex Head Injury Matrix (WHIM) main scale: a scale to assess and monitor patient's recovery after severe head injury. Clinical Rehabilitation 14:408–416.

Shumway-Cook A, Woollacott M 2007 Motor control: translating research into clinical practice, 3rd edn. Lippincott Williams & Wilkins, Philadelphia.

Soryal I, Sinclair E, Hornby J et al 1992 Impaired joint mobility in Guillain-Barré syndrome: a primary or secondary phenomenon? Journal of Neurology, Neurosurgery and Psychiatry 55:1014–1017.

Staub F, Bogousslavsky J 2001 Fatigue after stroke: a major but neglected issue. Cerebrovascular Diseases 12(2):75–81.

Taub E, Miller NE, Novak TA et al 1993 Technique to improve chronic motor deficit after stroke. Archives of Physical Medicine and Rehabilitation 74:347–354.

Taylor EW, Morris D, Shaddeau S et al 1993 Effects of water walking on hemiplegic gait. Aquatic physical therapy. Journal of Aquatic Section of the American Physical Therapy Association 1:10–13.

Teasdale GM, Jennett B 1974 Assessment of coma and impaired consciousness: a practical scale. Lancet 2:81–84.

Thornton H, Kilbride C 2004 Physical management of abnormal tone and movement. In: Stokes M (ed) Physical management in neurological rehabilitation, 2nd edn. Elsevier, Edinburgh, pp 431–450.

Tuckey J, Greenwood R 2004 Rehabilitation after severe Guillain Barré syndrome: the use of partial body weight support. Physiotherapy Research International 9(2): 96–103.

10

Tyrer S, Lievesley A 2003 Pain following traumatic brain injury: assessment and management. Neuropsychological Rehabilitation 13(1/2):189–210.

Tyson S, Nightingale P 2004 The effects of positioning on oxygen saturation in acute stroke: a systematic review. Clinical Rehabilitation 18:863–871.

Wade DT 1992 Measurement in Neurological Rehabilitation. Oxford: Oxford University Press.

Weber M, Birklein F, Neundarfer B 2001 Facilitated neurogenic inflammation in complex regional pain syndrome. Pain 91(3):251–257.

Wolf S, Winstein C, Miller J et al 2006 Effects of constraint-induced movement therapy of the upper extremity 3–9 months after stroke. The EXCITE randomised clinical trial. Journal of the American Medical Association 296(17):2095–2104.

Yekutiel K, Guttman E 1993 A controlled trial of the retraining of the sensory function of the hand in stroke patients. Journal of Neurology, Neurosurgery and Psychiatry 56:241–244.

Useful websites

Association of Chartered Physiotherapists Interested in Neurology (ACPIN): www.acpin.net.

Brain and Spine Foundation: www.bbsf.org.uk.

Headway: www.headway.org.uk.

United Kingdom Acquired Brain Injury Foundation (UKABIF): www.ukabif.org.uk.

Guillain–Barré Syndrome Support Group: www.gbs.org.uk.

The Stroke Association: www.stroke.org.uk.

Royal College of Physicians (London): www.rcplondon.ac.uk.

STEP: www.effectivestrokecare.org.

10.3 The acute patient with limited potential for recovery: complete spinal cord injury

Sue Paddison

INTRODUCTION

Spinal cord injury (SCI) is usually a sudden onset, life-transforming condition. SCI can be classified according to the degree of sparing of movement and sensation below the lesion as 'complete' (paralysis and loss of sensation below the level of the lesion with little prospect of further recovery) or 'incomplete' (variable levels of motor or sensory sparing with greater prospects of further recovery). The principles of assessment and treatment presented in subchapters 10.1 and 10.2 are directly applicable for the person with an incomplete lesion where recovery is anticipated. The focus of this section will be on the physiotherapy management of an adult with complete SCI where individuals will need to learn adaptive strategies to return to optimum control of their physical self and instigate their path to reintegration. An overview of the pathology and general management issues can be found in Chapter 6; for specific advice on the management of paediatric SCI patients refer to Short et al (1992).

This section aims to identify:

- Key areas of assessment of an acute spinal cord injured individual.
- Neurological deficits and early diagnosis of level of spinal cord lesion thus gaining insight into expected functional abilities.
- Key treatment objectives and management plan of the spinal cord injured person.

KEY ASSESSMENT INFORMATION

Comprehensive assessment is essential to identify key factors affecting the management of the SCI individual (Table 10.3.1). Spinal fractures and their stability must be established, as this will influence all therapeutic handling of an acutely injured SCI person (Harrison 2000, Grundy & Swain 2002). The overall aim of surgery is to minimize neurological deterioration, restore alignment and stabilization, to facilitate early mobilization, reduce pain, to minimize hospital stay and to prevent secondary complications (Johnston 2001). Key components of assessment specific to SCI are outlined in Table 10.3.2 (p. 150).

The American Spinal Injury Association (ASIA) Scale

On admission to hospital after a SCI, an ASIA chart should be completed with the patient in supine to provide a baseline assessment (ASIA 2002; see www.asia-spinalinjury.org). The chart comprises 10 key myotomes and 28 dermatomes. Pin prick and light touch are the two sensory tests for each myotome [see Box 10.3.1 for a summary of the ASIA Impairment Scale (AIS)]. See Fig. 10.3.1.

Box 10.3.1

A = Complete lesion, no S4–5 motor or sensory function.
B = Incomplete with sensory function not motor below the neurological level, must include S4–5.
C = Incomplete with motor activity below the neurological level, in more than half key muscles with less than grade 3.
D = Incomplete motor activity below the neurological level, in at least half or more key muscles with grade 3 or greater.

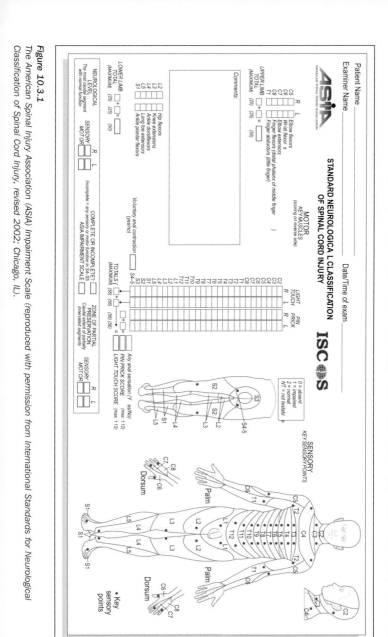

Figure 10.3.1
The American Spinal Injury Association (ASIA) Impairment Scale (reproduced with permission from International Standards for Neurological Classification of Spinal Cord Injury, revised 2002; Chicago, IL).

Table 10.3.1 Key factors for consideration in SCI management.

Spinal stability	● Takes account of structural and ligamentous damage ● Surgical or conservative management (bed rest/traction/bracing)
Orthotic bracing	● For conservative management or as an adjunct to the surgical fixation ● The Halo-Brace jacket for stabilizing the upper and lower cervical spine (Hossain et al 2004); thoraco-lumbar bracing systems vary extensively ● Timescales for wearing the brace depend on the surgical team's direction
Spinal shock	● Transient suppression and gradual return of reflex activity caudal to the SCI (Ditunno et al 2004)
Pain management	● May affect accuracy of assessment, respiratory effort and ability to participate in treatment ● Sources of pain: neurodynamics, central dysaesthesia, mechanical instability, fracture pain, muscle spasm pain, visceral pain, nerve root entrapment, syringomyelia (cyst formation within the spinal cord) and transitional zone pain (Nepomuceno et al 1979, Paddison & Middleton 2004)
Upper motor neurone (UMN) or lower motor neurone (LMN) lesions	● UMN injury involves the brain or spinal cord to the level of the cauda equina. The patient presents with spasticity and hyperreflexia ● LMN injury involves the lower spinal cord and peripheral nervous system. The conus originates from around spinal level T10 or below then becomes cauda equina
Autonomic dysreflexia	● A sympathetic nervous system dysfunction producing hypertension, bradycardia and headache with pilo-erection and capillary dilation and sweating, above the level of the lesion with lesions at T6 or above ● Can result from any noxious stimulus such as bladder or rectal distension ● A life-threatening condition that should be quickly identified and treated (Harrison 2000, Paddison & Middleton 2004)
Heterotopic ossification	● Calcification in denervated or UMN disordered muscle (David et al 1993) may result in loss of range in joints and impaired functional activities such as sitting ● May be confused in the early stages with DVT, when it presents as swelling, alteration in skin colour and increased heat, usually in relation to a joint

SCI, spinal cord injury.

Table 10.3.2 Key assessment information for SCI.

Database	● Spinal fractures ● Spinal level of lesion ● Spinal stability ● Associated injuries ● Respiratory status ● Spinal shock – transient suppression and gradual return of reflex activity caudal to the SCI (Ditunno et al 2004)
Subjective	● Pre-morbid musculoskeletal problems ● PMH: relevant respiratory factors
Objective	● Respiratory status (including FVC and cough) ● Passive range of movement of all joints ● Active movement ● Muscle strength: standard muscle chart (MRC 1982) and ASIA Chart (2002) ● Tone: Modified Ashworth Scale (Bohannon & Smith 1987) ● Sensory especially pin prick sensation (ASIA 2002) ● Joint range ● Other injuries

PMH, past medical history; FVC, forced vital capacity; MRC, Medical Research Council.

Age is a significant factor in indicating outcome (Burns & Ditunno 2001). With regard to incomplete lesions, pinprick preservation below injury level to S4/5 dermatomes is the best prognostic indicator for useful motor recovery with 75% of patients regaining ability to walk (Crozier et al 1991, Katoh & El Masry 1995, Poynton et al 1997). For incomplete paraplegia, studies show 85% of patients with muscles of grade 1 or 2 will recover to grade 3 or more, by one year post-injury. For 26% of patients with muscles grade 0, recovery to more than grade 3 was recorded (Waters et al 1993).

Spinal levels and functional independence

Physiotherapists need to be aware of the functional level patients can aspire to as outlined in Table 10.3.3.

Protecting the spine and preventing further damage

Maintaining spinal stability is crucial; spinal alignment can be maintained using orthotic devices, specialized turning beds and manual positioning with pillows. Physiotherapy intervention needs to be coordinated with positioning and protocols to determine the moving and turning of an SCI patient (Harrison 2000). Precautions are advised to limit joint range, to protect the spine during any

Table 10.3.3 Functional levels chart (adapted from Paddison & Middleton 2004, with permission).

Critical levels of innervation	Functional muscle activity	Functional activity
C1–C3	Neck control	● Ventilator dependant/phrenic stimulation ● Electric wheelchair ● Requires environmental control system
C3, 4, 5	Diaphragm function	● Independent/assisted breathing ● Electric wheelchair
C5	Biceps	● Limited upper limb function – feeding and self-propelling wheelchair on level surfaces ● Requires assistance from a caregiver for ADL and transfers
C6	Wrist extensors	● Adaptive hand function by learning to use a tenodesis grip (allowing the long flexors to shorten, thus producing finger flexion when the wrist is actively taken into extension) ● Manual wheelchair ● Independent feeding, grooming, and dressing top half
C7	Triceps	● Independent ADL, and transfers
T2 and below	Fully intact hand function	● Independent ADL, and transfers
T6–12	Abdominals	● Trunk control ● Coughing ● Ambulation with KAFO: swing to/ through gait pattern on crutches or rollator (T6–T9); may walk with crutches and manage stairs (T10–L1)

ADL, activities of daily living; KAFO, knee ankle foot orthoses.

intervention, and to work within pain limitations; these may be dependent on the surgeon or the orthotic device in situ (see Box 10.3.2).

Acute respiratory monitoring

The respiratory complications that can arise from SCI are outlined in Table 10.3.4 (see Chapter 13 for a more in-depth review of respiratory considerations). Respiratory failure remains one of the main causes of death in acute tetraplegia;

Box 10.3.2 Precautions (CSP, 1997)

Unstable paraplegia
● T9 and below limited to 30° hip flexion.

Unstable tetraplegia
● For unstable injuries at level of T4 and above, stabilize the head and neck for some upper limb movements using shoulder hold technique (the shoulders are held down onto the bed and the head stabilized between the forearms). Severity of spasticity will influence the decision to use a shoulder hold.
● Maintain full shoulder elevation with careful handling. May need to limit upper limb movements to 90 degrees if unable to adequately stabilize the neck during movements.
● Consider neural tension techniques for pain, where sensation is spared.
● No limit to straight leg raise (SLR). Patients are moved into flexion on bed rest but put into long sitting once up.

Table 10.3.4 Acute respiratory complications.

Spinal cord lesion	Complication	FVC % of normal
Lumbar and low thoracic	● Able to cough ● Decreased chest wall compliance	100–70%
High thoracic	● Unable to cough ● Further decrease in chest wall compliance ● Basal collapse ● Atelectasis ● Increased work of breathing ● Reduced expansion ● Autonomic dysfunction	30–50%
Low cervical	● Diapragm + accessory muscle fatigue ● Sputum retention – infection ● Collapse/consolidation ● Autonomic dysfunction	20%
Upper cervical	● Accessory only – ventilated	5–10%

FVC, forced vital capacity.

pneumonia is the leading cause of death in all persons with SCI (Jackson et al 1994). Patients with diminished or absent abdominal muscle activity will require assistance to cough and to clear secretions. This can be achieved using a manual assisted cough technique and by the Cough Assist Machine (JH Emerson Co). Patients require careful monitoring when FVC < 1L in an appropriate environment. Patients are at risk of cardiac arrest during initial suctioning due to unopposed vagal stimulation; having atropine ready for administration is advisable during this treatment.

TREATMENT CONSIDERATIONS IN THE ACUTE PHASE

Table 10.3.5 outlines acute physiotherapy management derived from Paddison & Middleton (2004).

Key interventions are:

- **Prophylactic chest care** especially for T6 and above; including assisted coughing, respiratory muscle training and positioning programme.
- **Maintenance of muscle length and joint range of movement.** This will include positioning in order to manage spasticity, hypertonia and prevent loss of range and the development of shoulder pain (Box 10.3.3). Some muscles are prone to contracture because of habitual positions adopted, muscle imbalance and weakness.
- **Active assisted and passive movements:** limbs are normally taken through range twice a day. No evidence-based rules for SCI are currently available; however, general principles can be adapted from guidelines for healthy individuals. The time spent on each joint movement will depend on the levels of spasticity, active strength available and pain.

Box 10.3.3 Maintenance of muscle length and joint range of movement (adapted from Paddison & Middleton 2004, pp. 136–139).

- The half crucifix position or bilateral shoulder external rotation.
- The 'frogged' position (for mass extensor spasticity) to maintain lower limbs in some flexion, abduction and external rotation.
- Full shoulder range of movement, elbow extension; essential for supported sitting.
- Production of the tenodesis grip (allowing the long flexors to shorten, thus producing finger flexion when the wrist is actively taken into extension; Whalley Hammell 1995, p 83).
- Hamstring length in order to achieve long sitting and calf length to enable standing.

Table 10.3.5 Treatment considerations in the acute phase (derived from Paddison & Middleton 2004).

	Paraplegia	Tetraplegia
Impairments	<ul><li>Respiratory compromise*</li><li>Weakness in affected muscle groups of trunk and lower limbs*</li><li>Altered tone – flaccid (cauda equina) or spasticity</li><li>Altered/loss sensation sense, cutaneous hypersensitivity*</li><li>Autonomic dysreflexia T6 and above* (Zejdlik 1992)</li><li>Muscle imbalance leading to contracture*</li><li>Other pathologies*</li></ul>	<ul><li>Greater respiratory compromise</li><li>Spasticity</li><li>Weakness of upper limbs and upper trunk</li><li>Other injuries e.g. brachial plexus lesion</li></ul>
Activity limitations	<ul><li>Pain* (Nepomuceno et al 1979)</li><li>Disrupted postural/balance systems*</li><li>Loss/impaired functional gait*</li><li>Compromised ability to cough*</li><li>Loss of bowel and bladder control*</li><li>Disrupted temperature control systems (Zejdlik 1992)</li><li>Pressure area considerations*</li></ul>	<ul><li>Loss/impaired function of upper limbs</li><li>Compromised ability to breath</li><li>Diminished ability for self care</li></ul>

10

Key aims & strategies		
	• FVC, respiratory muscle training* • Strengthen/maintain innervated muscles* • Passive and active-assisted movements* (CSP 1997) • Teach compensatory activities* • Prevent contractures* • Gait re-education with orthotics • Progressive standing programme: tilt table, with abdo binder • Anaesthetic skin prone to damage* and pressure stockings* • Address psychological issues • Education*	• Monitor/maintain respiratory function – respiratory support e.g.: IPPB (Van Houtte et al 2006) • Suction: be wary of vagal stimulation • Autonomic Dysreflexia T6 or above* (Zejdlik 1992) • Facilitate functional activity in all movements • Manage muscle imbalance: stretches, positioning, splinting • Compensatory activities e.g. tenodesis grip. (Whalley Hammell 1995, p 83)
Teamwork	• Medical/surgical/nursing team* • Occupational therapists • Orthotists* • Case manager/social worker* • Psychologist/psychiatrist*	• Anaesthetist/respiratory specialists • Liaise with speech and language therapist (SLT) for ventilated and high cervical cord injuries to assist with swallow and vocalization problems. • Breathing exercises can enhance work done with the SLT

*Denotes applies to paraplegia and tetraplegia.
FVC, forced vital capacity; IPPB, intermittent positive pressure breathing.

● Teaching **substitution movements** where active movement is lost, e.g. elbow extension using shoulder lateral rotation and gravity to assist. Splinting the hands of patients with C6 complete lesions, in order to produce an effective tenodesis grip.

● **Progressive mobilization up against gravity** using a tilt table is commonly used after flat bed rest. Patients will be hypotensive due to loss of venous tone and muscle pump. An abdominal binder and compression stockings are worn to assist in venous return. Pharmacological management will assist in the control of low blood pressure and complications of autonomic dysreflexia.

TREATMENT CONSIDERATIONS IN THE REHABILITATION PHASE
Breaking bad news

An inevitable part of each team member's role is to contribute to the patient's understanding of their condition and the implications of such. Patients will ask questions about their movement, sensation and the chances of recovery. A planned team approach is the best way to manage any in depth conversation regarding prognosis. This enables the patient to have an advocate with them, to help actively listen to the information they receive. During physiotherapy treatment it is best to rely on evidence-based information regarding possible chances of recovery, in general terms. There usually is never a clear answer. Factual reporting on the presentation today with a positive emphasis on the immediate goals, will help the patient to focus on each step at a time.

Physiotherapy intervention

Table 10.3.6 outlines the management of the rehabilitation phase.

Physiotherapy management (derived from Paddison and Middleton, 2004) in this phase will focus on:

● **Establishment of a standing programme:** progressing from tilt table to a standing frame.

● **Balance re-education:** progression from bilateral arm support to unilateral arm support to no arm support, e.g. reaching in different directions.

● **Basic level transfer techniques** from bed to wheelchair (see Table 10.3.7 for component breakdown; see more detailed guidance in Bromley (2006) pp. 185–214); progressing to varied level transfers and advanced transfers, e.g. chair to floor, car transfer (Bromley 2006, pp. 149–184).

Table 10.3.6 Treatment considerations in the rehabilitation phase (derived from Paddison & Middleton 2004).

	Paraplegia	Tetraplegia
Impairments	● Inability to sit or stand unaided* ● Skin prone to pressure marking* ● Disrupted postural control and balance systems*	● Loss of trunk stability
Activity limitations	● Postural hypotension* ● Heterotopic Ossification* (David et al 1998) ● Pain*	● Reduced exercise/activity endurance
Key aims & strategies	● Bed mobility* ● Balance re-education* ● Transfers* (Bromley 2006, pp. 185–214) ● Wheelchair training/seating* ● Splinting/orthotics* ● FES if lesion is UMN ● Botulinum toxin for spasticity* (Barnes et al 2001) ● Standing systems* ● Gait re-education with orthotics ● Self care education* ● Discharge planning*	● Long-term respiratory management – inspiratory muscle training, glossopharangeal breathing (Pryor & Webber 1998) ● Functional electrical stimulation (Johnston 2001)
Additional team involvement	● Urological team* ● Leisure/Sport coordinators* ● Community Health Care professionals* ● Work/Education authorities*	

*Denotes applies to paraplegia and tetraplegia.
FES, functional electrical stimulation; UMN, upper motor neurone.

10

Table 10.3.7 Initial level transfer components.

Legs up vs legs down	● Transfer initially with legs up for skin protection. The patients with trunk control may feel secure to practise legs down initially
Use of sliding board	● Always initiate transfers using a board and a towel over the wheel for skin protection
Position of front wheels	● Roll front castors forward to prevent the chair from tipping
Hand position	● Position hands with or without lifting blocks at the level of the greater trochanter of the hips ● Move one hand away onto the sliding board and the other beside the hip ● Lift and move towards the hand on the sliding board
Moving legs	● Once the lift has been performed and the patient moves onto the sliding board, the legs are moved by the patient or an assistant to allow the next lift to complete the transfer

Box 10.3.4 Bed mobility and mat activities

> ● **Rolling over:** using upper limbs to gain momentum and teaching self positioning of crossed legs to assist pelvis to roll.
> ● **Lying to sitting:** rolling into side lying, then push up into long sitting or sitting over the edge of the bed.
> ● **Long sitting:** hamstring stretching, lifting practice, e.g. push ups using blocks of different heights, moving around the plinth in different directions, manoeuvring legs.
> ● **Strength training:** using group exercise, free weights, sport, exercise equipment

● **Learning wheelchair mobility skills**, e.g. self propulsion, back wheel balance, kerbs and steps. This can be incorporated into sporting activities where appropriate. Wheelchair skills in power chair where appropriate.
● **Postural and wheelchair seating assessment** to facilitate an optimum pushing position and minimize upper limb joint pain.
● **General bed mobility and mat activities** (see Box 10.3.4).
● **Orthotics and gait training.** During rehabilitation, the patient may be assessed for suitability for walking with orthoses. See Box 10.3.5; for more detail see Bromley (2006) pp. 215–258. Depending on the fracture, gait

Box 10.3.5 Gait training

Spinal injury level and appropriate orthotic device

- **C7–L1**: ARGO (advanced reciprocal gait orthosis), RGO (reciprocal gait orthosis). Walkabout with rollator or crutches depends on level of function.
- **T6–T12**: Caliper walk with rollator; progress to crutches – depends on patient's function.
- **T9–L3**: Caliper walk with comfy handle crutches, HGO (hip guidance orthosis).
- **L3 and below**: Appropriate KAFO (Knee Ankle Foot Orthosis)/AFO or walking aid.

---

training will normally commence about a year after surgery, or earlier if no fixation surgery was indicated or if the patient is incomplete.

Reintegration

Although all the members of the MDT will play a role in supporting a patient, advice and guidance from a qualified psychologist is essential and, at times, one-to-one direct patient therapy by the psychologist is necessary. The process of adaptation to spinal paralysis, reflected as integration back into the community, is a gradual one. The process of case management has been found to be particularly important in supporting the complex process of reintegration of SCI patients. A key worker and case manager coordinate the many professional groups and agencies involved in the planning of discharge and return to home, work or school. This process is initiated almost as soon as the patient is medically stable. Early contact with local services and community health teams assists in cooperation and hopefully prevents unnecessary delays.

KEY CLINICAL MESSAGES

- SCI can be classified according to the degree of sparing of movement and sensation below the lesion. Prognostic indicators can be determined from S4/5 sparing.
- Key factors affecting the management of the SCI individual are: spinal stability; spinal shock; pain control; presence of spasticity; autonomic dysreflexia, skin integrity and heterotopic ossification.
- Physiotherapists need to be aware of the functional levels patients can aspire to according to their spinal injury level. Critical levels of innervation are: >C3

(ventilator dependant); C6 (tenodesis grip); <C7 (independent ADL and transfers), <T1 (intact hand function); >T6 (loss of abdominals).
- Acute respiratory monitoring is essential in lesions above T6 due to loss of abdominals leading to an ineffective cough.
- Teaching substitution movements where active movement is lost is essential.

References for subchapter 10.3

American Spinal Injuries Association (ASIA) 2002 International standards for neurological and functional classification of spinal cord injury. Chicago, ASIA; Revised 2002.

Barnes M, Bhakta B, Moore P et al 2001 The management of adults with spasticity using botulinum toxin. A guide to clinical practice. Ipsen Ltd.

Bohannon RW, Smith MB 1987 Interrater reliability of a modified Ashworth scale of muscle spasticity. Physical Therapy 67:206–207.

Bromley I 2006 Tetraplegia and paraplegia, 6th edn. Churchill Livingstone, London.

Burns AS, Ditunno JF 2001 Establishing prognosis and maximizing functional outcomes after spinal cord injury. Spine 26(24):S137–S145.

Chartered Society of Physiotherapy (CSP) 1997 Standards of physiotherapy practice for people with spinal cord lesions. CSP, London.

Crozier KS, Groziani V, Ditunno JF et al 1991 Spinal cord injury, prognosis for ambulation based on sensory examination in patients who are initially motor complete. Archives of Physical Medicine and Rehabilitation 72:119–121.

David O, Sett P, Burr RG et al 1993 The relationship of heterotopic ossification to passive movements in paraplegic patients. Disability and Rehabilitation 15:114–118.

Dittuno JF, Young W, Donovan WH 1994 The International Standards Booklet for neurological and functional classification of spinal cord injury. Paraplegia 32:70–80.

Dittuno JF, Little JW, Tessler A et al 2004 Spinal shock revisited: a four-phase model. Spinal Cord 42:383–395.

Grundy D, Swain A 2002 ABC of spinal cord injury, 4th edn. BMJ Publishers, London.

Harrison P 2000 Managing spinal injury: critical care. Spinal Injuries Association, London.

Hossain M, McLean A, Fraser MH 2004 Outcome of halo immobilisation of 104 cases of cervical spine injury. Scottish Medical Journal 49(3):90–92.

Jackson AB, Groomes TE 1994 Incidence of respiratory complications following spinal cord injury. Archives of Physical Medicine and Rehabilitation 75(3):270–275.

Johnston L 2001 Human spinal cord injury: new and emerging approaches to treatment. Spinal Cord 39:609–613.

Katoh S, El Masry WS 1995 Motor recovery of patients presenting with motor paralysis and sensory sparing following cervical spinal cord injury. Paraplegia 33(9):506–509.

Medical Research Council (MRC) of the United Kingdom 1982 Aids to the examination of the peripheral nervous system. Baillière-Tindall, Eastbourne.

Nepomuceno C, Fine PR, Richards JS et al 1979 Pain in patients with spinal cord injury. Archives of Physical Medicine and Rehabilitation 60:605–609.

Paddison S, Middleton F 2004 Spinal cord injury. In: Stokes M (ed) Physical management in neurological rehabilitation. Elsevier, London, pp 125–152.

Poynton AR, O'Farrel DA, Shannon F et al 1997 Sparing of sensation to pinprick predicts motor recovery of a motor segment after injury to the spinal cord. Journal of Bone and Joint Surgery Br 79:952–954.

Pryor JA, Webber BA 1998 Physiotherapy for respiratory and cardiac problems, 2nd edn. Churchill Livingstone, Edinburgh.

Short DJ, Frankel HL, Bergström EMK 1992 Injuries of the spinal cord in children. In: Vinken PJ et al (eds) Handbook of clinical neurology, vol 17(61): spinal cord trauma. Elsevier, London.

Van Houtte S, Vanlandewijke Y, Gosselink R 2006 Respiratory muscle training in persons with spinal cord injury: a systematic review. Respiratory Medicine 100(11):1886–1895 Epub 2006 Apr 12.

Waters RL, Adkins RH Yakura JS et al 1993 Motor and sensory recovery following complete tetraplegia. Archives of Physical Medicine and Rehabilitation 74:242–247.

Whalley Hammell K 1995 Spinal cord injury rehabilitation. Chapman & Hall, Canada.

Zejdlik CP 1992 Management of spinal cord injury, 2nd edn. Jones & Bartlett, Boston.

Essential reading

Bromley I 2006 Tetraplegia and paraplegia, 6th edn. Churchill Livingstone, London.

Paddison S, Middleton F 2004 Spinal cord injury. In: Stokes M (ed) Physical management in neurological rehabilitation. Elsevier, London, pp 125–152.

Useful web sites:

www.asia-spinalinjury.org.

Spinal Injuries Association: www.spinal.co.uk.

Multidisciplinary Association of Spinal Cord Injury Professionals: www.mascip.co.uk.

10.4 The patient with degenerative disease: multiple sclerosis

Jennifer A Freeman

INTRODUCTION

Degenerative long-term conditions, such as multiple sclerosis (MS), differ from recovering conditions, such as stroke, in a number of ways. In contrast to recovering conditions where the pathology is relatively stable, people with degenerative conditions develop an increasing number and range of new signs and symptoms over time as a consequence of continued (and usually irreversible) damage to the nervous system. This results in a progressive decline in their function and mobility. While recovery can occur, for instance after acute relapse in MS, the overall pattern is one of deterioration. Unfortunately the rate and pattern of this deterioration is not predictable and sometimes changes can occur quite suddenly and unexpectedly. These factors combine to make management very challenging.

The ever-changing nature of degenerative conditions requires the focus of physiotherapy to be placed on lifelong management (rather than lifelong 'hands on' treatment) whereby a partnership is developed with the person affected by the disorder to help them best manage its disabling consequences by adapting and readapting to their condition repeatedly over time. Box 10.4.1 summarizes some of the key management principles which can be helpful in achieving this.

Box 10.4.1 Key principles of management in degenerative long-term conditions.

- Comprehensive assessment and ongoing review
- Listening to and learning from patients
- Ensuring the patient and their family are central to planning and participating in their own management
- Clarifying the patient's perception of their main problems, their aims, and expectations of intervention
- Promoting self management
- Focusing therapy on maintaining activities within the context of the person's lifestyle
- Offering ongoing support with flexible service provision and intensive rehabilitation as appropriate at different times
- Adopting a coordinated multidisciplinary approach to management across services in various settings

KEY ASSESSMENT INFORMATION

The multiplicity of symptoms that may arise in MS means that its physical, cognitive and psychosocial consequences are often wide-ranging, variable and complex. Thorough and accurate assessment should be undertaken at the beginning of each new episode of care, in line with that described in Chapter 9. Table 10.4.1 summarizes key information which should be included specifically for people with MS.

The impact of MS on impairment, activity and participation differs markedly between individuals. Changes may be dramatic with a recent relapse; more gradual

Table 10.4.1 Key assessment information for people with MS.

Database For newly diagnosed patients	● Confirmation of diagnosis: a second neurological event is required for confirmation of diagnosis ● Awareness of diagnosis: the neurologist or GP should convey the diagnosis – not the physiotherapist's role
Database For people with established MS	● Classification of MS: benign, relapsing remitting, primary progressive, secondary progressive (McDonald et al 2001) ● Currently in relapse, or have they recently had a relapse? If so, how long ago was the relapse? ● Currently on a course of steroids? What is the steroid regimen? ● On disease-modifying drug therapy e.g. beta interferons? ● Using complementary medicine?
Subjective Since you were last assessed, or prior to this relapse, has any activity you used to undertake been limited, stopped or affected? (NICE 2003)	Prompts should be given regarding: ● mobility (including whether, when and how often they use a wheelchair) ● 'hidden' symptoms, which include: thinking and remembering; fatigue; vision; balance and falling; bladder and bowel control; sexual function; mood ● how fatigue impacts on daily life and exercise tolerance ● whether and how much their symptoms and function fluctuate over the course of a day. Predictable fluctuations (e.g. usually tired by mid afternoon) enable lifestyle modifications to accommodate this; unpredictable fluctuations are more difficult to manage
Subjective Specifically for people with a relapse	● How quickly are they recovering? ● How are they coping with these sudden changes? ● If the patient is currently on or has recently been on steroids, how have they responded to them?
Objective	● Assessment of impairments and activities should be undertaken ● Duration and nature of the physical assessment should take into account factors such as fatigability, emotional and cognitive status (see Chapter 9)
MS specific tools	● Fatigue Severity Scale (Fisk et al 1994) ● Multiple Sclerosis Spasticity Scale (Hobart et al 2006) ● The 12-item Multiple Sclerosis Walking Scale (Hobart et al 2003) ● Guys (UK) Neurological Disability Scale (Sharrack & Hughes 1999) ● Multiple Sclerosis Impact Scale (Hobart et al 2001) ● Multiple Sclerosis Quality of Life-54 Instrument (Vickrey et al 1995)

10

deterioration may occur in the progressive phase; or symptoms may remain virtually in status quo with benign disease. When changes have occurred, the reasons for these should be identified, considering impairments, and social and physical factors. When assessing people with MS it is essential to determine:

● fatigue levels in response to exercise and activities;
● ability to understand and recall discussions and instructions, and to problem solve at a functional level;
● whether any other co-morbidities are responsible for/contributing to the problems.

The life-long nature of MS makes it important to undertake re-assessments at appropriate intervals. NICE Guidelines (NICE 2003) recommend the use of a standardized review checklist at every new episode of care. These can act as a prompt, prevent duplication of questioning between health professionals, and provide a basis for future comparison. This is particularly useful where regular rotation of staff means that the person may often be reviewed by a different therapist.

KEY APPROACHES TO PHYSIOTHERAPY MANAGEMENT

In considering the needs of people with MS and how physiotherapy and multi-disciplinary rehabilitation should be incorporated throughout the course of the disease, it is helpful to divide the condition into four stages:

● Diagnosis
● Minimal disability
● Moderate disability
● Severe disability.

A practical framework for considering the key needs and main focus of care at each of these stages is presented in Table 10.4.2.

It is important to change the focus of physiotherapy management as the disease progresses. While there is clearly overlap, three main approaches are required:

● Health promotion
● Restorative rehabilitation
● Maintenance rehabilitation and palliative care.

When viewed together, these approaches provide a continuum of care in which a different emphasis is placed on different aspects of management throughout the disease course. Depending on individual needs and available resources, this can be provided within an inpatient (either acute hospital or a rehabilitation unit), outpatient or community setting.

Table 10.4.2 Key needs and interventions at different stages of MS (after Freeman et al 2003).

Stage of MS	Key needs	Focus of intervention by the multi-disciplinary team (MDT)
Diagnosis	<ul><li>Certain clear diagnosis</li><li>Appropriate support</li><li>Access to information</li><li>Continuing education</li><li>Disease-modifying drugs</li></ul>	<ul><li>Emphasis is on *health promotion* to maintain current levels of activities and participations by management of fatigue, regular exercise and a healthy lifestyle (Stuifbergen et al 2003)</li><li>Team working with the neurologist and nurse specialist to provide support, advice and information, either on an individual or group basis</li><li>Provision of physiotherapy on an outpatient basis as required</li></ul>
Minimal impairment	<ul><li>Advice, support and information</li><li>Self-management options</li><li>Treatment of relapses</li><li>Disease-modifying drugs</li><li>Management of symptoms</li></ul>	<ul><li>*Guided self management and health promotion* to facilitate regular exercise, maintain usual activities, and prevent complications (O'Hara et al 2002)</li><li>Symptomatic management by MDT (Kesselring & Beer 2005)</li><li>Relapse management alongside steroid treatment to improve residual deficits (Craig et al 2003)</li><li>Physiotherapy on an outpatient basis or in a hospital setting during relapse</li><li>Liaison with specialist professionals e.g. continence advisors, employment advisors</li></ul>

(continued)

Table 10.4.2 Key needs and interventions at different stages of MS (after Freeman et al 2003)—cont'd.

Stage of MS	Key needs	Focus of intervention by the multi-disciplinary team (MDT)
Moderate disability	• Rehabilitation and symptomatic management • Easy access to well co-ordinated services • Clear and consistent communication	• *Restorative rehabilitation and symptomatic management* to optimize activities and participations. Often achieved through comprehensive MDT rehabilitation programme, as an inpatient (Freeman et al 1997; Solari et al 1999) or within the community (Pozzilli et al 2002) • Liaison with specialist services, such as posture and seating clinics • Assess carer's needs; and provide education and support (McKeown et al 2003) • Implement/reinforce links with community care
Severe disability	• Access to information and expertise • Good communication and co-ordinated care within the community • Respite care • Palliative care	• *Maintenance rehabilitation* usually within the community, aimed at maintaining autonomy wherever possible • Management by all involved in care and throughout 24 hours of the day, rather than intensive 'hands on' physiotherapy • Emphasis on preventing or improving secondary complications such as pressure areas and contractures • Provision of appropriate equipment, environmental controls, wheelchairs, home adaptations and community mobility (NICE 2003) • Joint working between health and social care • Supportive care to increase comfort

MDT, multidisciplinary team.

ESSENTIAL PHYSIOTHERAPY MANAGEMENT STRATEGIES

Physiotherapy management strategies typically fall into two main categories:

1. Directly improving existing physical impairments, such as weakness, loss of range, altered tone and reduced cardio-respiratory fitness (Table 10.4.3).

2. Involving processes that include the acquisition of new skills and the changing of behaviour (Table 10.4.4, p. 170). These strategies are particularly important as the disease progresses, when impairments cannot be reversed.

The severity of deficits determines the types of exercise and activities undertaken. Weakness should be distinguished from altered tone, incoordination and fatigability (MS Society 2004). People with MS are less fit and active than normal sedentary subjects (Motyl et al 2005). No deleterious effects of exercise have been shown on disease activity, exacerbations, fatigue or spasticity (White & Dressendorfer 2004). Overheating should be minimized as it can result in conduction block. Useful advice includes:

● ensuring the environment is not hot
● drinking cold water before, during and after exercise
● pre-exercise cooling, such as a cool shower
● wearing light clothing
● working at a steady pace
● building in rest breaks to allow the body to cool down.

Management of ataxia and tremor is extremely difficult and is typically associated with a poor outcome. Education of helpful compensatory strategies (such as stabilization of upper limbs on supporting surfaces) can lessen the impact of ataxia and tremor on function, although this is often limited in success (Alusi et al 1999).

Interventions should always aim to improve activities and participation; focus on the function and goals of the individual, and never be simply aimed at improvement of impairments per se. These interventions should incorporate practice into daily routine – key when fatigue is a problem. Normal movement is not achievable as the disease progresses and the severity of impairments increases. Education of helpful compensatory strategies is vital to optimize function. It is essential to provide written information to support advice, as many people have cognitive difficulties.

The physiotherapist should always consider whether factors, other than physical impairment, may be interfering with mobility, such as fatigue, cognitive loss, sensory loss, deconditioning or unsuitable equipment (MS Society 2004). As the disease progresses people rely more heavily on walking aids and wheelchairs for mobility, particularly outdoors or over longer distances. Specialist wheelchairs are often required when disability is severe (NICE 2003). Discussions in relation to this should be undertaken with sensitivity (MS Society 2004). Liaison with

Table 10.4.3 Interventions focusing on improving impairments.

Core impairments	Interventions
Muscle weakness and fatigability	• For milder weakness, regimens include exercising major muscle groups using weights for 10–12 repetitions through full range for 2–3 sets, aiming for moderate fatigue by end of third set (De Bolt & McCubbin 2002) • Consider activating large muscle groups to avoid overload that may result in conduction block when weakness is present (White & Dressendorfer 2004) • Monitor fatigue during exercise
General fatigue	• Aerobic and endurance training (White & Dressendorfer 2004, Romberg et al 2004) • Energy conservation strategies (Mathiowetz et al 2001) • Ensure close liaison with the multidisciplinary team • Consider sleep, chronic pain, nutrition and daily routine
Cardiovascular deconditioning	• Endurance and aerobic training is effective in improving fitness, fatigue and function. Techniques include stationary cycling (Mostert & Kesselring 2002), treadmill training (Van den Berg et al 2006), Tai Chi (Wang et al 2004) and yoga (Oken et al 2004) • Aerobic exercise – at least 3 × per week at moderate level of perceived exertion (approximately 65% of VO_2 max) for 20–30 minutes (Petajan & White 1999) • Consider using group formats which can increase motivation and adherence to exercise, possibly because of added social benefits • Think about using local leisure centres

Spasticity and spasms	• Stretching, splinting and standing regimens (Boyd & Ada 2001) in combination with education and medication (Thompson et al 2005)
	• Education to avoid trigger and aggravating factors
	• Equipment such as posture and seating systems, wedges, rolls, and sleeping systems to incorporate within a 24 hour management approach
	• Relaxation and movement control inteventions such as Tai Chi, yoga and biofeedback
	• Referral for specialist advice to spasticity clinics may be required for people with more severe spasms and spasticity (Thompson et al 2005)
	• Consider if spasticity is masking weakness; and, if so, to what extent the person is using spasticity for function (MS Society 2004)
Ataxia and tremor	• Interventions to improve postural control and core stability, e.g. gymnastic ball (Jones et al 1996), pilates exercises and standing programmes
	• Aids and equipment to optimize function, e.g. rollator frames for walking or non-spill cups for drinking
	• Posture and seating equipment, e.g. head rest or high-backed chair, can reduce head titubation (head tremor; Alusi et al 1999)
Pain	• Transcutaneous electrical nerve stimulation (TENS – Al Smadi et al 2003) and thermal modalities
	• Ergonomic and environmental factors, e.g. working environment and wheelchair comfort should be evaluated
	• Referral to a musculoskeletal physiotherapist and specialist pain services may be appropriate to ensure effective management (NICE 2003)

Table 10.4.4 Interventions to improve activities and participation.

Core limitations and restrictions	Interventions
Gait	• Identify and treat reversible underlying impairments • Gait re-education to improve the safety, independence, pattern and efficiency of walking (Lord et al 1998; Wiles et al 2001). • Training with provision of equipment such as orthoses and walking aids • Functional Electrical Stimulation (FES) to improve the pattern and efficiency of gait in people with foot drop (Taylor et al 1999)
General mobility	• Task-related practice of mobility activities, e.g. transfers, stairs, using a wheelchair • Training with provision of equipment, e.g. transfer boards, wheelchairs • Teach others how to assist with tasks such as moving in bed or transferring
Daily functional activities	• Task-related practice of specific activities • Education of helpful compensatory strategies to maximize function • Appropriate aids, equipment and adaptations, in liaison with the occupational therapist (OT; Baker & Tickle-Dengen 2001) • Fatigue management through energy conservation strategies (Mathiowetz et al 2001) • Teaching others to assist, or take over activities that the person can no longer achieve independently
Maintenance of comfortable and functional postures	• 24 hour postural management: implementation and review of regimens for sleeping, sitting and standing postures • Positioning aids and equipment such as rolls, wedges, and sleeping systems
Leisure pursuits	• Teach techniques to enable maintenance of usual leisure pursuits or alternative pursuits
Occupational issues	• Identify whether any physical problems (motor, sensory, fatigue) impact on work ability • Vocational assessments within work environment • Advice, support, equipment and adaptations

specialist services such as mobility centres (driving assessment) (NICE 2003), functional electrical stimulation (FES) clinics, and orthotics clinics is important.

Close communication with the person with MS, their family and the health and social care team is crucial to reinforce a 24 hour management approach. This is central to prevent (wherever possible) or minimize secondary complications.

ONGOING REVIEW AND SUPPORT

In MS new symptoms can arise suddenly and unexpectedly; or alternatively can insidiously progress. Review systems (Table 10.4.5) are important to ensure the patient's health status is monitored, potential complications are identified, and progress is checked on implementation of the care plan. Co-ordination and

Table 10.4.5 Review and ongoing support systems.

Method of review	Issues to consider
Pre-scheduled appointments (e.g. at 6 or 12 months)	● Can help in managing insidiously progressive symptoms but of limited benefit in proactively managing symptoms or in responding to more intermittent, acute or complex needs ● Are any other professionals intending to review this person? If so, when is this scheduled?
Open access (self referral)	● Allows people flexibility in accessing services when their needs change, giving them the opportunity to take responsibility for self management ● To be effective, people need to know how, why, whom and when they should contact services ● Information leaflets, with flowchart of the decision-making process for contacting specific services, can help clarify these issues, also providing a prompt to people with memory difficulties
Open access supplemented by planned review	● Self-referral systems may not be suitable for people at risk of developing severe secondary complications or who are unable to engage effectively in decision making, e.g. those with cognitive problems or depression ● Planned face to face reviews to supplement the open access system provides an important safety net in these situations
Telephone reviews/help-lines	● These can be an efficient way to provide advice and support at times of need – enable easy access to systems within their usual lifestyles, e.g. if they are in work

10

where possible amalgamation of reviews can prevent duplication, unnecessary travel and inconvenience to the person with MS and their family. Table 10.4.5 summarizes different review and support systems and highlights issues to consider in their implementation.

Referral mechanisms differ between departments and health services. A local directory which provides contact and referral information about services relevant to MS and how they can be accessed can help all those involved in care to negotiate the complicated network of health and social service systems involved in the management of people with MS.

KEY CLINICAL MESSAGES

● People with MS develop an increasing number and range of new signs and symptoms over time as a consequence of continued (and usually irreversible) damage to the nervous system. The rate and pattern of this deterioration is not predictable.

● The life-long nature of MS makes it important to undertake re-assessments at appropriate intervals. Review systems are important to ensure the patient's health status is monitored, potential complications are identified, and progress is checked on implementation of the care plan.

● It is important to change the focus of physiotherapy management to suit the patient's level of disability as the disease progresses. Discussions in relation to the need for aids, adaptations and equipment should be undertaken with sensitivity (MS Society 2004).

References for subchapter 10.4

Alusi SH, Glickman S, Aziz TZ, Bain PG 1999 Tremor in multiple sclerosis. Journal of Neurology, Neurosurgery and Psychiatry 66:131–134.

Al Smadi J, Warke K, Wilson I et al 2003 A pilot investigation of the hypoalgesic effects of transcutaneous electrical nerve stimulation upon low back pain in people with multiple sclerosis. Clinical Rehabilitation 17:742–749.

Baker NA, Tickle-Dengen L 2001 The effectiveness of physical, psychological and functional interventions in treating clients with multiple sclerosis: a meta-analysis. American Journal of Occupational Therapy 55:324–331.

Boyd RN, Ada L 2001 Physiotherapy management of spasticity. In: Barnes M, Johnson G (eds) Upper motor neurone syndrome and spasticity: clinical management and neurophysiology. Cambridge University Press, chap 4, pp 96–120.

Craig J, Young CA, Ennis M et al 2003 A randomised controlled trial comparing rehabilitation against standard therapy in multiple sclerosis patients receiving intravenous steroid treatment. Journal of Neurology, Neurosurgery and Psychiatry 74:1225–1230.

De Bolt L, McCubbin J 2004 The effects of home based resistance exercises on balance, power and mobility in adults with multiple sclerosis. Archives of Physical Medicine and Rehabilitation 85:290–297.

Fisk JD, Ritvo PG, Ross L et al 1994 Measuring the functional impact of fatigue: initial validation of the fatigue impact scale. Clinical Infectious Diseases 18(suppl 1):S79-S83.

Freeman JA, Langdon DW, Hobart JC et al 1997 The impact of inpatient rehabilitation on progressive multiple sclerosis. Annals of Neurology 42(2):236–244.

Freeman JA, Ford H, Mattison P et al 2003 Developing multiple sclerosis healthcare standards: evidence-based recommendations for service providers. Multiple Sclerosis Society of Great Britain and Northern Ireland.

Hobart JC, Lamping DL Fitzpatrick R et al 2001 The Multiple Sclerosis Impact Scale (MSIS-29): a new patient-based outcome measure. Brain 124:962–973.

Hobart JC, Riazi A, Lamping DL et al 2003 Measuring the impact of MS on walking ability: the 12-item MS walking scale (MSWS-12). Neurology 60:31–36.

Hobart JC, Riazi A, Thompson AJ et al 2006 Getting the measure of spasticity in MS: the MS Spasticity Scale (MSSS-89). Brain 129:224–234.

Jones L, Lewis Y, Harrison J et al 1996 The effectiveness of occupational therapy and physiotherapy in multiple sclerosis patients with ataxia of the upper limb and trunk. Clinical Rehabilitation 10:277–282.

Kesselring J, Beer S 2005 Symptomatic therapy and neurorehabilitation in multiple sclerosis. Lancet Neurology 4(10):643–652.

Lord SE, Wade DT, Halligan PW 1998 A comparison of two physiotherapy treatment approaches to improve walking in multiple sclerosis: a pilot randomised controlled study. Clinical Rehabilitation 12:477–486.

Mathiowetz V, Matuska KM, Murphy ME 2001 Efficacy of an energy conservation course for persons with multiple sclerosis. Archives of Physical Medicine and Rehabilitation 82:449–456.

McDonald WI, Compston A, Edan G et al 2001 Recommended diagnostic criteria for multiple sclerosis: guidelines from the international panel on the diagnosis of multiple sclerosis. Annals of Neurology 50(1):121–127.

McKeown LP, Porter-Armstrong AP, Baxter GD 2003 The needs and experiences of caregivers of individuals with multiple sclerosis: a systematic review. Clinical Rehabilitation 17(3):234–238.

Mostert S, Kesselring J 2002 Effects of a short-term training program on aerobic fitness, fatigue, health perception and activity level of subjects with multiple sclerosis. Multiple Sclerosis 8:161–168.

Motyl RW, McAuley E, Snook EM 2005 Physical activity and multiple sclerosis: a meta-analysis. Multiple Sclerosis 11:459–463.

MS Society 2004 Translating the NICE MS Guideline into practice: a physiotherapy guidance document. London. MS Society, Chartered Society of Physiotherapy and Association of Physiotherapists in Neurology.

National Institute for Clinical Excellence 2003 Multiple sclerosis: management of multiple sclerosis in primary and secondary care. Clinical Guideline 8. 2003. National Institute for Clinical Excellence, London.

10

O'Hara L, Cadbury H, De Souza L et al 2002 Evaluation of the effectiveness of professionally guided self-care for people with multiple sclerosis living in the community: a randomised controlled trial. Clinical Rehabilitation 16:119–128.

Oken BS, Kishiyama S, Zajdel D et al 2004 Randomized controlled trial of yoga and exercise in multiple sclerosis. Neurology 62:2058–2064.

Petajan JH, White AT 1999 Recommendations for physical activity in patients with multiple sclerosis. Sports Medicine 27(3):179–191.

Pozzilli C, Brunetti M, Amicosante AMV et al 2002 Home based management in multiple sclerosis: results of a randomized controlled trial. Journal of Neurology, Neurosurgery and Psychiatry 73:250–255.

Romberg A, Virtanen A, Ruutianen J et al 2004 Effects of a six-month exercise programme on patients with MS. Neurology 63:2034–2038.

Sharrack B, Hughes RAC 1999 The Guy's Neurological Disability Scale (GNDS): a new disability measure for multiple sclerosis. Multiple Sclerosis 5(4):223–233.

Solari A, Filippini G, Gasco P et al 1999 Physical rehabilitation has a positive effect on disability in multiple sclerosis patients. Neurology 52:57–62.

Stuifbergen AK, Becker H, Blozis S et al 2003 A randomised clinical trial of a wellness intervention for women with multiple sclerosis. Archives of Physical Medicine and Rehabilitation 84:467–476.

Taylor PN, Burridge JH, Dunkerley AL et al 1999 Clinical use of the Odstock dropped foot stimulator: its effect on the speed and effort of walking. Archives of Physical Medicine and Rehabilitation 80(12):1577–1583.

Thompson AJ, Jarrett L, Marsden J et al 2005 Clinical management of spasticity (editorial). Journal of Neurology, Neurosurgery and Psychiatry 76:459–463.

Van den Berg M, Dawes H, Wade DT et al 2006 Treadmill training for individuals with multiple sclerosis: a pilot randomized trial. Journal of Neurology, Neurosurgery and Psychiatry 77:531–533.

Vickrey BG, Hays RD, Harooni R et al 1995 A health-related quality of life measure for multiple sclerosis. Qual Life Res 4:187–206.

Wang C, Collet JP, Lau J 2004 The effect of Tai Chi on health outcomes in patients with chronic conditions: a systematic review. Archives of Internal Medicine 164:493–501.

White LJ, Dressendorfer RH 2004 Exercise and multiple sclerosis. Sports Medicine 34(15):1077–1100.

Wiles CM, Newcombe RG, Fulller KJ et al 2001 Controlled randomized crossover trial of the effects of physiotherapy in chronic multiple sclerosis. Journal of Neurology, Neurosurgery and Psychiatry 70:174–179.

Key web sites

National (UK) clinical guideline on the management of MS in primary and secondary care (NICE 2003). Available at: www.nice.org.uk.

Physiotherapy guidance document on translating the MS national guideline into practice (MS Society 2004). Available at: www.mssociety.org.uk.

Charitable bodies provide useful up-to-date information for all people affected by MS. Fact sheets and expert consensus documents are available on many aspects of management; as are updates on recent research and reviews of the literature.

The National MS Society of Great Britain and Northern Ireland: www.mssociety. org.uk.

The MS Trust: www.mstrust.org.uk.

The National MS Society of America: www.nationalmssociety.org.

The Consortium of MS Centres: www.mscare.org.

10.5 The patient with degenerative disease: Parkinson's disease

Emma Stack

INTRODUCTION

In Parkinson's disease (PD), all types of movement (from postural control to fine dexterity) are impaired, as outlined in Chapter 6. Although primarily concerned with the motor features, physiotherapists need to be aware of the non-motor manifestations of the condition such as personality change, depression, sleep disturbance, and autonomic dysfunction including orthostatic hypotension, constipation and sexual dysfunction (Jankovic 1990).

As PD progresses:

● The efficacy of pharmacological management (largely dopamine replacement) diminishes;
● Disabling side-effects develop:
  ● 'On-Offs'(rapid fluctuations in motor function): Although able to move relatively freely when drugs work optimally, some patients are barely able to move at all when drug action is decreased or absent. These marked fluctuations are like a light switch going from 'on' to 'off'. They are initially predictable in relation to the timing of drug intake but become more random (Olanow & Hauser 1990)
  ● Dyskinesia (involuntary movement);
● Surgery, to disrupt pathological over-activity in the thalamus, globus pallidus or subthalamic nucleus, becomes an option (Hamani & Lozano 2003). Patients undergoing deep brain stimulation under local anaesthesia may benefit from physiotherapy (Chevrier et al 2006).

Physiotherapy is unlikely to impact on the three key motor signs of PD, i.e. bradykinesia (slowed movement), rigidity, and resting tremor; these are primary impairments – a direct result of the disease process; gait, balance, posture and transfers are the key domains for physiotherapy within PD. Supporting evidence is strongest for gait re-education (e.g. optimizing initiation, speed and stride length) and improving Activities of Daily Living (ADL) scores (Keus et al 2007). There is also some evidence to suggest that physiotherapy may help increase flexibility, strength and cardiovascular fitness, e.g. secondary complications/impairments. It would seem important to design therapy programmes which will hopefully prevent or at least slow down the development of these secondary impairments.

The key principles of management in degenerative long-term conditions outlined in Box 10.4.1 (p. 162) in relation to people with MS apply. A comprehensive multidisciplinary team (MDT), including specialist physicians and therapists, is required to meet the complex and progressive needs of people with PD. PD nurse specialists, where they exist, are key players. As well as helping people with PD to understand and manage their medication, they provide a constant point of contact for people living with PD, helping them to access the support and services they need. Within the MDT, physiotherapists maximize function (and minimize complications) through movement rehabilitation within a context of education and support for the whole person, using eclectic techniques (Ashburn et al 2004). According to Morris (2000), therapists need to:

1. Understand the pathogenesis of the presenting disorders (e.g. hypokinesia);
2. Manage the disorders according to disease stage (i.e. adjust intervention);
3. Problem-solve:
   - Tailor plans (to medication; cognition; environment; coexisting medical conditions)
   - Emphasize task-specific training within functional tasks (e.g. turning in bed).

KEY ASSESSMENT INFORMATION

Assessment in general is covered in Chapter 9 but there are PD specific aspects that the therapist should consider (see Table 10.5.1). It is preferable to perform the assessment in the patient's familiar surroundings in both the 'on' and 'off' states to reassess at the same point in the drug cycle record:

- Current medication
- Time of day
- Time since last dose
- 'On' or 'Off'.

Table 10.5.1 Key assessment information for people with Parkinson's disease (PD).

Database (from the records)	● Diagnosis (date and certainty) ● Neurological examination, including measures of PD severity and cognitive function ● Symptoms: some common symptoms will not be obvious at the time of assessment, e.g. depression and fatigue. Both impact on ability to perform ADL ● Sleep disorders: type of insomnia and contributory factors ● Pain (rigidity may present as painful stiffness)
Subjective	Falls history (Stack & Ashburn 1999) ● Ascertain the home situation and whether fear of falling restricts ADL ● Ask patient and/or carer to recall falls and near-misses over the previous 12 months: two or more falls is a risk factor for falling again. For each fall recalled, ascertain: ● Location (e.g. bathroom) ● Fall-related activity (e.g. turning, walking) ● Suspected cause (e.g. freezing, tripping) ● Saving reactions or landing
Objective	Observe and record movements and movement strategies, including: ● Walking (not just forward in straight lines) but steering and turning ● Attempting simultaneous tasks (e.g. walking while carrying or talking) ● Performing fall-related activities (e.g. reaching above shoulder level) ● Transferring (in and out of bed and chair) Use video (be careful not to introduce a trip hazard) to provide a lasting record that: ● Allows repeated observation ● Aids feedback to patient/carer

ADL; activities of daily living.

(*continued*)

Assessment also involves a detailed evaluation of the patient's functional difficulties (see Table 10.5.2); when assessing function, the key areas of assessment are:
● The fall history: falls information can be gathered at interview or by patient and/or carer completing a 'falls diary' at home between assessments
● Gait, balance, posture and transfers within everyday activities.

Table 10.5.1 Key assessment information for people with Parkinson's disease (PD)—cont'd.

Measurement tools	• Unified Parkinson's Disease Rating Scale (Lang & Fahn 1989)
	• Hoehn and Yahr Stages (Hoehn & Yahr 1967)
	• Parkinson's Activity Scale (Nieuwboer et al 2000) Effectiveness in activities, including bed mobility
	• Parkinson's Disease Questionnaire – PDQ-39 (Peto et al 1998)
	• Multiple Tasks Test (Bloem et al 2001) Simultaneous assessment of components of postural control
	• Functional Axial Rotation (Schenkman et al 2001) Measure of spinal rotation in sitting
	• Retropulsion Test (Visser et al 2003) Test for postural stability based on an unexpected shoulder pull
	• Standing Start 180° Turn Test (Stack and Ashburn, 2005) Video-based measure of turning
	• Turning in Bed (Stack & Ashburn 2006) Assess strategies in both directions in patient's own bed
	• Turning Step Count (Stack et al 2006) Count steps 'on-the-spot' and during functional turns

PHYSICAL INTERVENTION

The key options are (1) exercise, (2) cueing and (3) movement strategies. Exercise with cueing plus the development of cognitive strategies best improves function (Kamsma et al 1995, Viliani et al 1999), so techniques should be used together, e.g. use counting aloud and conscious control to teach structured movement sequences (Kamsma et al 1995, Nieuwboer et al 2002, Stack & Ashburn 2005). Guidelines for physiotherapy in PD have been published in the Dutch Journal of Physiotherapy (2004), by Keus et al (2007), and are available online (see useful websites).

Exercise

Physiotherapy should aim to promote function and general physical activity using exercise. People with PD reduce their habitual physical activity and lose the ability to pursue their exercise of choice, e.g. swimming, hiking (Fertl et al 1993).

Deficient trunk function (e.g. kyphosis; decreased range of movement – ROM) impacts on pulmonary function, leaving patients susceptible to chest infections and affecting ADL ability (Schenkman et al 2001). Fitness correlates with function and activity: maintaining activity is a step toward minimizing the cardio-respiratory complications of PD (Bridgewater & Sharpe 1996). Physiotherapists promote function through exercise programmes incorporating strength, flexibility,

Table 10.5.2 Assessment of functional difficulties

Gait	● Difficulty initiating gait (akinesia: poverty of movement) and reduced walking speed ● Diminished arm swing, trunk rotation, stride length, heel strike and ground clearance ● Some festinate (take increasingly rapid, short steps in a markedly flexed posture) ● Difficulty turning; patients turn the head and shoulders 'en bloc' and turn slowly, taking several steps on the spot ● Transient distractions in peripheral vision capture attention and impede movement (McDowell & Harris 1997), causing freezing (short duration breaks in motion), commonly when initiating gait, switching between activities, turning and at doorways (Giladi et al 1992)
Balance	● Patients are at high risk of falling; between 50–75% fall each year (Ashburn et al 2001a) ● A history of two or more falls over 12 months predicts further falls (Ashburn et al 2001b) ● Turning, reaching and rising from sitting are the activities that most commonly provoke postural instability (Stack & Ashburn 1999)
Posture	● Patients stand and walk stooped (in marked flexion, looking at the floor); they develop a narrow base (which compounds postural instability) as the distance between the heels diminishes
Transfers	● Difficulty transferring (e.g. bed; chair; bath; car) leading to dependence. ● Patients struggle if they lack leg power and/or flexibility and/or stability in the trunk (Inkster et al 2003, Nikfeker et al 2002)

10

coordination, balance and relaxation (Viliani et al 1999). Patients should be encouraged to continue a progressive exercise regimen that they can complete at home, unsupervised. A general programme could include:

● Exercise – Trunk and limbs (in lying, sitting and standing with particular emphasis on extension, rotation and large amplitude movements)
  – Face (see Katsikitis & Pilowsky 1996)
  – Speech
  – Breathing
  – Flexibility
● Training – Gait
  – Balance
  – Transfers
● Relaxation.

Interventions to modify impairments, activities and participation are identified in Table 10.5.3.

Cueing

Hypokinesia (slowness) is attributable to an inability to internally generate sufficiently large steps (Morris et al 1994a). Cues compensate for defective physiological mechanisms by utilizing cortical mechanisms to activate movement and overcome freezing (Lim et al 2005). Cues act like maps, signals and signposts when we are driving an unfamiliar route; when we do not know how fast to move or how far to go before turning off, we rely on external signals ('external cues') or have to recall the route we memorized consciously in advance ('internal cues'). In other words, we can bypass the under-performing basal ganglia (which ordinarily guide the tempo and magnitude of movements automatically) by using external

Table 10.5.3 Interventions to modify impairments, activities and participation.

Impairments, activity limitations and participation restrictions	Interventions
Strength	Hip and knee strength is related to ability to rise from sitting: patients have difficulty extending the hip and knee. These abnormalities may be amenable to change, as strengthening programmes prevent disuse weakness and increase motor unit recruitment in elderly people (Inkster et al 2003) ● Strength (knee extensors and flexors; ankle plantarflexors) can be improved by high-intensity resistance training (Hirsch et al 2003, Toole et al 2000) ● Patients can improve strength, stride length, walking velocity and posture through resistance training focused primarily on the lower limbs (Scandalis et al 2001) ● Participation in exercise classes incorporating trunk muscle training may improve trunk muscle performance (Bridgewater & Sharpe 1997)
Flexibility	Spinal ROM is impaired early in PD (Schenkman et al 2001). Turning 180° challenges postural stability: if patients lack head on neck rotation they cannot see where they are going as they start to turn (Stack 2004). ● Improvements in axial rotation and functional reach can be achieved with a flexibility programme (Schenkman et al 1998)

(*continued*)

Table 10.5.3 Interventions to modify impairments, activities and participation—cont'd.

Impairments, activity limitations and participation restrictions	Interventions
Flexed posture	● Unlike the other core areas of physiotherapy for PD (gait, balance and transfers) there is no evidence to demonstrate that physiotherapy improves flexed posture or even that it slows deterioration. Cognitive strategies (such as focusing on and practising standing up straight or 'walking tall') may help, as may positioning aids and equipment such as rolls, wedges, and sleeping systems
Gait	● Improvements in gait speed and stride length have been found with supervised treadmill training (Miyai et al 2000, 2002, Pohl et al 2003, Toole et al 2005)
Balance	History of falls or instability seen as the patient reaches, turns or rises may indicate need to improve balance control (Stack et al 2005) ● Balance classes, self-directed exercise and group Tai Chi improve balance (Kluding & Quinn McGinnis 2006) ● Balance exercises (challenging stable posture and increasing limits of stability) improve balance (Hirsch et al 2003, Toole et al 2000)
Functional activities	● Task-related practice of mobility activities e.g transferring, climbing stairs ● Teaching others to assist, or take over activities that the person can no longer achieve independently
Leisure pursuits	● Regular exercise (e.g. daily outdoor walking) promotes fitness and activity, prevents disuse decline and improves mood (Bridgewater & Sharpe 1996, 1997, Lokk 2000, Kuroda et al 1992) ● Patients maintain exercise capacity with regular aerobic exercise (Canning et al 1997) ● Strenuous cardiovascular, strength, flexibility and balance exercise improve fitness (Levine et al 2000)

10

or internal cues that are processed in the cortex. Therapists should identify activities that induce freezing and appropriate cues (see Box 10.5.1); those useful during walking may be less so during turning (Behrman et al 1998).

Movement strategies

Various types of strategies can be considered (see Table 10.5.4). However when attempting to modify the patient's movement strategies:

● Think before modifying posture or movement. Apparent 'abnormalities' (e.g. flexed posture; short stride) may be compensations for impaired postural stability; imagine yourself walking across an icy pavement!

● It may be necessary to promote further compensation, rather than to 'normalize' performance on a simple outcome measure (e.g. when turning, unsteady patients should slow down and take several small steps).

Box 10.5.1 Cueing.

● **Visual cues** – Strips of card/tape on floor; markers/prompts at eye level; strategically placed cue cards (Galletly & Brauer 2005, Marchese et al 2000, Nieuwboer et al 2001, Sidaway et al 2006)

● **Auditory cues** – Metronomes; audiotape with pulse embedded in music (Lim et al 2005, Marchese et al 2000, Morris et al 1994b, 1998, Nieuwboer et al 2001)

● **Proprioceptive cues** – A step backwards before starting to walk; rocking side to side, touch (Marchese et al 2000)

● **Auto-instruction/cognitive (or internal)** – Deliberately swinging the arms or taking large steps; walking fast; walking while counting aloud; concentrating on a movement component such as heel strike or long steps; memorizing parts of a movement sequence and rehearsing them mentally; visualizing appropriate step length and walking with steps that size (Behrman et al 1998, Lehman et al 2005, Nieuwboer et al 2001)

Multi-tasking

People with PD have difficulty with automatic movement and function better when consciously performing the components of an individual task sequentially, they find simultaneous tasks particularly challenging, e.g. gait deteriorates when carrying anything (Bond & Morris 2000; O'Shea et al 2002).

Table 10.5.4 Alternative movement strategies.

Falls management	● Review patient's falls history: tailor therapy to situations that provoke instability, e.g. turning, reaching, rising from chairs (Stack & Ashburn 1999, Yekutiel 1993)
	● Observe if appropriate compensations are used during everyday activities. If not, teach alternatives (e.g. break down movement components into steps; use support, widen base)
	 ● Each step should be a simple single movement or movement combination (Kamsma et al 1995)
	 ● Teach steps in logical sequence, each one:
	  Discrete (for rest between steps)
	  Consciously controlled (by undisturbed concentration)

To prevent injury after falls	● Modify environment (e.g. surfaces, clutter) ● Minimize need for hazardous activities (e.g. arrange furniture/belongings to lessen sharp turns) ● Lessen risk of injury on landing (sharp edges; hard floors; hip protection)
For turning	● Avoid dramatic changes of direction, confined spaces and carrying anything in both hands, so think ahead and plan before turning: ● Turn head first (to optimize vision) ● Slow down or turn in stages ● Choose a wide arc or preferred direction (one direction might be much safer) ● Use support (or keep a hand free) ● Perceive corners as curved trajectories rather than right angle turns (Yekutiel 1993)
For reaching (Stack et al 2005)	● Use support (from structure towards which person is reaching) ● Align forward (to optimize vision) ● Adopt stable, unchanging base (not step standing or squatting)

(*continued*)

Table 10.5.4 Alternative movement strategies—cont'd.

For moving in bed	● Teach alternatives when rolling unaided is no longer possible (Stack & Ashburn 2006) e.g.: 　● Pull or push on fixed external support (e.g. furniture; edge of mattress; rope ladder) 　● Hip-hitching (making repeated small repositioning movements of hips) 　● Sit up (to turn or get back into bed the other side) if rotational trunk movements severely limited. Sitting up may be less disruptive to sleep than struggling to roll ● Step-by-step methods (Kamsma et al 1995): 　● Into bed: (1) sit on bedside; (2) lift legs in one-by-one; (3) adopt optimal sitting position; (4) lower trunk 　● Out of bed: (1) move to bedside; (2) bring legs out; (3) push with arm to sit; (4) shift to bedside; (5) position feet; 6) stand 　● Turning: (1) pull knees up; (2) shift pelvis and shoulders; (3) rotate knees; (4) rotate trunk
Standing up and sitting down	● To overcome difficulty rising – greater trunk forward flexion and higher trunk velocity (forward momentum). Using an attentional mechanism, patients can develop increased muscle torque production to complete task (Nikfeker et al 2002) ● Step-by-step methods (Kamsma et al 1995) 　● Rising involves: (1) use of support; (2) feet close to chair; (3) sit on edge; (4) lean well forward; (5) extend legs and trunk aided by arms 　● Sitting involves: (1) come close to chair; (2) turn; (3) flex knees and trunk; (4) use support; (5) move to back of chair

Patients should:

● Avoid non-essential multiple simultaneous tasks, wherever possible;

● Be dissuaded from talking during complex tasks, including therapy session (to preserve attention);

● Practise essential dual-tasks and incorporate cues (Bloem et al 2001, Galletly & Brauer 2005).

MANAGEMENT CONSIDERATIONS
Referral to physiotherapy

Referral to physiotherapy is indicated when individuals have problems with gait, balance, posture or transfers. A positive response to 'do you have frequent difficulty turning' predicts freezing and/or falling, so should lead to further assessment (Stack et al 2006). Many argue for early referral, even from diagnosis, targeting mild disease (Nieuwboer et al 2002) with the objective of trying to prevent the secondary complications/impairments such as muscle length changes which may develop over time. Patients and carers should be able to make the referral. The need for individual vs group therapy should be considered (see Box 10.5.2).

Box 10.5.2

Individual vs group therapy

● Individuals need to:
      – Talk privately
      – Have their needs met
      – Be supervised exercising
      – Maximize therapy time

● Specialists advocate individual sessions (where personal needs are addressed) supplemented by groups (which provide social contact and motivation).

● Groups may target those newly diagnosed or in the later stages of PD. Mixed ability groups need particular attention.

● Most groups are multidisciplinary; key components are:
      – Monitoring
      – Exercise
      – Advice
      – Information sharing
      – Self-management

● Individuals like a choice of treatment context; carers may prefer to have their own group.

Involving carers

Involving carers is desirable, however the willingness of the patient to have any of their carers involved needs to be ascertained. Factors such as hospital transport and other commitments can be a barrier to carer involvement (see Box 10.5.3); most patients with PD are elderly and so are most of their carers.

Box 10.5.3

- Advise carers how best to assist the patient and facilitate movement while avoiding injury: teach moving and handling techniques and explain cueing strategies.
- Carers support many activities associated with core areas of physiotherapy. By explaining how PD affects movement, carers can feedback about symptoms and treatment response.
- Inform carers that they can ask for an assessment of *their needs* and about local support groups. Direct a carer who identifies a health need to an appropriate professional.

Duration of treatment

- Most intervention studies deliver one hour's treatment two to three times weekly over 4 to 12 weeks. In practice, physiotherapy is usually delivered once or twice weekly, over 6 to 8 weeks.
- Individuals should exercise and train at peak dose in the drug cycle (Dutch guidelines 2004, see Useful website, p. 190).

Follow-up

- Treatment effects disappear by six months and, left alone, patients may abandon exercise programmes through lack of motivation, difficulty finding time, forgetfulness, boredom and the need for carer support, so long-term management is desirable (Gage & Storey 2004, Hurwitz 1989).
- Repeated top-up programmes are required, particularly for elderly and cognitively impaired patients (Nieuwboer et al 2002).
- Regular home visits support continuation of exercise and maintenance of an active lifestyle (Fertl et al 1993, Hurwitz 1989).

KEY CLINICAL MESSAGES

- Patients may benefit from seeing a physiotherapist shortly after diagnosis but, for many, the onset of postural instability is an appropriate time for referral/ self-referral.
- Ascertaining a patient's full falls history, observing them perform everyday tasks they find challenging and evaluating their gait, balance, posture and transfers are the keys to assessment. If motor function fluctuates markedly throughout the drug cycle, assess patients in both the 'on' and 'off' phases.
- Therapists must take into account the patient's preference for participating in group therapy or for involving any carers when planning treatment.

● Teaching about exercise and how to use cueing and movement strategies to manage challenging tasks are the central themes of physiotherapy in PD; ongoing follow-up (to reinforce messages and to tailor the treatment to the progression of the disease) is essential.

References for subchapter 10.5

Ashburn A, Stack E, Pickering R et al 2001a A community-dwelling sample of people with PD: characteristics of fallers and non-fallers. Age and Ageing 30:47–53.

Ashburn A, Stack E, Pickering R et al 2001b Predicting fallers in a community-based sample of people with PD. Gerontology 47:277–281.

Ashburn A, Jones D, Plant R et al 2004 Physiotherapy for people with PD in the UK. International Journal of Therapy and Rehabilitation 11:160–167.

Behrman A, Teitelbaum P, Caurcaugh J 1998 Verbal instructional sets to normalise the temporal and spatial gait variables in PD. Journal of Neurology, Neurosurgery and Psychiatry 65:580–582.

Bloem B, Valkenburg V, Slabbekoorn M et al 2001 The multiple tasks test: strategies in PD. Experimental Brain Research 137:478–486.

Bond J, Morris M 2000 Goal-directed secondary motor tasks: their effects on gait in subjects with PD. Archives of Physical Medicine and Rehabilitation 81:110–116.

Bridgewater K, Sharpe M 1996 Aerobic exercise and early PD. Journal of Neurological Rehabilitation 10:233–241.

Bridgewater K, Sharpe M 1997 Trunk muscle training and early PD. Physiotherapy Theory and Practice 13:139–153.

Canning C, Alison J, Allen N et al 1997 PD: an investigation of exercise capacity, respiratory function and gait. Archives of Physical Medicine and Rehabilitation 78:199–207.

Chevrier E, Fraix V, Krack P et al 2006 Is there a role for physiotherapy during deep brain stimulation surgery in patients with PD? European Journal of Neurology 13:496–498.

Fertl E, Doppelbauer A, Auff E 1993 Physical activity and sports in patients suffering from PD in comparison with health seniors. Journal of Neural Transmission 5:157–161.

Gage H, Storey L 2004 Rehabilitation for PD: a systematic review of available evidence. Clinical Rehabilitation 18:463–482.

Galletly R, Brauer S 2005 Does the type of concurrent task affect preferred and cued gait in people with PD? Australian Journal of Physiotherapy 51:175–180.

Giladi N, McMahon D, Przedborski S 1992 Motor blocks in PD. Neurology 42:333–339.

Hamani C, Lozano A 2003 Physiology and pathophysiology of PD. Annals of the New York Academy of Science 991:15–21.

Hirsch M, Toole T, Maitland C et al 2003 The effects of balance training and high-intensity resistance training on persons with idiopathic PD. Archives of Physical Medicine and Rehabilitation 84:1109–1117.

Hoehn M, Yahr M 1967 Parkinsonism: onset, progression and mortality. Neurology 17:427–442.

Hurwitz A 1989 The benefit of a home exercise regimen for ambulatory PD patients. Journal of Neuroscience Nursing 21:180–184.

Inkster L, Eng J, MacIntyre D et al 2003 Leg muscle strength is reduced in PD and relates to the ability to rise from a chair. Movement Disorders 18:157–162.

Jankovic J 1990 Clinical aspects of PD. In: Marsden C, Fahn S (eds) The assessment and therapy of parkinsonism. Parthenon Publishing Carnforth, Lancs, England.

Kamsma Y, Brouwer W, Lakke J 1995 Training of compensational strategies for impaired gross motor skills in PD. Physiotherapy Theory and Practice 11:209–229.

Katsikitis M, Pilowsky I 1996 A controlled study of facial mobility treatment in PD. Journal of Psychomotor Research 40:387–396.

Keus S, Bloem B, Hendriks E et al 2007 Evidence-based analysis of physical therapy in Parkinson's disease with recommendations for practice and research. Movement Disorders 22(4):451–460.

Kluding P, Quinn McGinnis P 2006 Multidimensional exercise for people with PD: a case report. Physiotherapy Theory and Practice 22:153–162.

Kuroda K, Tatara K, Takatorige T et al 1992 Effect of physical exercise on mortality in patients with PD. Acta Neurologica Scandinavia 86:55–59.

Lang A, Fahn S 1989 Assessment of PD. In: Munsat T (ed) Quantification of neurological deficit. Butterworth. Stoneham MA, USA.

Lehman D, Toole T, Lofald D et al 2005 Training with verbal instructional cues results in near-term improvement of gait in people with PD. Journal of Neurologic Physical Therapy 29:2–8.

Levine S, Brandenberg P, Pagels M 2000 A strenuous exercise program benefits patients with mild to moderate PD. Clinical Exercise Physiology 2:43–48.

Lim I, van Wegen E, de Goede C et al 2005 Effects of external rhythmical cueing on gait in patients with PD: a systematic review. Clinical Rehabilitation 19:695–713.

Lokk J 2000 The effects of mountain exercise in parkinsonian persons – a preliminary study. Archives of Gerontology and Geriatrics 31:19–25.

Marchese R, Diverio M, Zucchi F et al 2000 The role of sensory cues in the rehabilitation of parkinsonian patients. A comparison of two physical therapy protocols. Movement Disorders 15:879–883.

McDowell S, Harris J 1997 Irrelevant peripheral visual stimuli impair manual reaction times in PD. Vision Research 37:3549–3558.

Miyai I, Fujimoto Y, Yoshishige U et al 2000 Treadmill training with body weight support: its effect on PD. Archives of Physical Medicine and Rehabilitation 81:849–852.

Miyai I, Fujimoto Y, Yamamoto H et al 2002 Long-term effect of body-weight supported treadmill training in PD: a randomised controlled trial. Archives of Physical Medicine and Rehabilitation 83:1370–1373.

Morris M 2000 Movement disorders in people with PD: a model for physical therapy. Physical Therapy 80:578–597.

Morris M, Iansek R, Matyas T et al 1994a The pathogenesis of gait hypokinesia in PD. Brain 117:1169–1181.

Morris M, Iansek R, Matyas T et al 1994b Ability to modulate walking cadence remains intact in PD. Journal of Neurology, Neurosurgery and Psychiatry 57:1532–1534.

Morris M, Iansek R, Matyas T et al 1998 Abnormalities in the stride length-cadence relation in parkinsonian gait. Movement Disorders 13:61–69.

Nieuwboer A, de Weerdt W, Dom R et al 2000 Development of an activity scale for individuals with advanced PD: reliability and 'on-off' variability. Physical Therapy 80:1087–1096.

Nieuwboer A, de Weerdt W, Dom R et al 2001 The effect of a home physiotherapy program for persons with PD. Journal of Rehabilitation Medicine 33:266–272.

Nieuwboer A, de Weerdt W, Dom R et al 2002 Prediction of outcome of physiotherapy in advanced PD. Clinical Rehabilitation 16:886–893.

Nikfeker E, Kerr K, Attfield S et al 2002 Trunk movement in PD during rising from seated position. Movement Disorders 17:274–282.

Olanow C, Hauser R 1990 The treatment of early Parkinson's disease. In Marsden C, Fahn S (eds) The assessment and therapy of parkinsonism. Parthenon Publishing Carnforth, Lancs, England.

O'Shea S, Morris M, Iansek R 2002 Dual task interference during gait in people with PD: effects of motor versus cognitive secondary tasks. Physical Therapy 82:888–897.

Peto V, Jenkinson C, Fitzpatrick R 1998 PDQ-39: A review of the development, validation and application of a Parkinson's disease quality of life questionnaire and its associated measures. Journal of Neurology 245(supplement 1):S10–S14.

Pohl M, Rockstroh G, Ruckriem S et al 2003 Immediate effects of speed-dependent treadmill training on gait parameters in early PD. Archives of Physical Medicine and Rehabilitation 84:1760–1766.

Scandalis T, Bosak A, Berliner J et al 2001 Resistance training and gait function in patients with PD. American Journal of Physical Medicine and Rehabilitation 80:38–43.

Schenkman M, Cutson T, Kutchibhatla M et al 1998 Exercise to improve spinal flexibility and function for people with PD: a randomized, controlled trial. Journal of the American Geriatric Society 46:1207–1216.

Schenkman M, Clark K, Xie T et al 2001 Spinal movement and performance of a standing reach task in participants with and without PD. Physical Therapy 81:1400–1411.

Sidaway B, Anderson J, Danielson G et al 2006 Effects of long-term gait training using visual cues in an individual with PD. Physical Therapy 86:186–194.

Stack E 2004 When gait isn't 'straight forward', how do you assess the ability to turn? Synapse – Journal and Newsletter of ACPIN (Spring) 6–7 ISSN 1369-958X.

Stack E, Ashburn A 1999 Fall-events described by people with PD. Physiotherapy Research International 4:190–200.

Stack E, Ashburn A 2005 Early Development of the Standing Start 180° Turn Test. Physiotherapy 91:6–13.

Stack E, Ashburn A 2006 Impaired bed mobility and disordered sleep in PD. Movement Disorders 21:1340–1342.

Stack E, Ashburn A, Jupp K 2005 Postural instability during reaching movements in people with severe PD. Physiotherapy Research International 10:146–153.

Stack E, Ashburn A, Jupp K 2006 Turning strategies demonstrated by people with PD during an everyday activity. Parkinsonism and Related Disorders 12:87–92.

Toole T, Hirsch M, Forkink A et al 2000 The effects of a balance and strength training program on equilibrium in parkinsonism: a preliminary study. Neurorehabilitation 14:165–174.

Toole T, Maitland C, Warren E et al 2005 The effects of loading and unloading treadmill walking on balance, gait, fall risk and daily function in parkinsonism. Neurorehabilitation 20:307–322.

Viliani T, Pasquetti P, Magnolfi S et al 1999 Effects of physical training on straightening-up. Disability and Rehabilitation 21:68–73.

Visser M, Marinus J, Bloem B et al 2003 Clinical tests for the evaluation of postural instability in patients with PD. Archives of Physical Medicine and Rehabilitation 84:1669–1674.

Yekutiel M 1993 Patients' fall records as an aid in designing and assessing therapy in parkinsonism. Disability and Rehabilitation 15:189–193.

Essential reading

Gage H, Storey L 2004 Rehabilitation for PD: a systematic review of available evidence. Clinical Rehabilitation 18:463–482.

Keus S, Bloem B, Verbaan D et al 2004 Physiotherapy in Parkinson's disease: utilisation and patient satisfaction. Journal of Neurology 251:680–687.

Useful web site

KNGF Guidelines for physiotherapy in patients with Parkinson's disease. Supplement (in English) to the Dutch Journal of Physiotherapy 114 (vol 3) 2004 https://www.fysionet.nl/dossier_files/uploadFiles/Eng_RichtlijnParkinsonsdisease_251006.pdf?PHPSESSID = c203f3fced349276c53cad77001bcc7a.

CHAPTER 11

Outcome measurement

Emma K Stokes

WHY MEASURE?

The use of standardized outcome measures (SOMs) in physiotherapy practice has increased significantly in the past 10–15 years, from a time when information about the change of status in a patient was not usually recorded or outcome being described in terms of the patient getting better, improving or being discharged (Partridge 1982).

In the current climate, using SOMs is a requirement for 'best' physiotherapy practice and is one of the core standards of practice adopted by all members of the European Region of the World Confederation for Physical Therapy in May 2002 (ER-WCPT 2002) (Box 11.1). Using SOMs, as well as the evidence from research and clinical guidelines, is part of evidence-based practice (EBP) (Herbert et al 2005, Parker-Taillon 2002; also see Chapter 1 of this book).

It is important to understand the distinction between measurement and assessment. Measurement is the application of standard scales or instruments to variables, giving a numerical score, which may be combined for each variable to give an overall score, while assessment is the process of understanding a measurement in a specific context (McDowell & Newell 1996). A variety of different functions, which are not exclusive and can co-exist in one measurement instrument, have been identified (Feinstein 1989) (Box 11.2).

It is possible to measure the effects of intervention for the individual patient or client, for groups of patients with similar diagnoses and at a larger scale for services. An outcome measurement may be used to answer a variety of different questions (Box 11.3).

WHAT TO MEASURE?

The International Classification of Functioning, Disability and Health (ICF) (WHO 2001) is a classification system, the overall aim of which is to 'provide unified and standard language and framework for the description of health and health related states.' It may be used as a clinical tool in rehabilitation and outcome evaluation and in addition, it is used as a model to consider and inform the choice of outcome

Box 11.1

European Region of the World Confederation for Physical Therapy Core Standards

Standard 6   Taking account of the patient's problems, a published, standardized, valid, reliable and responsive outcome measure is used to evaluate the change in the patient's health status.

Criterion 6.1 The physiotherapist selects an outcome measure that is relevant to the patient's problem.

Criterion 6.2 The physiotherapist ensures the outcome measure is acceptable to the patient. The physiotherapist selects an outcome measure that he/she has the necessary skill and experience to use, administer and interpret.

Criterion 6.6 The result of the measurement is recorded immediately.

Criterion 6.7 The same measure is used at the end episode of care.

Box 11.2

Functions of measurement instrument

Identify the presence or absence of a state, e.g. depression

Denote a change due to intervention

Predict an outcome, e.g. discharge destination, functional ability

Offer a guideline, e.g. may require assistance or assistive device

Communication aid, e.g. alerts other staff to particular requirements of patient

Teaching tool

Provide a problem list

Box 11.3

What an outcome measurement can tell us . . .

Is a particular set of activities assisting the patient during a given treatment session?

Has your physiotherapy intervention over a period of time, e.g. from admission to discharge, made any difference to your client/patient?

Does a group programme have an effect on outcome in a group of patients?

What is the effect of the physiotherapy component of a multi-disciplinary team intervention?

---

measured (Finch et al 2002, Salter et al 2005a, b). The health and health-related domains within the ICF are described as they relate to the body, the individual and society – 'Body Structures and Functions' and 'Activities and Participation'. It has two parts – 'Functioning and Disability' and 'Contextual Factors'. Table 11.1 gives examples of ICF domains and specific ICF codes.

The choice of outcome measurement depends on the question being asked – see Box 11.3. Finch et al (2002) have proposed three levels in relation to rehabilitation targets and matching these with outcome measurements – strategy, intervention, and programme, as outlined in Table 11.2 (for more in-depth reading see Finch et al 2002).

CHOOSING A MEASURE

Having considered the issues raised in Boxes 11.1, 11.2 and 11.3, the other aspect of choosing an outcome measure is that it should be a published, standardized, valid and reliable measure. A significant amount of research is required to design, develop and evaluate an outcome measure hence in clinical practice it is best to use measures that are published rather that creating your own. There are two main sources of information about measurement properties – the primary peer-review publications relating to the SOM, of which there may be many in a diversity of journals and secondary sources such as textbooks, journal papers and databases that collate SOMs and provide a review of the measurement properties (Bowling 2001, 2005, Finch et al 2002, McDowell & Newell 1996, Portney & Watkins 2000, Wade 1992). Table 11.3 (p. 196) outlines the properties of reliability and validity and how these properties inform clinical utility and decision making.

WHAT MEASUREMENTS TO USE?

Linking the ICF categories exactly with standardized outcome measures is not precise; linking rules have been created (Cieza et al 2005) and Table 11.4 (p. 197) lists some commonly used standardized, valid and reliable outcome measures for use with people who have a neurological diagnosis. They are listed under the headings of impairments, activities and participation, and where overlap exists it is because the SOM includes both. For additional details, use the references listed beside the SOM.

Table 11.1 The International Classification of Functioning, Disability and Health (ICF) (WHO 2001).

Definitions of components of ICF	ICF domains	ICF categories	Definition of categories
Impairments are problems with body functions and/or structures	Body functions – physiological functions	b110 Consciousness functions	State of awareness and alertness
	Body functions – sensory functions and pain	b280 Pain	Sensation of pain
	Body functions – movement functions	b7651 Tremor	Functions of alternating contraction and relaxation of a group of muscles around a joint
	Body structures – structures of the brain	s1103	Basal ganglia and related structures
Limitations in activity are difficulties associated with performing an activity	Activities & participation – mobility	d410 Changing basic body position	Getting into and out of a body position and moving from one location to another
Restrictions in participation are challenges that a person may have in a life situation	Activities & participation – carrying, moving and handling objects	d430 Lifting and carrying objects	Raising up an object or taking something from one place to another
	Activities & participation	d450 Walking	Moving along a surface on foot

11

Table 11.2 Using the International Classification of Functioning, Disability and Heath (ICF) to inform choice of Standardized Outcome Measures (SOMs) (adapted from Finch et al 2002).

Levels		Structure/function	Example SOM	Activity/participation	Example SOM
Strategy Target is an organ, cell, tissue e.g. muscle, joint	Increase range of motion of a joint	Joints of the wrist and hand	Goniometry	Hand function	Frenchay Arm Test
Intervention Target is the individual patient	Motor re-learning of upper extremity function post-stroke	Person with stroke	Specific arm function measurement	Hobbies involving arm function	Canadian Occupational Performance Measure
Programme Target is a group of people	Group exercise intervention			People with MS with fatigue, mobility difficulties	Fatigue Severity Scale, Hauser Ambulation Index

Table 11.3 Measurement properties and how they inform choice and decision making.

Measurement property	Component of property	Definition	What does it tell us?
Reliability	Relative – inter and intra	Agreement between raters or two points in time made by the same rater	Indicates amount of random error in standardized outcome measure (SOM)
	Absolute reliability	Indication of reliability expressed in units of the original measurement	Amount of change needed to ensure change is greater than measurement error
	Internal consistency	Measurements taken at one point in time – indicating the homogeneity of the outcome measure	Relationship between individual items in the SOM and the overall score
Validity	Face and content	Indication of whether, on the surface, the outcome measure measures what it intends to measure	Is the measure suitable for the purpose you have in mind, i.e: intervention, client group etc.
	Criterion – concurrent and predictive	Comparing the new outcome measure to a 'gold standard', at one point (concurrent) or at a future point in time (predictive)	How the new measure performs against a more established measure
	Criterion – diagnostic	Accuracy of the outcome measure in identifying whether or not a condition is present	Using scores on the SOM to predict a future event, e.g: falls
	Construct – including convergent and discriminant validity	Deeper evaluation of the outcome measure. Developer proposes ideas or constructs about the measure and evaluates the construct	Could be that the SOM measures one or more domains, that it differentiates between groups of subjects
	Responsiveness	The ability of the outcome measure to capture change over time. Often under-reported	Is the instrument useful to use over a period of time when an intervention has taken place?
	Sensitivity	A test's ability to obtain a positive result when the target condition is present (true positive)	Probability of a positive test result among patients with a disorder
	Specificity	A test's ability to obtain a negative result when the target condition is not present (true negative). A highly specific instrument rarely tests positive when a disorder is absent (false positive)	Probability of a negative test result among patients without a disorder

Table 11.4 Examples of linking outcome measures to the International Classification of Functioning, Disability and Health (ICF).

Impairments, limitations of activity and restrictions in participation	Standardized outcome measures
A. Impairments	
Pain	Visual analogue scale (Finch et al 2002), 11 point numeric rating scale for pain (Finch et al 2002)
Mental state	Mini-mental state examination (Folstein et al 1975) Glasgow Coma Scale (Teasdale & Jennett 1974) Nottingham sensory assessment (Lincoln et al 1998)
Exercise tolerance	Timed walking tests (Wade 1992)
Fatigue	Fatigue Impact Scale (Fisk et al 1994) Multi-dimensional Fatigue Inventory (Smets et al 1995) Fatigue Severity Scale (Krupp et al 1989)
Mobility of joints	Goniometry
Muscle power and tone	Dynamometry (Bohannon & Smith 1987), Medical Research Council Scale (Gregson et al 2000) Modified Ashworth Scale (Pomeroy et al 2000, Gregson et al 2000)
Movement – Gait pattern	Gait analysis systems
B. Impairments & limitations in activities	Chedoke-McMaster Stroke Assessment (Gowland et al 1995) Rivermead Motor Assessment (Lincoln & Leadbitter 1979) Motor Assessment Scale (Carr et al 1985) Fugl-Meyer Assessment of Motor Recovery (Fugl-Meyer et al 1975) SCOPA (Martinez-Martin et al 2005) Kurtze Extended Disability Status Scale (Noseworthy 1994) Action Research Arm Test (Lyle 1981) Timed Up & Go (Podsialdlo & Richardson 1991)

(continued)

Table 11.4 Examples of linking outcome measures to the International Classification of Functioning, Disability and Health (ICF)—cont'd.

Impairments, limitations of activity and restrictions in participation	Standardized outcome measures
C. Limitations of activities	Barthel Index (Mahoney & Barthel 1965)
	Functional Independence Measure (Granger 1998)
	Berg Balance Scale (Berg et al 1989)
	Functional Reach Test (Duncan et al 1990)
	Activities-specific Balance Confidence Scale (Powell & Myers 1995)
	Postural Assessment Scale for Stroke Patients (Benaim et al 1999)
	Hauser Ambulation Index (Hauser et al 1983)
	Frenchay Arm Test (Heller et al 1987)
	Frenchay Activities Index (Holbrook & Skilbeck 1983)
	Rivermead Mobility Index (Collen et al 1991)
D. Limitations of activities & restriction of participation	Canadian Occupational Performance Measure (Law et al 1998)
	Reintegration to Normal Living Index (Wood-Dauphinee et al 1988)
	Stroke Impact Scale (Duncan et al 1999)
	EuroQol (Shrag et al 2000)
	SF-36® (McDowell & Newell 1996) www.sf-36.com

SCOPA, SCales for Outcomes in PArkinson's disease (Martinez-Martin et al 2005).

KEY MESSAGES

● Always use an SOM – do not invent your own.
● Decide what you need to measure (it is not necessary to measure everything) and how you will use the information.
● Make your choice of measure based on why you are measuring, e.g. to see if your treatment is effective.
● If a measure you have chosen does not meet your needs overall, consider using another measure.

References

Benaim C, Perennou DA, Villy J, Rousseaux M, Pelissier JY 1999 Validation of a standardized assessment of postural control in stroke patients. Stroke 30:1862–1868.

Berg KO, Wood-Dauphinee SL, Williams JI et al 1989 Measuring balance in the elderly: preliminary development of an instrument. Physiotherapy Canada 41:304–311.

Bohannon RW, Smith MB 1987 Assessment of strength deficits in eight paretic upper extremity muscle groups of stroke patients with hemiplegia. Physical Therapy 67:522–555.

Bowling A 2001 Measuring disease: a review of disease-specific quality of life measurement scales, 2nd edn. Open University Press, Buckingham.

Bowling A 2005 Measuring health: a review of quality of life measurement scales. Open University Press, Berkshire.

Carr JH, Shepherd RB, Nordholm L et al 1985 Investigation of a new motor scale for stroke patients. Physical Therapy 65:175–180.

Cieza A, Geyh S, Chatterji et al 2005 ICF linking rules: an update based on lessons learned. Journal of Rehabilitation Medicine 37:212–218.

Collen FM, Wade DT, Robb GF, Bradshaw CM 1991 The Rivermead Mobility Index: a further development of the Rivermead Motor Assessment. International Disability Studies 13:50–54.

Duncan PW, Weiner DK, Chandler J et al 1990 Functional reach: a new clinical measure of balance. Journal of Gerontology 45:M192–M197.

Duncan PW, Wallace D, Lai SM et al 1999 The Stroke Impact Scale Version 2 Evaluation of reliability, validity and sensitivity to change. Stroke 30:2131–2140.

European Region of the World Confederation for Physical Therapy (2002) European Core Standards of Physiotherapy Practice. http://www.physio-europe.org/index.php?action=81 25 Sept 2006.

Feinstein A 1989 Clinimetrics. Yale University Press, New Haven.

Finch E, Brooks D, Stratford P, Mayo E 2002 Physical rehabilitation outcome measures – a guide to enhanced clinical decision making, 2nd edn. Decker, Ontario, BC.

Fisk JD, Ritvo PG, Ross L et al 1994 Measuring the impact of fatigue: initial validation of the Fatigue Impact Scale. Clinical Infectious Diseases 18(suppl 1):S79–83.

Folstein MF, Folstein SE, McHugh PR 1975 Mini-mental state: a practical method of grading the cognitive state of patients for the clinician. Journal of Psychiatric Research 12:189–198.

Fugl-Meyer AR, Jaaslo L, Leyman et al 1975 The post stroke hemiplegic patient 1. A method for evaluation of physical performance. Scandinavian Journal of Rehabilitation Medicine 7:13–31.

Gowland C, van Hullenaar S, Torresin W et al 1995 Chedoke–McMaster Stroke Assessment: development, validation and administration manual. School of Rehabilitation Science, McMaster University, Hamilton, ON, Canada.

Granger CV 1998 The emerging science of functional assessment: our tool for outcomes analysis. Archives of Physical Medicine and Rehabilitation 79:235–240.

Gregson JM, Leathley MJ, Moore AP et al 2000 Reliability of measurements of muscle tone and muscle power in stroke patients. Age and Ageing 29:223–228.

11

Hauser SL, Dawson DM, Lehricj JR et al 1983 Intensive immuno-suppression in progressive multiple sclerosis: a randomised, three-arm study of high dose intravenous cyclophosphamide, plasma exchange and ACTH. New England Journal of Medicine 308:173–180.

Heller A, Wade DT, Wood VA et al 1987 Arm function after stroke: measurement and recovery over the first three months. Journal of Neurology, Neurosurgery and Psychiatry 50:714–719.

Herbert R, Jamtvedt G, Mead J et al 2005 Outcome measures measure outcomes, not effects of intervention. Australian Journal of Physiotherapy 51:3–4.

Holbrook M, Skilbeck CE 1983 An activities index for use with stroke patients. Age and Ageing 12:166–170.

Krupp LB, LaRocca NG, Muir-Nash J, Steinberg AD 1989 The Fatigue Severity Scale: application to patients with multiple sclerosis and systemic lupus erythematosus. Archives of Neurology 46:1121–1123.

Law M, Baptiste S, Carswell-Opzoomer et al 1998 Canadian Occupational Performance Measure. 3rd edn. Ottawa, ON: CAOT Publications.

Lincoln NB, Leadbitter D 1979 Assessment of motor function in stroke patients. Physiotherapy 65:48–51.

Lincoln NB, Jackson JM, Adams SA 1998 Reliability and revisions of the Nottingham sensory assessment for stroke patients. Physiotherapy 84:358–365.

Lyle RC 1981 A performance test for assessment of upper limb function in physical rehabilitation and research. International Journal of Rehabilitation Research 4: 483–492.

Mahoney FI, Barthel DW 1965 Functional evaluation: the Barthel Index. Maryland State Medical Journal 14:61–65.

Martinez-Martin P, Benito-Leon J, Burguera J et al 2005 The SCOPA-Motor Scale for assessment of Parkinson's disease is a consistent and valid measure. Journal of Clinical Epidemiology 58:674–679.

McDowell I, Newell C 1996 Measuring health. A guide to rating scales and questionnaires, 2nd edn. Oxford University Press, New York.

Noseworthy JH 1994 Clinical scoring methods for multiple sclerosis. Annals of Neurology 36(suppl):S80–S85.

Parker-Taillon D 2002 CPA initiatives put the spotlight on evidence-based practice in physiotherapy. Physiotherapy Canada 12:15–24.

Partridge CJ 1982 The outcome of physiotherapy and its measurement. Physiotherapy 68:362–363.

Podsiadlo D, Richardson S 1991 The Timed 'Up & Go' a test of basic functional mobility for frail elderly. Journal of the American Geriatric Society 39:142–148.

Pomeroy VM, Dean D, Sykes L et al 2000 The unreliability of clinical measures of muscle tone: implications for stroke therapy. Age and Ageing 29:229–233.

Portney LG, Watkins MP (eds) 2000 Foundations of clinical research: applications to practice. 2nd edn. Prentice-Hall Health, London.

Powell LE, Meyers AM 1995 The Activities-specific Balance Confidence (ABC) Scale. Journal of Gerontology 50A:M28-M34.

Salter K, Jutai JW, Teasell R et al 2005a Issues for selection of outcome measures in stroke rehabilitation: ICF Body Functions. Disability and Rehabilitation 27: 191–207.

Salter K, Jutai JW, Teasell R et al 2005b Issues for selection of outcome measures in stroke rehabilitation: ICF Activity. Disability and Rehabilitation 27:315–340.

Shrag A, Selai C, Jahanshahi M et al 2000 The EQ-5D a generic quality of life measures is a useful instrument to measure quality of life in patients with Parkinson's disease. Journal of Neurology, Neurosurgery and Psychiatry 69:67–73.

Smets EM, Garssen B, Bonke B, De Haes JC 1995 The multi-dimensional fatigue inventory (MFI) psychometric qualities of an instrument to assess fatigue. Journal of Psychosomatic Research 39:315–325.

Teasdale G, Jennett B 1974 Assessment of coma and impaired consciousness. A practical scale. Lancet 2:81–83.

Wade D 1992 Measurement in neurological rehabilitation. Oxford University Press, Oxford.

Wood-Dauphinee SL, Opzoomer MA, Williams JI 1988 Assessment of global function: the Reintegration to Normal Living Index. Archives of Physical Medicine and Rehabilitation 69:583–590.

World Health Organization 2001 International classification of functioning, disability and health. WHO, Geneva.

11

CHAPTER 12

Continuity of care

Fiona Jones

INTRODUCTION

The term 'Continuity of Care' is used when referring to patients experiencing some form of transition or transfer of care. Patients with neurological conditions may experience many different types of transitions or transfer of care, which might include:

- **Discharge home from hospital** following a period of acute care;
- **Transfer of care** from acute hospital services to intermediate care or to a rehabilitation centre e.g. post stroke;
- **Admission to hospital from home** for neurological investigation and management at the initial stage of diagnosis of progressive neurological conditions, e.g. multiple sclerosis;
- **Reintegration back into the community** from specialist rehabilitation centres e.g. following spinal cord injury;
- **Discharge from all physiotherapy services** and transition towards long-term self-management.

Many healthcare providers see patients only at key stages, which can cause fragmentation of care. Living with a neurological condition presents a diversity of symptoms and experiences, which require close collaboration between services to support the patient's health, social and psychological needs effectively. Continuity of care for patients with neurological conditions includes transfer of information and case management, and is discussed in this chapter with reference to two core elements:

- Enabling the integration of healthcare services for the individual patient (Haggerty et al 2006)
- Transition towards self-management (Jones 2005).

Box 12.1

Standard 11 (CSP core standards 2005)
- Arrangements for transfer of care are recorded in the patient's notes.
- Information relayed to those involved in ongoing care in the most appropriate manner and format.
- Discharge summaries sent to referrers on completion of the episode of care.
- Discharge information sent to the patient's GP for those who self-refer to physiotherapy.
- All transfer of information should respect requirements of consent and confidentiality.

ENABLING INTEGRATION OF HEALTHCARE SERVICES FOR THE INDIVIDUAL

The Chartered Society of Physiotherapy (CSP) Core Standards (2005) provide guidance on transfer of care or discharge (see Box 12.1).

In the UK, the government has provided guidance for multidisciplinary teams on meeting the needs of patients and carers over time; for example, see the National Institute for Clinical Excellence guidelines for management of MS in acute and secondary care (NICE 2003) and the National Service Framework (NSF) for long-term neurological conditions (DoH 2005). The NSF contains 11 quality requirements which emphasize: the need for an integrated service of assessment, recognition of needs, diagnosis, acute and longer term support, and high quality timely access to rehabilitation and equipment (DoH 2005). Factors that will help facilitate greater continuity of care over time are identified in Table 12.1.

Therapists can help to address some of these quality requirements and improve continuity of care by transferring information from one healthcare provider to another using the International Classification of Functioning, Disability and Health (ICF) nomenclature (WHO 2001), and through Integrated Care Pathways (ICPs), especially when complex interdisciplinary care is required over time. Therapists need to think carefully about when to use ICPs, for example a Cochrane review of in-hospital care pathways for stroke did not advocate their routine use based on the rationale that a rigid pathway may reduce clinical reasoning and individual reassessment (Kwan & Sandercock 2005). The CSP (2002) states that ICPs, which are designed to describe expected progress of a specific patient group, should be multidisciplinary, locally agreed and evidence based. ICPs can be helpful

Table 12.1 Enabling factors for continuity of care (adapted from DoH 2003, and NICE 2003).

Accurate knowledge and understanding of the condition	● Knowledge about current guidelines for the prescription of drugs or the medical and surgical interventions available.
Regular discussions with the patient and family	● Sharing information, ideas and concerns. ● Discussions including the patient and their family in an open, non-threatening and collaborative way.
Regular interdisciplinary team meetings and discussions	● To aid effective communication of treatment goals and short- and long-term management. ● To share information using clear terminology avoiding profession-specific jargon. ● To agree timelines to plan for efficient use of resources and strengthen team working.
Careful co-ordination of services	● Minimizing input from different numbers of professionals e.g. use of key workers. ● Joint notes to reduce repetition of information and enable effective audit of notes and interventions.
Regular re-assessment	● To monitor change over time and predict and respond to level of support as required. ● Using validated, sensitive outcome measures.
Knowledge and understanding of psychological and social factors	● Factors which might be acting as both facilitators and barriers to rehabilitation. ● Psychological factors which could include depression, anxiety, self-efficacy, helplessness and apathy. ● Social factors which could include family and community support, spiritual support, work-based issues.
Awareness of range of services	● To offer support to the patient and their family at different stages and times of need. ● To understand the patient's expectations of service provision. ● To promote community resources, such as support groups, services available from the voluntary sector, educational and vocational courses.
Risk assessment of manual handling and equipment needs	● For regular assessment of equipment needs and reappraisal of support for carer, particularly when an individual has a progressive neurological condition.

12

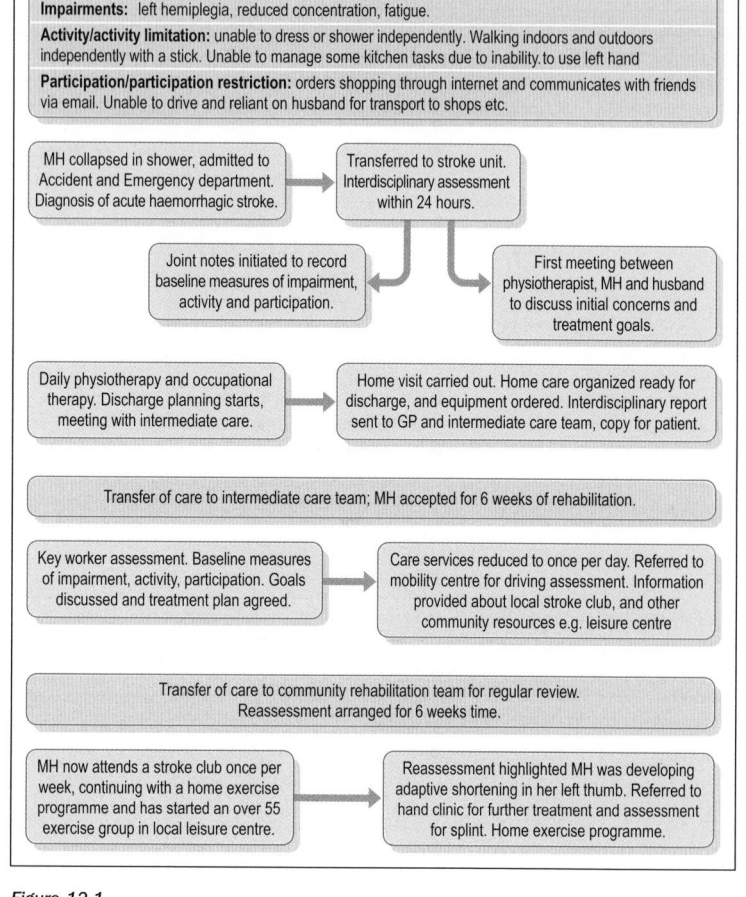

MH: 69-year-old woman, right hemisphere haemorrhagic stroke. Lives in 2-storey house with her husband.

Impairments: left hemiplegia, reduced concentration, fatigue.

Activity/activity limitation: unable to dress or shower independently. Walking indoors and outdoors independently with a stick. Unable to manage some kitchen tasks due to inability.to use left hand

Participation/participation restriction: orders shopping through internet and communicates with friends via email. Unable to drive and reliant on husband for transport to shops etc.

MH collapsed in shower, admitted to Accident and Emergency department. Diagnosis of acute haemorrhagic stroke.

Transferred to stroke unit. Interdisciplinary assessment within 24 hours.

Joint notes initiated to record baseline measures of impairment, activity and participation.

First meeting between physiotherapist, MH and husband to discuss initial concerns and treatment goals.

Daily physiotherapy and occupational therapy. Discharge planning starts, meeting with intermediate care.

Home visit carried out. Home care organized ready for discharge, and equipment ordered. Interdisciplinary report sent to GP and intermediate care team, copy for patient.

Transfer of care to intermediate care team; MH accepted for 6 weeks of rehabilitation.

Key worker assessment. Baseline measures of impairment, activity, participation. Goals discussed and treatment plan agreed.

Care services reduced to once per day. Referred to mobility centre for driving assessment. Information provided about local stroke club, and other community resources e.g. leisure centre

Transfer of care to community rehabilitation team for regular review. Reassessment arranged for 6 weeks time.

MH now attends a stroke club once per week, continuing with a home exercise programme and has started an over 55 exercise group in local leisure centre.

Reassessment highlighted MH was developing adaptive shortening in her left thumb. Referred to hand clinic for further treatment and assessment for splint. Home exercise programme.

Figure 12.1
Care pathway of an individual following acute stroke.

for complex cases. See case example using the ICF and an individual care pathway in Figure 12.1.

Many national neurological support groups have developed or contributed to specific protocols and checklists for managing patients with specific and complex needs; see the Motor Neurone Disease Society (2005) for an example. Therapists should consult such documents when planning service provision aiming to prevent crises and emergency hospital admissions. Physiotherapists can play a role in the requirements of the NSF for patients with rapidly progressing conditions by:

- Anticipating care needs and co-ordinating services between health and social care, and in some instances may adopt the role as key worker or case manager;
- The prompt and timely provision of equipment and adaptations;
- Regular monitoring of respiratory status (forced vital capacity, FVC), at least every 3 months;
- Supporting patients to decide on the use and timing of non-invasive ventilation, as required;
- Contributing to palliative care arrangements, as necessary;
- Supporting family and carers in their day-to-day caring role, carrying out a regular risk assessment of manual handling needs, and providing advice and support as required.

TRANSITION TOWARDS SELF-MANAGEMENT

Living with a neurological condition presents a number of challenges and individual needs will change over time. This is the case whether living with a single incident condition such as stroke, or a progressive condition such as Parkinson's disease.

A number of core skills underpin successful self-management, which may help an individual to cope with the transition of discharge from therapy services to effective self-management (see Box 12.2).

Successful self-management is supported by many condition-specific guidelines. Patients should be encouraged to play an active part in making informed decisions in all aspects of their healthcare (see Chapters 2 and 3); this should involve relevant and accurate information. Physiotherapists can enhance patients' self-management skills by incorporating the following strategies for good communication and confidence building (Table 12.2).

Box 12.2

Core self-management skills (Lorig & Holman 2003)
- Problem solving.
- Decision making.
- Resource utilization.
- Collaboration.
- Taking action.

Table 12.2 Strategies for good communication and confidence building.

Good communication strategies (from NICE guidelines for management of MS in acute and secondary care, 2003).	Confidence-building strategies (adapted from sources of self-efficacy by Bandura 1997).
• Privacy and quiet to encourage useful and meaningful interaction. • Ensuring family are present if requested. • Starting by asking the person what they know and understand already. • Establishing the nature and extent of information required. • Considering the balance between the risks and benefits of giving information. • Tailoring the communication to individual ability, situation and culture. • Clarifying specific options/choices. • Offering back-up information in different ways (written, pictures, audio or video). • Providing information about the range of relevant community resources. • Considering the need for emotional support. • Documenting all interactions and informing other healthcare workers about what has been communicated.	• Encouraging the individual to set small achievable targets. • Using targets with real personal value, rather than rehabilitation tasks. • Keeping a record or diary of successful achievements. • Watching and learning from other patients who have been through similar experiences. • Encouragement to interpret changing signs and symptoms such as spasms, pain and fatigue, and working out ways of self-management. • Learning how the disease may progress and using methods of preventing secondary problems, such as adaptive shortening, postural deformity. • Finding ways of keeping active that do not necessarily require equipment or attendance at gym or health club. • Encouraging family and friends to give appropriate support and encouragement.

MS, multiple sclerosis.

Self-management is enhanced when a person has strong self-efficacy; a psychological construct defined as 'the belief that a person has in their capability to organize and execute a certain course of action required to produce given attainments' (Bandura 1997). Self-efficacy can be raised or lowered through different experiences (Lorig & Holman 2003), and can influence: the course of action; how long a person will persevere; resilience to adversity; whether thought processes are negative or positive; and the amount of stress and depression experienced when coping with different demands.

Effective ways of strengthening an individual's self-efficacy include: experiences of success in rehabilitation; encouraging patients to problem solve, make plans, set targets and reflect on individual successes, however small (Jones 2005). These

Box 12.3

> **Designing effective home exercise programmes (HEP)**
> - Decide together on main aims and priorities.
> - Encourage 'ownership' of HEP, by personalizing where possible, e.g. using real life pictures, relating to personal targets.
> - Consider individual learning and cognitive styles, e.g. visual or auditory information.
> - Provide ideas for exercise progression and recognizing need and ways to adapt programme.
> - Practise methods of integrating exercises and activities into normal daily routine.
> - Discuss how to recognize decline and when to seek further help and advice.
> - Provide extra tips on keeping active, be creative and encourage the patient to fully utilize all practice opportunities.
> - Make sure all written information is clear.
>   - Use >14 font
>   - Embolden key information
>   - Use boxes to highlight specific instructions
>   - Use pictures and photographs wherever possible
>   - Avoid large blocks of unbroken text

12

ways of developing self efficacy can be implemented by physiotherapists when designing home exercise programmes (see Box 12.3).

SUMMARY

Continuity of care for patients with neurological conditions includes transfer of information and case management. Enabling integration of healthcare services and the patient's transition towards self-management is a key element of continuity of care (Jones 2005). To achieve a co-ordinated and smooth progression of care from the patient's point of view, a rehabilitation service needs (Freeman et al 2000):

1. Excellent information transfer which follows the patient.
2. Effective communication between professionals and services and patients.
3. Flexibility to adjust to the needs of the individual over time.
4. Care from as few professionals as possible, consistent with needs.
5. Named individual professionals (e.g. key workers) who can assist with information provision, emotional support and liaison with other agencies, and build a lasting therapeutic relationship.

References

Bandura A 1997 The nature and structure of self-efficacy. In: Bandura A (ed) Self-efficacy: the exercise of control. New York, WH Freeman.

Chartered Society of Physiotherapists 2002 Integrated Care Pathways. PA46. Accessed: www.csp.org.uk.

Chartered Society of Physiotherapists 2005 Core Standards of Physiotherapy. Accessed: www.csp.org.uk.

Department of Health (DoH) 2003 Discharge from hospital: pathway, process and practice. Health and Social Joint Unit and Change Agent Team. DoH, London.

Department of Health (DoH) March 2005 The National Service Framework for Longer Term Conditions. DoH, London.

Freeman GS, Robinson I, Ehrich K et al 2000 Continuity of care: report of a scoping exercise for the SDO Programme of NHS R & D. Accessed: www.ReFeR.nhs.uk.

Haggerty JH, Reid RJ, Freeman GK et al 2006 Continuity of care: a multidisciplinary review. BMJ 327:1219–1221.

Jones F 2005 Strategies to enhance chronic disease self-management: how can we apply this to stroke? Disability & Rehabilitation 8:841–847.

Kwan J, Sandercock P 2005 In-hospital care pathways for stroke. Stroke 36: 1348–1349.

Lorig K, Holman H 2003 Self-management education: history, definition, outcomes and mechanisms. Ann Beh Med 26(1):1–7.

Motor Neurone Disease Society 2005 The National Service Framework for long-term conditions: delivering the NSF for rapidly progressing conditions.

National Institute for Clinical Excellence 2003 Multiple sclerosis: management of multiple sclerosis in primary and secondary care. Clinical Guideline 8.

World Health Organization 2001 International Classification of Functioning, Disability and Health. WHO, Geneva.

Essential information sources

Department of Health, March 2006 Supporting people with long term conditions to self-care: a guide to developing local strategies and good practice.

Website: www.longtermconditions.csip.org.uk.

Website: http://www.des.emory.edu/mfp/self-efficacy.html.

OTHER CONSIDERATIONS

CHAPTER 13

Respiratory considerations

Adrian Capp

INTRODUCTION

Neurological disease or trauma may affect ventilation by altering rate, depth and pattern of breathing. Associated muscle weakness and fatigue will also contribute to respiratory compromise and dysfunction. Initially, this will result in dysfunction of gas exchange which can, if left uncorrected, lead to respiratory failure. If swallowing, cough and secretion clearance are also affected then airway protection will be compromised resulting in possible aspiration. It is, therefore, vital that a full respiratory assessment is completed and close liaison with the medical team and other members of the multi-professional team, e.g. speech and language therapists, is sought. This chapter covers:

- Respiratory assessment of the neurological patient
- Respiratory considerations for specific neurological conditions.

AIMS OF PHYSIOTHERAPY

The acute phase

Many neurological conditions have a direct influence on the respiratory system, leading to an acute deterioration of respiratory function. As neurological deterioration can occur quickly, careful monitoring is essential during the acute phase.

The management aim in this phase is to ensure adequate oxygenation to the brain and vital organs to avoid secondary ischaemic changes; therefore, physiotherapy treatment aims should be directed at:

- Prevention of sputum retention
- Optimizing lung volume
- Maintenance of a patent airway
- Ensuring adequate ventilation.

The rehabilitation phase

After the acute phase has stabilized early rehabilitation can commence. It is important to ensure that oxygenation is maximized to avoid ischaemia. The balance between rehabilitation activity and the demands on the cardiorespiratory system from any residual neurological deficit must be maintained. If there has been a period of immobility due to the neurological insult, then systemic changes will have occurred. This includes cardiorespiratory deconditioning, muscle weakness from immobility, alignment changes of joints and muscle plus potential secondary conditions not associated with the primary illness such as critical illness poly-neuropathy. It is, therefore, important to monitor patients for signs of fatigue or deterioration during early mobilization. This may indicate that the intervention is not being tolerated and needs to be adapted.

Progressive disorders may exhibit a gradual deterioration in function, including the respiratory system; therefore, physiotherapy intervention should be aimed at maximizing available function within the limits of the cardiorespiratory system.

ASSESSMENT

In conjunction with a full respiratory assessment, particular attention should be given to the following assessment areas.

Lung function

Inspiratory muscle weakness leads to a reduction in vital capacity (VC). Significant diaphragm weakness is associated with a fall in VC by >25% when going from an upright to a supine position (Howard & Davidson 2003). This is due to the abdominal contents pushing up on the weakened diaphragm. It should be noted that in mild muscle weakness lung function might be normal (Pryor & Prasad 2002).

Monitoring of VC is useful in progressive conditions, such as Guillain–Barré syndrome, indicating when ventilatory support is required. Mechanical ventilation is usually required when VC falls below 15 mL/kg body weight (Polkey et al 1999).

Functional residual capacity (FRC) will be reduced if there is weakness in the respiratory muscles that keep the chest wall expanded at the end of expiration (Pryor & Prasad 2002).

Arterial blood gases

Hypercapnia (increased levels of carbon dioxide) and associated acidosis (increased acidity) will often develop in the presence of significant respiratory muscle weakness with associated hypoventilation (Pryor & Prasad 2002). For those with chronic hypoventilation, a raised arterial bicarbonate level is often found. This is a compensating mechanism and may be more pronounced in the morning or after periods of sleep (Howard & Davidson 2003).

Chronic nocturnal hypoventilation may occur in patients with neuromuscular and chest wall disease. Symptoms suggestive of nocturnal hypoventilation include poor sleep quality, hypersomnia, morning headaches, nightmares, waking with breathlessness and enuresis (urinary incontinence). A patient with a VC of less than 50% of predicted may be at risk of nocturnal hypoventilation and may benefit from further investigation and instigation of non-invasive ventilation (NIV). If effective, resolution of clinical symptoms is expected. Overnight respiratory sleep study will assist in diagnosis by showing derangement of arterial blood gases and reduced oxygen saturations (Annane et al 2000, Ward et al 2005).

Chest radiographs

Chest radiographs will show volume loss associated with generalized weakness. A raised hemi-diaphragm may indicate unilateral diaphragm weakness (Howard & Davidson 2003).

Respiratory pattern

Respiratory pattern is subjective; however, it may give an indication of the degree of respiratory muscle weakness. Respiratory pattern can be affected by damage to the respiratory centres in the pons and upper midbrain; respiratory muscle weakness and fatigue; or abnormal alterations in arterial blood gas tensions. If respiratory pattern changes during mobilization, it may indicate deterioration in respiratory function (Stiller & Phillips 2003).

Respiratory reserve (PaO_2/FiO_2 ratio) (Stiller & Phillips 2003)

The partial pressure of oxygen (PaO_2) in arterial blood falls steadily with age, reaching approximately 10.3 kPa by the age of 60 years (West 2001). The fraction of inspired oxygen (FiO_2) can assist in the assessment of suitability for rehabilitation. This should be taken into account in conjunction with PaO_2 and reflects the respiratory reserve (Fig. 13.1). The ratio between PaO_2/FiO_2 can be calculated easily and used to give an indication of a patient's ability to tolerate rehabilitation (Stiller & Phillips 2003).

$$\frac{\text{Partial Pressure of Arterial Oxygen kPa (PaO}_2)}{\text{Fraction of Inspired Oxygen (FiO}_2)} \times 7.5 = \text{Respiratory Reserve}$$

Examples

Normal breathing room air

$$\frac{13.3\ kPa}{0.21} \times 7.5 = 475 \quad \text{High Respiratory Reserve}$$

Head injury with tracheostomy

$$\frac{10.2\ kPa}{0.30} \times 7.5 = 255 \quad \text{Marginal Respiratory Reserve}$$

Figure 13.1
Calculation for respiratory reserve (Stiller & Phillips 2003). Examples are shown for a healthy person breathing room air and a head-injured patient.

13

A PaO_2/FiO_2 ratio:

- above 300 indicates that a patient is likely to have sufficient respiratory reserve to tolerate rehabilitation
- between 200 and 300 indicates marginal respiratory reserve
- below 200 indicates low respiratory reserve.

If the benefit of mobilizing a patient who has marginal respiratory reserve outweighs the potential risks, then increasing respiratory support or additional supplemental oxygen should be considered. The use of respiratory reserve should be used in conjunction with all available parameters to assess suitability for early rehabilitation.

RESPIRATORY FUNCTION IN NEUROLOGICAL CONDITIONS

Examples are given for each type of neurological condition:

Central conditions (Table 13.1)

- Cerebrovascular disease
- Multiple sclerosis
- Lateral medullary syndrome.

Table 13.1 Central nervous system conditions (Howard & Davidson 2003, Howard et al 1992, Polkey et al 1999).

Common respiratory problems in:	Respiratory considerations	Treatment considerations
Unilateral or bilateral tegmental infarcts in the pons	Apneustic breathing (deep, gasping inspiration with a pause at full inspiration, followed by brief insufficient release) Impairment of carbon dioxide responsiveness	Reduced response to demands on cardiorespiratory systems during exercise
Lateral medullary syndrome	Acute failure of automatic respiration	Requires mechanical ventilation
Basal pons infarcts Pyramids and adjacent ventral portion of the medulla	Irregular breathing pattern Inability to initiate volitional breathing	Inability to effectively cough to command Inability to deep breathe to command Inability to breath hold
Lesion in anterior pathways	Loss of automatic control Apnoea (cessation of breathing)	Requires mechanical ventilation

Neural control of respiration depends on three pathways:

1. Automatic (metabolic) respiration – to maintain acid–base balance (Howard & Davidson 2003).
2. Voluntary (behavioural) respiration – allows modulation of ventilation in response to voluntary acts such as speaking, singing, breath hold and straining (Howard & Davidson 2003).
3. Limbic (emotional) control – allows respiratory modulation to emotion such as laughing, coughing and anxiety (Howard & Davidson 2003).

Subarachnoid haemorrhage

Specific blood pressure parameters should be set by the neurosurgeon/intensive care specialist stating the desired systolic and diastolic pressure to maintain adequate cerebral perfusion. In the presence of an unprotected aneurysm, this will be to reduce the risk of rupture. Any intervention that may increase blood pressure should be used with caution. These include coughing, straining (Valsalva's manoeuvre) and manual techniques if they cause a pain response. It is essential to ensure the patient has adequate pain relief prior to intervention. If the patient is already sedated then bolus sedation may be indicated.

If vasospasm is present, then blood pressure will need to be maintained to minimize ischaemia of brain tissue. In this case, interventions that drop blood pressure should be used with caution. These will include manual hyperinflation (MHI), intermittent positive pressure breathing (IPPB), non-invasive ventilation (NIV) and changes in posture from supine to upright. Patients must be monitored for any changes in their neurological status e.g. limb weakness, changes in conscious levels or a drop in their Glasgow Coma Score (GCS). Patients with vasospasm will usually be on a level of a vasopressor to increase blood pressure. This will prohibit mobilization.

Spinal cord

● Traumatic spinal cord injury
● Transverse myelitis

Respiratory function and treatment will depend on the neurological level and whether the lesion is complete or incomplete (Table 13.2).

Note. Incomplete injuries have a mixed picture of functional level due to areas of respiratory muscle preservation.

Spinal injuries above the level of T6 are at risk of haemodynamics instability due to the loss of sympathetic outflow. This results in hypotension and bradycardia on suctioning. Intravenous atropine should be available.

Table 13.2 Spinal cord level and respiratory function (Clapham 2004, Howard & Davidson 2003, Pryor 1999).

Level of lesion	Affected respiratory muscles	Respiratory Considerations	Treatment considerations
C2	Diaphragm, intercostals, abdominals and accessory muscles	No respiratory effort Ventilator dependent No cough Fatigue	Suction Manual Hyperinflation Manual techniques
C4	Partial diaphragm, partial accessory muscles, intercostals and abdominals	Ventilator independent but may require nocturnal ventilation Paradoxical breathing Ineffective cough Fatigue	Glossopharyngeal breathing Assisted cough Intermittent positive pressure breathing (IPPB)
C6	Partial accessory muscles, intercostals and abdominals	Ventilator independent Ineffective cough Fatigue	As for C4
T1	Intercostals and abdominals	Ineffective cough Fatigue	As for C6
T12	None	Effective cough	All respiratory physiotherapy techniques

13

In patients with diaphragm and respiratory muscle involvement, continuous positive airway pressure (CPAP) will not improve ventilation or carbon dioxide retention (Winslow & Rozovsky 2003).

Anterior horn cell
- Poliomyelitis
- Motor neurone disease
- Proximal spinal atrophy

Respiratory insufficiency occurs due to respiratory muscle weakness or associated bulbar weakness leading to aspiration and bronchopneumonia (Howard & Davidson 2003; also see Table 13.3).

Neuropathy (Table 13.4)
- Guillain–Barré syndrome
- Neuralgic amyotrophy

Table 13.3 Anterior horn cell (Howard & Davidson 2003, Howard & Orwell 2002, Polkey et al 1999, Winslow & Rozovsky 2003).

Common respiratory problems in:	Respiratory considerations	Treatment considerations
Poliomyelitis	Respiratory muscle weakness Fatigue	All respiratory physiotherapy interventions appropriate
Motor neurone disease	Respiratory muscle weakness Bulbar weakness Fatigue	May require ventilatory support e.g. non- invasive ventilation (NIV) All respiratory physiotherapy interventions appropriate

Table 13.4 Neuropathy (Howard & Davidson 2003).

Common respiratory problems in:	Respiratory considerations	Treatment considerations
Guillain–Barré syndrome	Primarily inspiratory muscle weakness Weakness of abdominal muscles Weakness of accessory muscles Bulbar weakness Retained secretions Aspiration pneumonia Atelectasis (collapsed lung) Fatigue	1/3 will require mechanical ventilation A drop in tidal volume of <15 mL/kg indicates the need for ventilatory support May require prolonged weaning All physiotherapy techniques appropriate

Respiratory insufficiency occurs due to respiratory muscle weakness or associated bulbar weakness leading to possible respiratory failure, aspiration or broncho-pneumonia (Howard & Davidson 2003). The use of vital capacity monitoring is useful in determining both deterioration and resolution of respiratory function.

Neuromuscular junction
- Myasthenia gravis
- Lambert–Eaton myasthenic syndrome
- *Clostridium botulinum*

Muscle fatigue may occur in patients with pathologies affecting the neuromuscular junction (Table 13.5). A graded regimen of rehabilitation should be used with additional ventilatory support when rehabilitating in the early stages.

Muscle conditions
● Muscular dystrophies
● Metabolic myopathies

Respiratory insufficiency due to respiratory muscle weakness or associated bulbar weakness can lead to possible respiratory failure, aspiration or bronchopneumonia (Howard & Davidson 2003). Associated skeletal changes may further affect respiratory function and compliance of the chest wall (Table 13.6).

Table 13.5 Neuromuscular junction (Howard & Davidson 2003).

Common respiratory problems in:	Respiratory considerations	Treatment considerations
Myasthenia gravis	Diaphragm weakness may occur with mild peripheral weakness Fatigue	Long-term ventilation All physiotherapy techniques appropriate

Table 13.6 Muscle (Howard & Davidson 2003, Howard et al 1993, Polkey et al 1999).

Common respiratory problems in:	Respiratory considerations	Treatment considerations
Duchenne muscular dystrophy	Respiratory failure develops late Intercostal and expiratory muscle weakness Scoliosis Kyphosis Bulbar weakness Fatigue	Aspiration (the entry of secretions or foreign material into the trachea or lungs) Reduced lung compliance All physiotherapy techniques appropriate
Becker's muscular dystrophy	Scoliosis Respiratory muscle weakness Fatigue	All physiotherapy techniques appropriate
Fascioscapulohumeral dystrophy	May have selective diaphragm weakness Fatigue	All physiotherapy techniques appropriate
Acid maltase deficiency	Early selective diaphragm weakness Fatigue	All physiotherapy techniques appropriate

MANAGEMENT OF TRAUMATIC BRAIN INJURY

The classification of the pathophysiology of brain injury is shown in Table 13.7. In reality both primary focal and diffuse brain injury coexist.

Primary brain injury occurs at the time of injury and is irreversible. The management of traumatic brain injury is aimed at prevention of secondary brain injury (Coles 2004, Marik 2002).

Secondary damage occurs to neurones, due to physiological responses, following the initial injury leading to cerebral ischaemia (Marik 2002). Terminology associated with cerebral pressures and blood flow, with normal ranges, are shown in Table 13.8.

Due to the limited space within the cranial vault, if there is a rise in volume (e.g. from a haematoma, space-occupying lesion or increase in cerebral blood volume), then there will be a subsequent rise in intracranial pressure (ICP). In Figure 13.2, the point marked on the curve indicates the point when the brain's

Table 13.7 Classification of brain injury.

Primary brain injury	Secondary brain injury
Focal:	Extracranial causes:
Disruption of brain vessels	Systemic hypotension
Haematoma formation	Hypoxaemia (reduced oxygen levels)
Contusions	Hypercarbia (excess carbon dioxide)
Traumatic subarachnoid haemorrhage	Disturbances of blood coagulation
Diffuse:	Intracranial causes:
Diffuse axonal injury	Haematoma
	Brain swelling
	Disturbances in the microvascular circulation
	Infection

Table 13.8 Definition and normal values relating to cerebral haemodynamics (Clapham 2004, Coles 2004).

Term	Definition	Normal range
Intracranial pressure (ICP)	Pressure within the cranial cavity	0–10 mm Hg
Cerebral perfusion pressure (CPP)	The net pressure of blood flow to the brain	70–100 mm Hg
Cerebral blood flow (CBF)	The amount of blood that passes through the brain per minute	50 mL/100 g/min of brain tissue

13

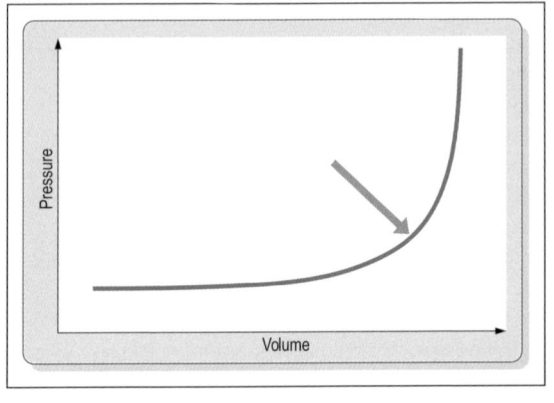

Figure 13.2
Monroe Kellie doctrine. Graph showing the normal volume–pressure relationship within the cranial vault. Arrow indicates point where brain compliance is lost due to all compensatory mechanisms within the cranial vault being exhausted. After this point on the graph, a small rise in intracranial volume will cause an exponential rise in intracranial pressure. (From Lindsay & Bone 2004, with permission.)

Table 13.9 Signs and symptoms of raised intracranial pressure (ICP).

Early signs and symptoms	Late signs and symptoms
Headache	Severe headache
Confusion	Projectile vomiting
Convulsions	Reduced level of consciousness
Irritability	Irregular breathing
Lethargy	Abnormal limb posturing
Restlessness	Flexion/extension
Focal neurology	Cushing's response
Pupil dysfunction	Impaired brainstem function

compliance stops, leading to a large increase in pressure with a small increase in volume (Lindsay & Bone 2004). The signs and symptoms of raised ICP are shown in Table 13.9.

It is important for the physiotherapist to consider any potential effects an intervention may have on cerebral perfusion pressure (CPP), as a rising ICP or a falling

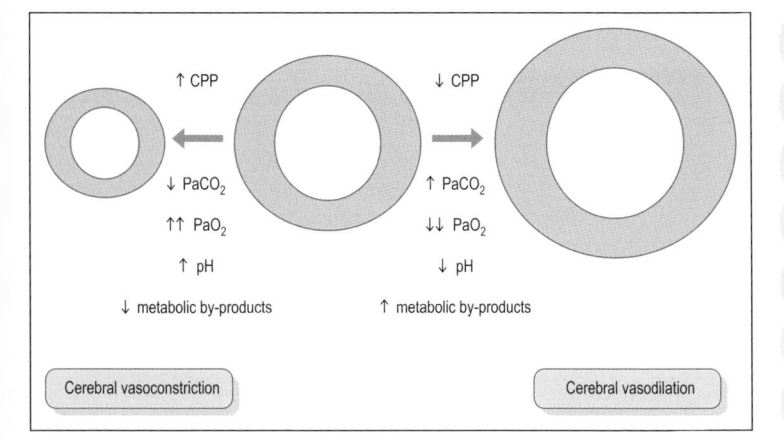

Figure 13.3
Factors affecting cerebral vasculature. Diagram showing the effect of the reactivity of the cerebral vasculature to the partial pressure of carbon dioxide (PaCO$_2$), partial pressure of oxygen (PaO$_2$), blood acidity/alkalinity (pH) and metabolic by-products. (From Lindsay & Bone 2004, with permission.)

mean arterial pressure (MAP) can have detrimental effects which, if sustained, will lead to cerebral ischaemia (CPP = MAP − ICP). The cerebral vasculature is highly responsive to changes in the partial pressure of carbon dioxide (PaCO$_2$), metabolic by products, level of blood acidity or alkalinity and partial pressure of oxygen (PaO$_2$). This can result in increased cerebral blood volume leading to an increase in ICP or cerebral ischaemia (Fig. 13.3).

PHYSIOTHERAPY INTERVENTIONS IN PATIENTS WITH ACUTE TRAUMATIC BRAIN INJURY

Patients who have undergone a traumatic brain injury commonly present with a reduced level of consciousness (LOC); respiratory problems associated with this are outlined in Table 13.10.

Physiotherapy cardiorespiratory interventions may themselves have a detrimental effect on cerebral oxygenation which could potentially contribute to the secondary cerebral ischaemia. Therefore, a brief risk assessment prior to respiratory interventions should be carried out involving ICP and CPP (Table 13.11). Liaising with the staff caring can give important information regarding patient response to handling or interventions. Local policies should be checked regarding monitors, equipment, patient parameters and post-surgical procedures.

Table 13.10 Common problems with reduced consciousness level (Clapham 2004, Pryor & Prasad 2002).

Common problems	Treatment considerations
Reduced airway protection	● Use of airway protection techniques
Sputum retention	● Insertion of nasopharyngeal airway [if non intubated or had a tracheostomy (opening through the trachea to create an airway)] ● Insertion of oral airway (if non intubated or had a tracheostomy) ● Suction ● Gravity-assisted positioning ● Manual hyperinflation ● Manual techniques, e.g. chest vibrations/shaking, percussion ● Intermittent positive pressure breathing (IPPB) ● Neurophysiological facilitation of respiration techniques
Hypoventilation	● Manual hyperinflation ● IPPB ● Non-invasive ventilation (NIV)
Atelectasis (collapsed lung)	● Manual hyperventilation ● IPPB
Type II respiratory failure (low oxygen, with high carbon dioxide)	● Liaise with critical care specialist ● May require intubation or NIV

Table 13.11 Risk assessment (Clapham 2004).

Intracranial pressure (ICP)	Cerebral perfusion pressure (CPP)	Risk
<15 mm Hg	70 mm Hg (stable)	LOW
15–20 mm Hg	70 mm Hg (settles quickly after treatment within 5 minutes)	MODERATE
>20 mm Hg	Low	HIGH

If physiotherapy is indicated and the risk of treatment is deemed acceptable, the potential detrimental effects associated with individual treatment modalities need to be carefully considered (Table 13.12). Remember in order to minimize the detrimental effects of physiotherapy intervention:

● Keep treatment time short (Clapham 2004)
● Increase the patient's level of sedation.

Table 13.12 Effects of Physiotherapy Intervention (Clapham 2004, Paratz & Burns 1993, Pryor & Prasad 2002).

Physiotherapy technique	Potential treatment effects
Manual hyperinflation (MHI)	↑ intrathoracic pressure leading to: ↓ venous return to the heart leading to ↑ cerebral blood volume and ↑ intracranial pressure (ICP) ↓ filling pressure to the right atrium from the inferior vena cava leading to ↓ in stroke volume and drop in blood pressure (see Figure 13.2) The depth and rate of manual hyperventilation will affect the cerebral vasculature as a result of carbon dioxide retention or removal. This can either reduce or increase intracranial pressure. If intracranial pressure is high, then rapid small volume breaths will reduce ICP by removal of CO_2 to allow intermittent manual hyperinflation breaths. Intersperse this with large volume MHI breath for therapeutic effect.
Positioning	Treatment position may be limited to 15–30 degrees head up position to reduce ICP. Head must be kept aligned in midline (chin in line with sternum) to reduce pooling of venous blood within the brain from neck vein obstruction in patients with a raised ICP. Patients may not tolerate turning. Bolus sedation may be required. When changing patients' position do so slowly in patients with raised ICP. Risk of aspiration if bulbar weakness.
Manual techniques (shaking, vibrations, percussion)	Noxious stimulation. Ensure adequate analgesia. May require bolus sedation. N.B. Bolus sedation may drop blood pressure Bronchospasm Slow single-handed percussion may reduce ICP
Intermittent positive pressure breathing (IPPB) /The Bird/non-invasive ventilation (NIP)	↑ intrathoracic pressure therefore may have similar effects to MHI May reduce mean arterial pressure (MAP)

(*continued*)

Table 13.12 Effects of Physiotherapy Intervention (Clapham 2004, Paratz & Burns 1993, Pryor & Prasad 2002)—cont'd.

Physiotherapy technique	Potential treatment effects

Suction	Hypoxia
	Hypercapnia leading to ↑ ICP
	  ↑ intrathoracic pressure due to coughing leading to increased ICP
	  Valsalva's manoeuvre (forced exhalation against closed vocal cords)
	  Vasovagal response (cardioinhibitory and vasodepressor responses) leading to bradycardia (heart rate under 60 beats per minute)

References

Annane D, Chevrolet JC, Chevret S, Raphaël JC 2000 Nocturnal mechanical ventilation for chronic hypoventilation in patients with neuromuscular and chest wall disorders (review). Cochrane Database of Systematic Reviews 2000, Issue 1. Art. No.: CD001941. DOI:10.1002/14651858.CD001941.

Clapham L 2004 Calls to the neurology/neurosurgical unit. In: Beverley Harden (ed) Emergency physiotherapy. Churchill Livingstone, Edinburgh.

Coles J 2004 Regional ischemia after head injury. Neuroscience 10:120–125.

Howard RS, Davidson C 2003 Long term ventilation in neurogenic respiratory failure. Journal of Neurology, Neurosurgery and Psychiatry 74(suppl III):iii24–iii30.

Howard RS, Orwell RW 2002 Management of motor neurone disease. Postgraduate Medical Journal 78:736–741.

Howard RS, Wills CM, Hirsh NP et al 1992 Respiratory involvement in multiple sclerosis. Brain 115:479–494.

Howard RS, Wills CM, Hirsh NP, Spencer GT 1993 Respiratory involvement in primary muscle disorders: assessment and management. Quarterly Journal of Medicine 86:175–189.

Lindsay K, Bone I 2004 Neurology and neurosurgery illustrated. Churchill Livingstone, New York.

Marik P 2002 Management of head trauma. Chest 122(2):699.

Paratz J, Burns Y 1993 The effect of respiratory physiotherapy on intracranial pressure, mean arterial pressure, cerebral perfusion pressure and end tidal carbon dioxide in ventilated neurosurgical patients. Physiotherapy Theory and Practice 9:3–11.

Polkey MI, Lyall RA, Moxham J, Leigh PN 1999 Respiratory aspects of neurological disease. Journal of Neurology, Neurosurgery and Psychiatry 66:5–15.

Pryor J 1999 Physiotherapy for airway clearance. European Respiratory Journal 14:141–1424.

Pryor J, Prasad SA 2002 Physiotherapy for respiratory and cardiac problems. Adults and paediatrics, 3rd edn. Churchill Livingstone, Edinburgh.

Stiller K, Phillips A 2003 Safety aspects of mobilising acutely ill inpatients. Physiotherapy Theory and Practice 19:239–257.

Ward S, Chatwin M, Heather S, Simonds AK 2005 Randomised controlled trial of non-invasive (NIV) for nocturnal hypoventilation in neuromuscular and chest wall disease patients with daytime normocapnea. Thorax 60:1019–1024.

West J 2001 Pulmonary physiology and pathophysiology. An integrated, case-based approach. Lippincott Williams & Wilkins, Philadelphia.

Winslow C, Rozovsky J 2003 Effects of spinal cord injury on the respiratory system. American Journal of Physical Medicine and Rehabilitation 82(10):803–814.

CHAPTER 14

Cognitive perceptual considerations

F Colin Wilson

INTRODUCTION

Clinical neuropsychologists aim to identify and interpret disorders of cognitive function such as memory, language, learning, and thinking and reasoning; this also includes perceptual (integration of information from the environment), emotional and behavioural disorders arising from neuropathology.

Therapists need to have an understanding of the above disorders in order to screen patients for cognitive perceptual dysfunction, and address these deficits as part of their planned therapy intervention. This chapter provides an overview of common cognitive disorders arising following acquired brain injury (ABI) as well as current treatment approaches. This chapter offers therapists' suggestions for minimizing the impact of these deficits on therapy activity and rehabilitation delivery.

In neurorehabilitation, it is important to appreciate the distinction between **focal injuries** such as stroke and **diffuse insults** such as traumatic brain injury (TBI); diffuse injuries are associated with widespread tearing and shearing of neuronal connections. The effects of these acquired injuries can affect cognitive functioning, mood, motivation and engagement in rehabilitation. Examples are given related to TBI, stroke or cerebrovascular accident (CVA), and anoxic injury (lack of oxygen to the brain). Refer to Chapter 6 for an overview of common neurological conditions.

COGNITIVE EFFECTS

Traumatic brain injury (TBI)

Following TBI after emergence from coma and post-traumatic amnesia, individuals may experience a range of post-concussion symptoms (PCS) (see Table 14.1). After severe or very severe traumatic brain injury [prolonged coma (Glasgow Coma Scale: GCS < 8) and/or post-traumatic amnesia greater than 1 week], there is likely to be both primary and secondary damage (Box 14.1).

Table 14.1 Common symptoms following traumatic brain injury (TBI).

Post-concussional symptoms (PCS)	Mild to moderate TBI (GCS: mild = 13–15; moderate = 9–12)	Severe TBI (GCS <8 for 6+hours)
• Dizziness • Persistent headaches • Reduced stamina • Fatigue/sleep disturbance • Noise/light sensitivity • Blurred/double vision • Tinnitus • Slowed thinking • Reduced concentration • Poor memory	• Impaired speed of processing (thinking speed) • Poor divided attention • Poor memory • Reduced 'frustrative' tolerance • Low mood (depression) • Marked anxiety • Post-traumatic stress disorder (PTSD)	• Reduced speed of thought/ information processing • Overall decline in intellectual functioning • Difficulties with word finding and sentence construction • Impaired divided attention and marked distractibility • Limited concentration • Poor memory and new learning ability • Reduced independent planning, problem solving and reasoning • Reduced or total lack of initiation • Poor self-regulation (verbal, physical or sexual disinhibition) • Mood swings, irritability • Limited insight or awareness of their acquired neurological deficits

GCS, Glasgow Coma Scale; severity levels from Campbell (2004) p. 106.

Box 14.1

Primary damage

Diffuse white matter damage (tearing of axonal connections), contusions along the frontal-temporal plane and ruptured blood vessels (haemorrhage) causing reduced oxygen supply to the brain

Secondary damage

May result from cerebral haemorrhage leading to anoxic/hypoxic damage (loss or reduced oxygen supply), cerebral swelling and/or the build-up of cerebrospinal fluid (hydrocephalus) leading to increased intracranial pressure (ICP).

Cerebrovascular accident (CVA)

Following focal injury such as CVA, the pattern of cognitive deficits is dependent on the site of the stroke and its severity. In the acute setting, confused or disordered speech, reduced ability to process information, impaired alertness/arousal and poor attention/concentration are commonly observed regardless of stroke localization. Typical deficits and suggested practical rehabilitation approaches are outlined in Table 14.2. Depending on the deficits identified, specialist assessment by speech and language therapy (SLT), occupational therapy (OT) and clinical neuropsychology will be required (British Psychological Society 2002). Refer to Chapter 15 in this pocketbook on communication considerations. See national clinical guidelines for stroke (section 4.2) by Intercollegiate Working Party for Stroke (IWPS) (2004).

HYPOXIC/ANOXIC INJURY

Following hypoxic/anoxic injury which can occur in association with TBI or separately following cardiac/respiratory arrest or carbon monoxide poisoning, the pattern of cognitive deficits is dependent on the nature and duration of the period of loss or reduction of cerebral blood supply. The neuropathology associated with hypoxic/anoxic injury is often widespread involving the basal ganglia, thalamus, white matter projections and diffuse cortical areas (Caine & Watson 2000). Acquired deficits can include ataxia, extra-pyramidal symptoms, 'mental slowness', memory problems, a combination of memory and executive difficulties, dysarthria, dyspraxia, naming difficulties, impaired visual recognition including agnosia (inability to recognize objects) and prosopagnosia (inability to recognize faces) and limited attentional control (Peskine et al 2004, Wilson et al 2003a).

Guiding principles for cognitive disorders

Some suggestions in relation to how therapists can minimize the impact of these deficits on therapy activity are provided in Box 14.2 (p. 235), which outlines guiding principles to consider in assessment and when planning intervention(s) particularly in acute and post-acute settings.

BEHAVIOURAL AND EMOTIONAL DISORDERS

Following acquired brain injury (ABI), patients in general are at increased risk of developing a range of emotional and behavioural disorders. Emotional disturbance with a mixture of reactive anxiety and depression is particularly common and can influence patient engagement with therapy and rehabilitation outcome unless addressed. Bipolar disorders, mania, obsessive-compulsive disorder (OCD) and psychotic episodes unless presenting prior to the acquired brain injury are

Table 14.2 Common cognitive and behavioural deficits after stroke.

Arterial lesion	Observed deficits	Assessment	Rehabilitation strategies
Anterior cerebral artery (ACA)	Severe hemiplegia Sensory loss (affected lower limb)	Neurological examination Somatosensory exam	Limb care and positioning Facilitated movement repetitive training
ACA Damage to supplementary motor area (SMA)	Poor initiation/control of voluntary movement Limited speech Ideomotor apraxia (disorder of skilled voluntary movements)	Ability to follow verbal or gestural commands Assess ability to demonstrate actions on request	Errorless learning [Hand-over-hand facilitation to shape series of movement(s) in sequence, Wilson et al 2003b]
ACA mesial/orbital frontal areas	Personality change Apathy Marked disinhibition	Employ patient and family interviews and self-report measures	Information to family members and staff Structure environment to minimize opportunities for disinhibited behaviour
Anterior communicating artery aneurysms (AcoA)	Acute/chronic confusion Impaired memory and new learning Confabulation (includes events or details in conversation which have not occurred)	Orientation Ability to recall new information Safety awareness Route finding	Supervision Provide environmental cues Structure activity Minimize risks of wandering e.g. alarms/sensor switches

Middle cerebral artery (MCA)	Contralesional hemiplegia Visual field loss Global dysphasia (DOM) Unilateral neglect (disorder of visuo-spatial awareness usually NON-DOM)	Visual fields testing Tests for neglect and sustained attention (concentration) Establish level of comprehension and awareness Promote use of neglected side via visual/auditory cues, positioning of therapy tasks, use of prism lenses
Superior MCA	Upper limb and facial paresis Poor expression Poor speech prosody (deficit in rate of speech) Ideomotor apraxia (DOM) Unilateral neglect (NON-DOM)	Ability to copy movements via instruction or gesture Personal and extra-personal neglect tests (Comb-Razor Test, Line Cancellation etc.) Repetitive practice Intensive SLT programme involving shaping of speech sounds Affected limb activation
Inferior MCA	Homonymous hemianopia (deficit of nasal and temporal visual field on same side of hemiplegia) Receptive understanding Dysgraphia (problems with writing) Dyscalculia (DOM-problems with numbers) Unilateral neglect Anosognosia (lack of awareness of illness) Constructional and dressing dyspraxia Agitation (NON-DOM)	Visual fields testing Pen and paper neglect tests Interview and self-report measures to establish level of awareness/insight Copying gestures, use of objects Interview – identify possible sources of agitation Advice to visually scan into affected visual field Establish mode of communication Establish 'real life' use of memory via errorless learning. Use compensatory aids Visual scanning training and limb activation Directive feedback to patient and family. Provide opportunities to learn and adapt to acquired deficits Frequent practice using shaping of affected limb Commence ABC behavioural records

(continued)

14

233

Table 14.2 Common cognitive and behavioural deficits after stroke—cont'd.

Arterial lesion	Observed deficits	Assessment	Rehabilitation strategies
Posterior cerebral artery (PCA)	Cortical blindness (total or partial loss of vision with intact pupil response to light) Confusion Impaired memory Poor shape, size and colour perception Ability to perceive moving but not static objects	Visual fields testing Orientation Ability to recall new information Visuo-spatial/Visuo-perceptual assessments such as Cortical Vision Screening Test – CORVIST, The Visual Object and Space Perception Battery – VOSPB	Establish level of visual field deficit and patient awareness Consistently orientate to task/activity Organize environment to minimize real life perceptual difficulties
PCA (DOM)	Alexia without agraphia (impaired ability to read but not write) Visual agnosia (impaired ability to identify objects)	Pencil and paper tasks of writing and reading prose Able to identify and use common and uncommon objects	Consider talking books Consider use of visual markers or anchors placed on commonly employed objects Provide opportunities to learn and adapt to acquired deficits
PCA (NON DOM)	Unilateral neglect Constructional dyspraxia Agitation/confusion	Visual fields testing Pen and paper neglect tests Tests for dyspraxia	Establish level of visual field deficit and patient awareness Consistently orientate to task/activity Organize environment to minimize real life perceptual difficulties

ABC, antecedents, behaviours, consequences; CORVIST, Cortical Vision Screening Test (James et al 2001); DOM, dominant; NON DOM, non dominant; SLT, speech & language therapist; VOSPB, Visual Object and Space Perception Battery (Warrington & James 1991).

Box 14.2 Guiding cognitive principles for rehabilitation.

1. Establish nature, site and extent of ABI.
2. Assess level of responsiveness/orientation to current environment.
3. Assess patient understanding of their current problems/deficits (awareness).
4. Alter environment (minimize noise, distractions) and promote active attention to therapy activity, which may require employing a set number of repetitions.
5. Tailor therapy to maximize patient understanding of therapy demands within the context of interdisciplinary team working context.
6. Implement errorless learning (learning without errors: Wilson (2004) provides details) as part of holistic therapy practice and ward-based activity.
7. Employ SMART goals (specific, measurable, achievable, realistic and timed goals, Cott & Finch 1990) in therapy (to minimize patient confusion and anxiety).
8. Provide concise feedback to patient and family to promote positive engagement (consider the use of agreed tangible rewards to reinforce engagement; e.g. watching a chosen favourite DVD after physiotherapy).
9. Facilitate multiple opportunities for practice across functional contexts (skill generalization) from therapy to ward to home setting.

quite rare (1–2%; Brown 2004) and require consultation and referral to neuropsychiatry.

Individuals with emerging insight of their acquired physical, communicative and cognitive deficits are probably more at risk of depression particularly over time. Those surviving TBI have also an increased risk of suicide, which remains fairly constant over time after injury (1%: at least three times the standard mortality rate; Fleminger et al 2003), which may be associated with ongoing alcohol/drug abuse. Table 14.3 provides an overview of frequently occurring emotional and behavioural difficulties within the first year following TBI, stroke and hypoxic/anoxic injury [for more details, see Brown (2004), Williams et al (2003)].

Behavioural problems can directly interfere with therapy engagement and compliance such as kicking directed towards staff, biting or indirectly reduced participation resulting from use of verbal aggression or use of inappropriate/disinhibited language throughout therapy. Nonetheless, often behaviour problems can be relatively easily addressed in the context of good interdisciplinary team working including regular communication between neurorehabilitation team members as well as the patient and their family. In addition, it is important that all interdisci-

Table 14.3 Common emotional-behavioural difficulties following ABI (Brown 2004).

TBI	Apathy (46%) Depression (20–40%) Anxiety (10–25%) Pain (50+%): headaches, spasticity, contractures, heterotopic ossification, complex regional pain syndromes Reduced anger control PTSD (19–26%) Reduced community involvement Reduced relationship satisfaction and quality Inability to return to work or previous enjoyed leisure pursuits Severe behavioural disorders (verbal, physical and sexual disinhibition, aggression)
Stroke	Apathy (57%) Depression (20–40%) Anxiety (30%) Pain (spasticity, contractures, complex regional pain syndromes)
Hypoxia/anoxia	Apathy (79%) Depression Anxiety Agitation Reduced anger control Affective dysregulation (inability to control internal emotional state) Egocentric or childish behaviour Poor psychosocial and vocational reintegration Severe behavioural disorders (lack of initiation, disinhibition, loss of judgement)

PTSD, post-traumatic stress disorder.

plinary staff can commence and complete structured behavioural observation(s) records with antecedent (A), behaviour (B) and consequence (C) sections at the very least [see Table 14.4; Wilson et al (2003b, p. 46)].

Such recording methods permit patient–staff/family interactions to be reviewed and possible triggers for behaviour to be identified. Without these, it is very difficult to reliably identify reductions or escalations in behaviour patterns or to establish whether or not a planned behavioural management plan is effective.

Behavioural management approaches

There are a variety of treatment strategies, which can be applied to increase or decrease behaviour. Methods such as chaining (teaching a series of task steps

Table 14.4 Sample ABC behavioural record.

Date/time	A (Antecedents)	B (Behaviour)	C (Consequences)	Possible options
4th May 2006 8.30 am	Two staff were with John helping him to get washed and dressed before breakfast	John started shouting at Sharon (Nurse) and then attempted to hit me (Physio) as we were standing him from his wheelchair	I told John to 'stop shouting' and helped John to return to sitting in his wheelchair	• Discuss with other team members re: alternatives • Inform John about care task and how he can be involved • Ignore shouting • Temporarily withdraw and return to John when he is calmer • Establish reward for John when he doesn't shout or isn't attempting to hit out at staff

together), modelling (initiating and demonstrate the activity), shaping (rewarding gradually closer approximations to the desired therapy task) and systematic desensitization (gradually increasing task demand with use of relaxation) can be employed to increase involvement or teach new skills (Wilson et al 2003b).

Positive reinforcement is undoubtedly one of the most influential methods for improving behaviour employing praise, rest breaks, positive social attention or meaningful (tangible) rewards including increased access to enjoyable activities (Wilson et al 2003b, p. 56). Fear or increased anxiety when attempting to develop new skills after ABI is not uncommon (such as walking with an aid or transferring with unfamiliar staff) and frequently benefits from the combined use of planned (step-by-step) desensitization while also employing on-the-spot applied relaxation techniques [see Matthies et al (1997) for more information]. Therapists are recommended to seek advice in relation to behavioural management protocols from a clinical psychologist (with neurorehabilitation experience) or a clinical neuropsychologist before implementing behavioural programmes especially if any potentially aversive technique(s) are being employed.

Severe behavioural problems

While less common, severe behavioural problems can contribute to treatment disruption, staff injury as well as family stress or distress. Severe verbal and physical aggression can occur as an individual regains consciousness but remains agitated and confused. Unfortunately, in busy acute medical and surgical wards, difficult patterns of behaviour may be unintentionally reinforced or reward; typical behavioural approaches for disruptive behaviour are identified in Box 14.3 (Wilson et al 2003b).

Alternatively, depending on the patient's own level of cognitive functioning (ability to remember and concentrate) as well as insight/awareness in relation to presenting behavioural difficulties, approaches such as anxiety or anger management which involves developing awareness of anxiety or anger triggers, learning and select alternative ways of coping including relaxation and using these new methods when required can be employed (O'Leary 2000, Wilson et al 2003b).

Box 14.3

Behavioural approaches
- Decreasing stimulation
- Increasing staff/task predictability including signalling when an activity will start and finish
- Reinforcing appropriate behaviour (when it occurs)
- Ignoring the unwanted behaviour (such as spitting at staff)
- Rewarding an alternative behaviour (such as participating in a conversation during a board game without shouting at staff): differential reinforcement
- Response cost based on negative reinforcement involving the withdrawal of something meaningful <u>every time</u>, an unwanted behaviour occurs
- Time Out On The Spot (TOOTS) which involves complete withdrawal from interaction after an unwanted behaviour occurs for a set amount of time

---

EMOTIONAL PROBLEMS

After ABI, emotional problems can arise directly from neurological injury (disruption or loss of specific neural connections (for instance pathological laughing and crying) or can combine with internal psychological factors such as attitudes towards disability and the self to reduced quality of life. Alternatively they may arise as a result of the impact of functional impairments on social involvement (Gainotti 1993). Clearly, where marked emotional difficulties are affecting rehabilitation engagement or day-to-day functioning, then referral to an appropriately qualified clinical psychologist or clinical neuropsychologist should be actively considered.

After brain injury, structured psychotherapy often requires adaptation in order to minimize the impact of cognitive deficits [Khan-Bourne & Brown (2003) provides useful advice], while cognitive behaviour therapy is increasingly recognized as being of clinical value in the management of anxiety (Williams et al 2003), depression (Khan-Bourne & Brown 2003), irritability (Alderman 2003) and post-traumatic stress disorder (McMillan et al 2003). Undoubtedly, the use of cognitive behaviour approaches requires more investigation in larger multi-centre trials of psychosocial outcome after ABI.

KEY CLINICAL MESSAGES

● Changes in cognitive functions following ABI can be subtle as well as profound.
● Cognitive-perceptual, emotional and behavioural changes require skilled comprehensive cognitive assessment within an interdisciplinary team context.
● Clinical psychologists or neuropsychologists are key members of the interdisciplinary neurorehabilitation team (IWPS 2004, Royal College of Physicians and British Society of Rehabilitation Medicine 2003).
● There is limited access to psychologists in everyday practice. Therapists need to have an understanding of cognitive disorders in order to screen patients for cognitive dysfunction, and address these deficits as part of their planned therapy intervention.

Acknowledgements

The helpful comments and suggestions of Avril Law, Carrie Spence and Laura Wheatley-Smith, Clinical Specialist Physiotherapists at the Regional Acquired Brain Injury Unit, Belfast in relation to earlier drafts of this chapter are gratefully acknowledged.

References

Alderman N 2003 Contemporary approaches to the management of irritability and aggression following traumatic brain injury. In: Williams WH, Evans JJ (eds) Biopsychosocial approaches in neurorehabilitation. Psychology Press, Hove (UK), pp 211–240.

British Psychological Society 2002 Psychological services for stroke survivors and their families. British Psychological Society, Leicester (UK).

Brown R 2004 Psychological and psychiatric aspects of brain disorder: nature, assessment and implications for clinical neuropsychology. In: Goldstein L H, McNeil J E (eds) Clinical neuropsychology: a practical guide to assessment and management for clinicians. John Wiley & Sons, Chichester, England, pp 81–98.

Caine D, Watson DG 2000 Neuropsychological and neuropathological sequelae of cerebral anoxia: a critical review. Journal of International Neuropsychological Society 6:86–99.

Campbell M 2004 Acquired brain injury: trauma and pathology. In: Stokes M (ed Physical management in neurological rehabilitation, 2nd edn. Elsevier, London, pp 103–124.

Cott C, Finch E 1990 Goal setting in physical therapy practice. Physiotherapy Canada 43:19–22.

Fleminger S, Oliver DL, Williams WH, Evans J 2003 The neuropsychiatry of depression after brain injury In: Williams WH, Evans JJ (eds) Biopsychosocial approaches in neurorehabilitation. Psychology Press, Hove (UK), pp 65–87.

Gainotti G 1993 Emotional and psychosocial problems after brain injury. Neuropsychological Rehabilitation 3:259–277.

Intercollegiate Working Party for Stroke (IWPS) 2004 National clinical guidelines for stroke, 2nd edn. Royal College of Physicians, London.

James M, Plant GT, Warrington EK 2001 Cortical vision screening test. Thames Valley Test Company, Bury St Edmunds, England.

Khan-Bourne N, Brown RG 2003 Cognitive behaviour therapy for the treatment of depression in individuals with brain injury. In: Williams WH, Evans JJ (eds) Biopsychosocial approaches in neurorehabilitation. Psychology Press, Hove (UK), pp 89–107.

Matthies BK, Kreutzer JS, West DD 1997 The behaviour management handbook. The Psychological Corporation, San Antonio.

McMillan TM, Williams WH, Bryant R 2003 Post-traumatic stress disorder and traumatic brain injury: a review of causal mechanisms, assessment, and treatment. In: Williams WH, Evans JJ (eds) Biopsychosocial approaches in neurorehabilitation. Psychology Press, Hove (UK), pp 149–164.

O'Leary CA 2000 Reducing aggression in adults with brain injuries. Behavioural Interventions 15:205–216.

Peskine A, Picq C, Pradat-Diehl P 2004 Cerebral anoxia and disability. Brain Injury 18(12):1243–1254.

Royal College of Physicians and British Society of Rehabilitation Medicine 2003 Rehabilitation following acquired brain injury: National Clinical Guidelines. RCP, BSRM, London.

Warrington EK, James M 1991 The visual object and space perception battery. Thames Valley Test Company, Bury St Edmunds, England.

Williams WH, Evans JJ, Fleminger S 2003 Neurorehabilitation and cognitive-behaviour therapy of anxiety disorders after brain injury: an overview and a case illustration of obsessive-compulsive disorder. In: Williams WH, Evans JJ (eds) Biopsychosocial approaches in neurorehabilitation. Psychology Press, Hove (UK), pp 133–148.

Wilson BA 2004 Management and remediation of memory problems in brain-injured adults. In: Baddeley AD, Kopelman MD, Wilson BA (eds) The essential handbook of memory disorders for clinicians. John Wiley & Sons, Chichester (UK), pp 199–226.

Wilson FC, Harpur J, Watson T et al 2003a Adult survivors of severe cerebral hypoxia – case series and comparative analysis. Neurorehabilitation 18:291–298.

Wilson BA, Herbert CM, Shiel A 2003b Behavioural approaches in neuropsychological rehabilitation. Psychology Press, Hove (UK).

Useful websites

Headway: www.headway.org.uk.
International Brain Injury Association: www.internationalbrain.org.
Stroke Association: www.stroke.org.uk.

CHAPTER 15

Communication considerations

Linda Armstrong

INTRODUCTION

In this chapter four adult-acquired neurological communication disorders (dysarthria, articulatory dyspraxia, aphasia and right hemisphere brain damage communication disorder) and their impact on neurological physiotherapy practice are considered. Their effects on clinical communication are described using case examples, with particular emphasis on physiotherapist/client interactions; compensatory strategies to improve clinical conversations are suggested. Types of communication aid and their usefulness are outlined. The possible side-effects of some drugs on communication are listed. The chapter starts below with definitions of speech and language, verbal and nonverbal communication and the aetiology of adult-acquired neurological communication disorders.

SPEECH VERSUS LANGUAGE

A most important basic distinction in understanding neurological communication disorders is that of speech versus language (see Table 15.1). These are separate motor and linguistic functions, which may be separately affected in an individual or may both contribute to a person's reduced communicative effectiveness.

Speech (or spoken language) is generally the preferred method of expressing ourselves in words, i.e. of verbal communication (phonetics, phonology, syntax, semantics, pragmatics: see Table 15.1 for definitions). However, written language is another possible method of verbal communication for both clients and therapists, especially when spoken language is difficult to understand or use. Non-verbal methods of communication (i.e. not word-based) are also powerful and can be significantly exploited when an individual has severe speech and/or language difficulties. These include body language, facial expression, vocalizations, tone of voice and gesture. For example, a vocalization, such as 'ah' said with varying intonation patterns can convey whether an individual is agreeing or disagreeing, making a statement or asking a question.

Table 15.1 Definitions of speech and language.

Term	Definition	Level for academic study
Speech	The sound produced by co-ordinated movements of the lips, tongue, soft palate and vocal cords	Phonetics: study of the sounds of human speech
Language	Understanding and expression of words and sentences (using speech or writing)	Phonology: selection and sequencing of sounds Semantics: meaning Syntax: grammar Pragmatics: interactional aspects

AETIOLOGY OF ACQUIRED NEUROLOGICAL COMMUNICATION DISORDERS

The main medical diagnoses associated with neurological communication disorders are outlined in Table 15.2.

Table 15.2 Main medical diagnoses associated with acquired neurological communication disorders.

Medical diagnosis	Dysarthria	Articulatory dyspraxia	Aphasia	Right hemisphere communication disorder
Stroke	X	X	X	X
Head injury	X	X	X	x
Cerebral tumour	X	X	X	X
HIV and AIDS	X	X	X	
Parkinson's disease	X			
Motor neurone disease	X			
Multiple sclerosis	X			
Huntington's disease	X			
Myaesthenia gravis	X			

Dysarthria

Dysarthria is a disorder of speech production, caused by weakness, slowness, altered tone and/or incoordination of the muscles used in speech. It is 'a difficulty in producing or sustaining the range, force, speed and coordination of the movements needed to achieve appropriate breathing, phonation, resonance and articulation for speech' (Royal College of Speech and Language Therapists 2006, p. 249). It can range from mild to severe, with symptoms varying according to the locus of damage. Speech intelligibility will either gradually improve or deteriorate over time, dependent on the aetiology. The main symptoms and effects of dysarthria are listed in Table 15.3 (for a fuller description see Yorkston et al 1999). (See also Boxes 15.1 and 15.2.)

Table 15.3 Symptoms of dysarthria and their effects on communication.

Symptom	Effect
Reduced articulatory accuracy	'Slurred' speech – person may sound drunk
Altered rate	Speech is slower/faster than normal, or festinant (accelerating)
Reduced intonation/altered stress	Speech sounds 'boring' or staccato
Altered volume	Speech is quieter or louder than normal
Altered nasality	Person will sound as if they have a cold
Reduced effectiveness of breathing for speech	Speech flow is interrupted for top-up breaths

Box 15.1

An example of mild dysarthria:

Mr A has recently been diagnosed with motor neurone disease. His speech is normal for most of the day, but becomes slurred in the evening. If he has a quiet day, speech fatigue is less obvious.

Box 15.2

An example of severe dysarthria:

Mrs B has had Parkinson's disease for the past twelve years. Her articulation is very limited by reduced lip and tongue movements and her voice is very quiet. People who know her well can follow what she says as long as there is no background noise.

Impact of dysarthria on clinical communication

Dependent on the severity, an individual's dysarthria may have either little or significant impact on clinical conversations during physiotherapy sessions. Some possible effects include:

- Increased time required to understand what the individual is saying
- Increased time for individual to convey messages via a communication aid
- Altering clinical environment to reduce background noise
- Possible re-scheduling of appointment time.

Compensatory strategies for dysarthria (helping clinical conversations)

- Liaise regularly with the individual's speech and language therapist on the most useful compensatory strategies – likely to change over time and differ according to type and severity of dysarthria
- Most people with dysarthria will understand what you say, so there is no need to speak louder or otherwise adapt what you say
- Ask the individual what they find most helpful and most unhelpful, e.g. giving the individual extra time to respond is most helpful
- If you have not fully understood:
  - repeat back the part of the message you have understood, rather than the individual having to repeat the whole message
  - or ask yes-no questions for clarification
- If the person is able to write, provide a pencil and paper to supplement or replace speech attempts, if required
- Ensure that the individual's communication aid is available, if appropriate
- Sometimes very simple compensations are adequate, e.g. ensuring you are face-to-face with the person to gain the maximum from all non-verbal information, as well as spoken component.

Communication aids

Communication aids are probably most helpful for people with dysarthria and provide 'methods of communicating which supplement or replace speech and handwriting' (Royal College of Speech and Language Therapists 2006, pp. 229–230). They represent one branch of augmentative and alternative communication (AAC). The other is unaided AAC, e.g. body movements, gesture, signing or eye-pointing. This has the advantage of being present without any gadgets but a disadvantage in difficulty conversing about topics out of the immediate context. Some people with acquired neurological disorders find some methods of unaided AAC difficult, e.g. because of hemiplegia, dyspraxia or bradykinesia.

Communication aids can broadly be divided into two categories, both with advantages and disadvantages (see Table 15.4):

- Low-tech – generally paper-based (e.g. Figures 15.1 and 15.2)
- High-tech – usually electronic with voice output (e.g. Figure 15.3). For more detailed information, see Beukelman et al (2000).

Table 15.4 Communication aids used by people with acquired neurological communication disorders.

	Low-tech communication aids	High-tech communication aids
Examples	Alphabet chart, communication book/passport	Lightwriter (see Figure 15.3) TalksBac (predictive communication device for adults with non-fluent aphasia)
Advantages	Easily replaced, portable, cheap	Flexibility in message composition, messages may be pre-programmed
Disadvantages	Slow, limited by contents, demanding on listener concentration	Break-downs, require high level of manual dexterity and relatively intact cognition, lengthy training, tuning in to synthetic voice quality

Helping an individual to use a communication aid
● Ensure the communication aid is to hand during physiotherapy sessions
● Conversation using all communication aids will be slower than normal speech, especially while the individual is learning its use, so clinical conversations will take longer
● Continue to focus on the individual as well as the communication aid, so you do not miss any non-verbal communication
● Modify your questioning to enable a short but informative response.

Articulatory dyspraxia
The theory related to acquired articulatory dyspraxia is controversial. Some authors define it as a motor (speech) disorder in its own right; others construe it as part of aphasia (see later) and so include it among language (linguistic) symptoms. Using the former theoretical stance, articulatory dyspraxia arises from 'deficits in the planning or programming of movement for speech, although movement of the same musculature for non-speech tasks is normal' (Yorkston et al 1999, p. 72). It can range in severity from mild to severe. Symptoms are described in Table 15.5, p. 250. (See also Boxes 15.3 and 15.4.)

Impact of articulatory dyspraxia on clinical communication
The impact will vary with severity and possible co-existence of dysarthria and aphasia. Some possible effects include:
● Increased time required to understand what the individual is saying
● Frustration caused by inconsistency of speech production.

15

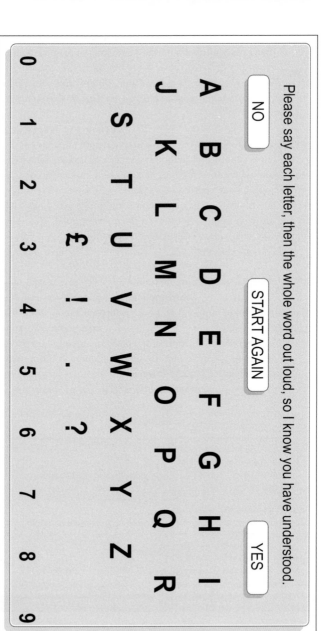

Please say each letter, then the whole word out loud, so I know you have understood.

NO   START AGAIN   YES

A B C D E F G H I
J K L M N O P Q R
S T U V W X Y Z
£ ! . ?
0 1 2 3 4 5 6 7 8 9

Figure 15.1
An alphabet chart.

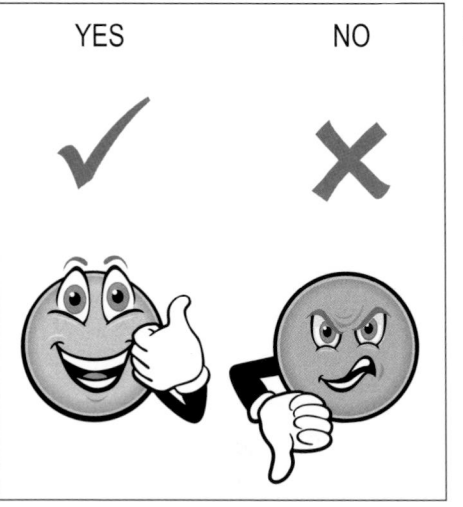

Figure 15.2
A yes-no chart.

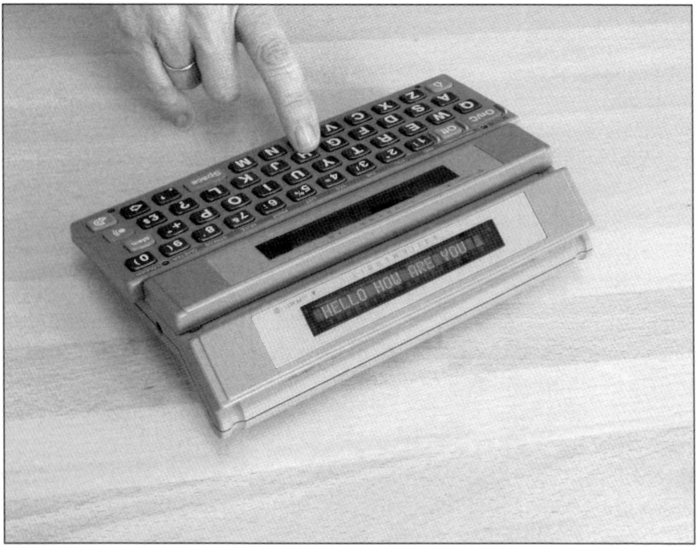

Figure 15.3
A Lightwriter. Reproduced with permission of Toby Churchill Ltd.

Table 15.5 Symptoms of articulatory dyspraxia and their effects on communication.

Symptom	Effect
Articulatory errors and inconsistencies	Reduced speech intelligibility
Articulatory groping and re-trials	Reduced speech intelligibility, increased message time
Difficulty in initiating articulations	Problems starting the message
Secondary effect on speech rhythm and intonation	Altered pattern of speech

Box 15.3

An example of mild articulatory dyspraxia:
Mrs C had a stroke nine months ago. When she uses long words, she sometimes misarticulates sounds and misprogrammes the order of the sounds, for example, 'umlebela' for 'umbrella'. She knows as soon as she has said something incorrectly and can usually correct herself if she slows down.

Box 15.4

An example of severe articulatory dyspraxia:
Mr D had a stroke two months ago. He can be stimulated easily to saying 'automatic sequences', such as the days of the week and the months of the year, and can finish off a phrase that someone else starts, such as 'fish and . . .' but is unable to say anything spontaneously. He is extremely frustrated and his family cannot understand why he can sing songs he knew before his stroke but cannot tell them what he wants.

Compensatory strategies for articulatory dyspraxia
The strategies listed above for people with dysarthria are also effective for people with articulatory dyspraxia.

Aphasia
Aphasia is a linguistic disorder, which can affect both language comprehension and production so that the individual with aphasia may have difficulty with:
● understanding of the spoken word/spoken sentences
● understanding of the written word/written sentences

- word finding/sentence construction
- spelling/writing sentences
- gesture/time/money.

It is usually associated with damage to the dominant cerebral hemisphere. The severity and nature of symptoms will vary with the extent and location of the brain damage. For a fuller description see Chapey (2001) and for current research on aspects of aphasia, see the journal Aphasiology. The terms 'dysphasia' and 'aphasia' are now used interchangeably, with 'aphasia' currently the dominant term. Aphasia can co-exist with dysarthria and articulatory dyspraxia. Aphasia is usually a chronic disorder, although spontaneous recovery is usually apparent for some months after the stroke. The main symptoms of aphasia and their effects on communication are shown in Table 15.6. (See also Boxes 15.5 and 15.6.)

Box 15.5

> **An example of mild aphasia:**
> Ms E is able to hold normal conversations in a one-to-one situation but finds it difficult to understand when watching her favourite soap operas on television. She avoids family parties as she gets very tired trying to follow conversations in noisy places. She occasionally says 'son' when she means 'daughter', which produces some misunderstandings. She now has some difficulty in writing words with irregular spellings, such as 'shoe' and 'heart'.

Box 15.6

> **An example of severe aphasia:**
> Following a stroke six months ago, Mr F watches only sport on television now as he cannot follow other programmes. His wife has to simplify what she says so that he can understand her. His spontaneous spoken output is a four-letter swear word, produced with varying emphasis, depending on whether Mr F is asking a question, making a statement or exclamation. He can copy his name and address with 75% accuracy but cannot write anything he wants to say.

Impact of aphasia on clinical communication

Dependent on the severity, an individual's aphasia may have either little or significant impact on clinical conversations during physiotherapy sessions. Possible effects include:

Table 15.6 Symptoms of aphasia and their effects on communication.

Symptom	Effects
Phonology – difficulty deciphering sounds in others' spoken words or incorrect selection of sounds in words or incorrect order of sounds when using spoken language	● Difficulty in understanding what is being said ● Phonemic paraphasias, e.g. 'float' → 'toat', 'purple' → 'purckle' ● Neologisms, e.g. 'skatch' 'snookle' (i.e. sound selection so distorted that target word is not recognizable) ● Jargon – meaningless strings of sounds but with appropriate rhythm
Semantics – word meaning affected – difficulty in understanding others or expressing self	● Difficulty understanding the meaning in what others say or written material ● Semantic paraphasias, i.e. a word close in meaning to the target is expressed, e.g. 'yes' for 'no', 'mother' for 'wife', 'children' for 'grandchildren', 'pen' for 'pencil', 'shoes' for 'socks' ● Verbal paraphasia, i.e. a real word unrelated to the target is expressed, 'dog' for 'chair', 'bag' for 'milk', 'jumper' for 'aeroplane', 'clock' for 'horse' ● Recurrent utterance or stereotype, i.e. same inappropriate word or phrase expressed whenever the person tries to speak – may be a swear word ● Word finding difficulty, i.e. cannot think of the exact word to express. They may have partial knowledge, e.g. 'it's a long word', 'it starts with p'. The word may be 'at the tip of the tongue' ● Circumlocution to try to overcome word finding difficulty, e.g. 'wrote lots of plays, old man, tragedies' (target – Shakespeare) – may use a gesture
Syntax – sentence grammar affected	● Difficulty understanding others' spoken sentences or written material ● Agrammatism – difficulty using grammatical words in sentences, e.g. 'dog dug mud bone' for 'the dog dug in the mud for the bone', 'have tea?' for 'would you like some tea?' ● Paragrammatism, i.e. errors in grammar, e.g. 'the dog is digged by the bone'

- Difficulty following spoken or written therapy instructions or explanations
- Increased time required to understand what the individual is trying to tell you, e.g. symptom description, questions about exercises provided
- Altering clinical environment is required to reduce background noise.

Compensatory strategies for auditory comprehension problems

- Ensure that you have the individual's attention before you start speaking
- Use gesture and demonstration to aid comprehension with those who have difficulty in following spoken language
- If you are a fast speaker, try to speak slightly slower to give the person more time to process what you are saying
- Use short simple sentences and instructions. Do use adult words though
- Check that the person has understood. If not, repeat and rephrase as necessary
- Avoid changing the topic too abruptly and mark it with, e.g. 'now I want to speak about your leg'
- Even when an individual has severe auditory comprehension problems, some of what is said will be understood, so be very careful that you always say things that you would be happy for the individual to understand
- Shouting is **not** a useful compensatory strategy for auditory comprehension deficits.

Aphasia-friendly information (compensating for reading comprehension deficits)

Aphasia-friendly written information is modified to help the individual understand it better and is most helpful for people with moderate aphasia. People with mild reading comprehension problems will usually manage to understand health educational materials with extra time and effort. People with severe reading comprehension problems will not usually understand written text however much it is modified. Current research evidence indicates that useful principles for adapting written information include (Worrall et al 2005):

- essential information only
- use simple words and clear/big print
- use white space
- perhaps use symbols or pictures – but these may actually be distracting.

Some people with aphasia do not like pictures or symbols because of the associated child-like stigma. Aphasia-friendly written information is also much longer than normal written text. See Figure 15.4 for an example.

15

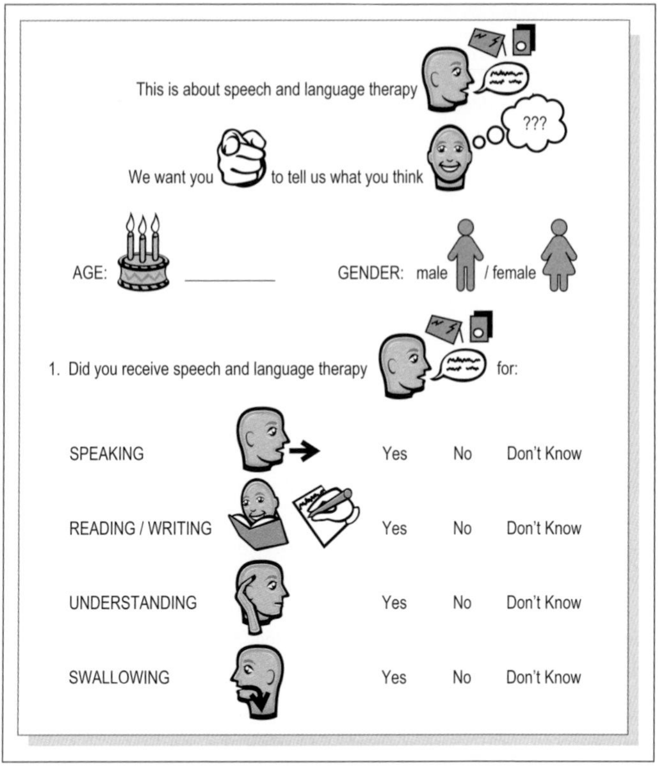

Figure 15.4
An example of aphasia-friendly material. Reproduced with permission of Victoria Gall.

Compensatory strategies for spoken language expression problems

● If you have understood what the individual has said, there is no need to correct any sound or word selection, or grammatical errors
● If the person uses one or two words instead of a full grammatical sentence, accept this if you have understood the meaning
● Encourage use of non-verbal means when spoken language problems are severe, e.g. gesture, pointing, communication book or drawing
● Check for 'yes'-'no' confusion

● Phrase your questions carefully – can the person answer reliably with 'yes' or 'no', e.g. 'have you been doing your exercises every day'? or is offering a choice more reliable, e.g. 'have you done your exercises once or seven times?' or will an open question be appropriate, e.g. 'tell me how you've been getting on with your exercises'.

Compensatory strategies for written language expression problems
● Check that the person is able to use written language expression before asking for written feedback, e.g. exercise diaries
● If they have significant difficulties, adapt feedback sheets for minimal written language input, e.g. use tick box responses.

Box 15.7

Useful aphasia web-sites and further reading about the experience of having aphasia:

www.ukconnect.org

www.speakability.org.uk

www.aphasiahelp.org

www.aphasianow.org

Parr et al 2003 & 2004

Right hemisphere communication disorder

A range of communication problems has relatively recently been identified in some people with right (non-dominant) hemisphere brain damage (RHBD). These are usually much more subtle than those experienced by people with aphasia and most can be labelled as pragmatic deficits, i.e. problems with the interactional aspects of communication. See Table 15.7 for a list of symptoms and their effects, and Myers (1999) for a fuller description. This list describes current understanding of this communication disorder, evidence about which continues to be published. (See also Boxes 15.8 and 15.9.)

It is important with this communication disorder to distinguish changes in the above aspects of communication from the individual's pre-morbid conversation style.

Impact of RHBD communication disorder on clinical communication
● Symptoms are more subtle than with other communication disorders and RHBD is still controversial in the research literature
● Any impact of this disorder is likely to affect the interactional aspects of clinical communication.

15

Table 15.7 Symptoms of right hemisphere brain damage (RHBD) and their effects on communication.

Symptom	Effect
Verbosity or taciturnity (habitual silence/reserve in speaking)	Speaks much more or much less than previously, with negative impact on conversational turn-taking
Difficulty in making inferences	Does not understand when parts of the message are implied rather than clearly stated
Difference in appreciation of humour	May take a literal meaning and so not get your jokes!
Lack of subtle use of language	May offend people
Disorganized verbal information	Symptom description less clear, difficulty keeping to the point and providing the appropriate type and amount of detail
Turn-taking	May interrupt while you are explaining what you would like done
Eye contact	May not look at you as you explain exercises
Monotonous verbal output	May sound bored

Box 15.8

An example of mild RHBD communication disorder:

Mr G's wife tells you that since his stroke, Mr G never seems to get to the point of a story. She thinks that this is why some of his friends have stopped visiting him.

Box 15.9

An example of severe RHBD communication disorder:

Mrs H comes to your gym for physiotherapy to improve her left leg function. She never stops speaking so it is very difficult to engage her in the work you have planned. She never looks at you and so you find it very difficult to initiate a turn in the conversation.

Compensatory strategies for RHBD communication disorder
- Find out whether conversational style and pragmatic abilities have changed post-stroke – wide range of normality in these aspects of communication
- Be explicit about when you require the person to look and/or listen to you during sessions
- Check that the individual has understood any more abstract instructions or explanations that you give.

WHAT SPEECH AND LANGUAGE THERAPY HAS TO OFFER PEOPLE WITH ACQUIRED NEUROLOGICAL COMMUNICATION DISORDERS
- Assessment
- Differential diagnosis
- Direct therapy to allow the person to maximize communicative effectiveness, e.g. exaggerating articulation, re-educating speech rate, therapy for semantic deficits or grammatical deficits
- Indirect intervention, e.g. suggestions on modifying environment for maximal communicative effectiveness, educating significant others and other members of the healthcare team regarding the nature of the communication disorder and useful compensatory strategies
- Provision of and training in use of communication aids: low-tech paper-based aids (e.g. alphabet charts) or high-tech aids (i.e. electronic voice output aids).

Referring to speech and language therapy
Speech and language therapy services operate an open referral system for people with communication disorders. Referrals for assessment can be made if you are concerned about a client's communication ability or if you feel that there has been a significant change in someone with a long-standing communication difficulty.

SIDE-EFFECTS OF MEDICATIONS ON COMMUNICATION
Some medications, e.g. those for Parkinson's disease, will often have a beneficial effect on communicative effectiveness. The side-effects of others will adversely affect communication (see Table 15.8 for examples).

KEY MESSAGES
- Neurological damage can affect speech and/or language
- Four different adult-acquired communication disorders have been presented in this chapter (dysarthria, articulatory dyspraxia, aphasia and right

15

hemisphere brain damage communication disorder). Communication disorders deriving from mainly cognitive problems are not included

● Each one can be mild, moderate or severe
● Depending on the locus of neurological damage, these disorders may co-occur
● Depending on medical diagnosis, the severity of the disorder(s) will decrease or increase over time
● Liaise regularly with speech and language therapy colleagues over individuals with severe difficulties in particular, so that up-to-date compensatory strategies are used to enhance the effectiveness of physiotherapy.

Table 15.8 Medications with possible adverse side-effects on communication.

Medication type	Adverse side-effect
Opioids, anticholinergics and some antidepressants, antipsychotics and antihistamines	Dry mouth
Anxiolytics, some antidepressants and anticonvulsants	Dysarthria
Anxiolytics, opioids, antipsychotics and some antidepressants, antihistamines and anticonvulsants	Drowsiness
Anticholinergics, antidepressants, anticonvulsants, hypnotics, anxiolytics – many commonly used drugs	Confusion (especially in elderly)

References

Beukelman DR, Yorkston KM, Riechle J 2000 Augmentative and alternative communication for adults with acquired neurologic disorders. Paul H Brookes Publishing Co, Baltimore.

Chapey R (ed) 2001 Language intervention strategies in aphasia and related communication disorders. Lippincott Williams and Wilkins, Philadelphia.

Myers P 1999 Right hemisphere damage: disorders of communication and cognition. Singular Publishing Group, San Diego.

Parr S, Duchan J, Pound C 2003 Aphasia inside out. Open University Press, Maidenhead.

Parr S, Pound C, Byng S 2004 The stroke and aphasia handbook. Connect Press, London.

Royal College of Speech and Language Therapists 2006 Communicating Quality 3. Royal College of Speech and Language Therapists, London.

Worrall L, Rose T, Howe T et al 2005 Access to written information for people with aphasia. Aphasiology 19:923–929.

Yorkston K M, Beukelman DR, Strand EA et al 1999 Management of motor speech disorders in children and adults, 2nd edn. Pro-ed, Austin.

Acknowledgement

Many thanks to Sheila MacLaren, physiotherapy colleague in the Kinross Locality Community Rehabilitation Team, and to colleagues in the Perth and Kinross CHP Speech and Language Therapy Service for reading and commenting on early drafts of this chapter.

15

CHAPTER 16

Orthotic management

Paul T Charlton

INTRODUCTION

The International Standards Organisation defines an orthosis as an external device used to modify the structural or functional characteristics of the neuromuscular system (ISO 8549-1:1989). This includes all splints, calipers, braces, supports, trusses, casts. The current terminology of orthoses is based on a 1976 publication (Training Council of Orthotists 1976) but only describes the sections of the body the orthosis covers; common examples are set out in Table 16.1. Matters are further complicated by use of trade or manufacturer names, or names limited to certain localities; orthoses are best described by function.

Evidence for the use of orthoses is abundant but inconclusive. There are many small studies considering effects on gait and tempo-spatial parameters (de Wit et al 2004, Franceschini et al 2003, Hesse et al 1996, Hesse 2003). While the findings are generally positive, they are too variable to provide strong clinical evidence. There is less research on the subjective effects of orthoses, such as muscle activity and motor learning, with some indications of benefit (Hesse et al 1999, Leung & Moseley 2002). The 2004 report of a consensus conference on the orthotic management of people after stroke (Condie 2004) concluded that the scientific literature on orthotic management of stroke was generally poor in terms of quality and quantity. As with physiotherapy, lack of research should not negate intervention and clinical reasoning based on sound principles should lead to patient benefit.

Basic principles

Orthoses are based on a minimum of three point force systems; an example for controlling foot plantar flexion is provided in Figure 16.1 and Table 16.2. By considering where to apply forces for the desired effect we can ensure our orthosis is designed and applied appropriately and where potential pressure problems may arise.

Orthoses act as levers; the longer the lever, the more comfortable and effective the orthosis. Short knee braces require considerable force to achieve the same turning effect as full length orthoses.

Table 16.1 Classification of orthoses.

Abbreviation	Type of orthosis	Description
FO	Foot orthosis	Insole, shoe
AFO	Ankle foot orthosis	Any orthosis covering the ankle and foot, below knee plaster, anklet, below knee stocking
KAFO	Knee ankle foot orthosis	Any orthosis covering the knee ankle and foot, commonly refers to full leg caliper
LSO	Lumbar sacral orthosis	Corset or spinal brace
WHO	Wrist hand orthosis	Any orthosis covering the wrist and hand

Table 16.2 Control of plantar flexion.

Force	Orthotic design	Therapist as an orthosis
1	Footplate or shoe	Push foot up
2	Heel strap or shoe fastening	Push heel down
3	Top posterior edge of calf band or orthosis	Keep calf forward by having patient on a stable base

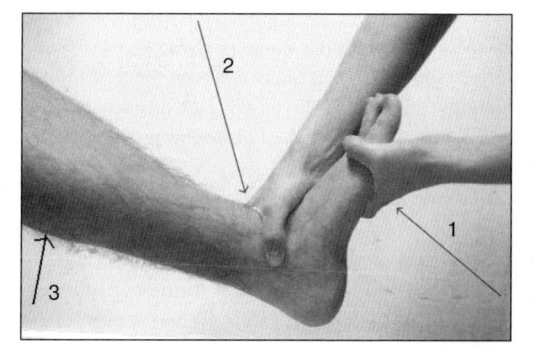

Figure 16.1
Control of plantar flexion:
Force 1 indicates pushing
the foot up while 2
demonstrates the force
required to keep the heel
down and 3 the
counterforce from the
patient on a stable base.

16

In assessing potential to correct or achieve alignment, it is important to consider the force required and the patient's ability to tolerate this. Degree of force will also influence design of orthosis which must have sufficient rigidity to apply correction and withstand deforming forces.

POTENTIAL AIMS AND LIMITATIONS OF INTERVENTION

Orthoses may be used to achieve the following therapeutic aims:
● Stretch or prevent contractures
● Provide stability
● Improve alignment
● Optimize alignment
● Challenge stability.

Orthoses always have an input to the sensory as well as the motor system. Some orthoses, such as silicone and Lycra, provide compression, sensory input and some limitation on joint movement but are not based on biomechanical principles. It is not fully understood how these work and research continues.

In early rehabilitation, patients will often adopt abnormal alignment to achieve stability in the absence of normal control. Early rehabilitation may involve challenging stability by improving alignment to elicit normal anti-gravity recruitment (Shumway-Cook & Woollacott 2001). It is suggested that combining appropriate orthotic intervention to optimize alignment and therapy intervention to access and recruit appropriate muscle groups could be the ideal intervention. Orthoses can improve safety, efficiency and reduce compensatory movements (Table 16.3).

Table 16.3 Common compensations and orthotic solutions.

Common compensation	Common cause	Orthotic solution
Circumduction	Lack of ankle dorsiflexion	Maintain dorsiflexion
Excessive knee and hip flexion	Lack of ankle dorsiflexion	Maintain dorsiflexion
Hip hitching	Lack of ankle dorsiflexion	Maintain dorsiflexion
Knee hyperextension	Lack of ankle dorsiflexion	Maintain dorsiflexion
Knee hyperextension	Lack of quadriceps activity	Optimize alignment and challenge stability to induce appropriate recruitment
Knee hyperextension	Lack of quadriceps activity	Optimize alignment and provide stability
Knee hyperextension	Lack of hamstring activity	Optimize alignment

16

Limitations of orthotic intervention include preventing normal movement and inducing weakness by non use of muscles. It should be recognized and accepted that normal movement is not possible within an orthosis provided to mechanically limit range. If there is potential to access useful movement at such joints, then a regimen should be adopted to include periods outside the orthosis to develop control of the joint. This should obviously be within a safe environment and preferably in normal alignment, possibly under supervision.

Orthotic management in upper motor neurone syndromes

With increased tone, the force required to achieve and maintain alignment is greater than in its absence. Care must be taken as discomfort and pain from corrective pressure could exacerbate the abnormal tone. However, the principles of optimizing alignment with a view to maximizing normal movement and function still apply. Success will depend on identifying influencing factors and intervening accordingly.

It is strongly recommended that a systematic approach is used to identify orthotic intervention rather than seeking orthoses claiming to be 'tone inhibiting' (Table 16.4).

Orthotic management in lower motor neurone syndromes

A common challenge with slow progressive neuropathies, such as Charcot–Marie–Tooth disease and muscular dystrophies, is gradual lack of range at joints in the presence of muscle imbalance. Orthoses can be used to limit loss of range. Contracture correction devices apply low load prolonged stretch to reverse contracture. Care is needed when trying to normalize alignment, as it may interfere with compensations that patients depend on for function.

Table 16.4 Factors affecting abnormal tone and potential orthotic intervention.

Factors which may influence increased tone	Potential orthotic intervention
Specific movements	Limit movement to optimal alignment
Movement within a certain range	Limit range
Poor alignment	Realign
Weakness/instability	Provide stability
Fatigue	Optimize efficiency
Pain	Optimize weight-bearing surfaces
Confidence	Sensory input

16

Assessment

Assessment should involve identifying the aim of intervention and how it would fit within a treatment regimen. This involves simulating orthotic intervention by handling or positioning the patient to ensure the change in alignment is tolerable and effective. This will also allow assessment of the force required to achieve the desired effect and any negative effects of intervention. Consideration of sensation, oedema, compliance and cosmesis should then be used to identify orthotic design and materials required.

In the early stages, an orthosis may only be required to facilitate recovery, in which case a permanent orthosis may not be practical and a temporary orthosis could be made using synthetic plaster. Combination casts and plaster back-slabs are all forms of orthosis (Edwards & Charlton 2002). The importance is in fabrication and material selection to achieve the required function and alignment in the presence of any deforming forces such as bodyweight or spasticity. It is possible to integrate orthotic intervention into all stages of neuro-rehabilitation (Butler 1997, Butler & Major 1992, Butler et al 1992) and enabling function in optimal alignment thereby reducing compensations (Table 16.5).

Whenever a change in alignment can facilitate improved function or recruitment then there is a potential for orthotic intervention. While therapists may prefer to do this manually, they cannot always be present or maintain alignment during function. With care, this may be achieved with an orthosis. Time and cost may be

Table 16.5 Timing of intervention and role of orthoses.

Timing of intervention	Use of orthosis	Time worn	Treatment regime
Early weight bearing	Optimize alignment and provide distal stability	During therapy sessions	Facilitate recruitment against gravity in controlled environment
Early walking	Optimize alignment and provide distal stability	Between therapy sessions	Maintain alignment and stability between treatment sessions
Functional walking	Optimize alignment and provide distal stability	Between therapy sessions	Maintain alignment and stability between treatment sessions
Long term	Optimize alignment and provide distal stability	Permanently	Manage a deficit in the absence of recovery

16

prohibitive for short-term intervention but orthotic principles can be used with temporary orthoses or plasters.

Many patients will recover so that the need for orthotic control reduces or is eliminated, hence the need for regular review and re-assessment. Others will be left with a deficit requiring long-term maintenance and management. The danger of not addressing these deficits at the end of the rehabilitation process is the potential for contracture and adoption of compensatory strategies which may be difficult to reverse if identified later. It may still be possible to change alignment and learned patterns but may require considerable commitment of resource from both the service and the patient (Baker & Charlton 2005).

TYPES OF ORTHOSES AND APPLICATIONS
Foot and ankle problems
Common foot and ankle postures, their potential proximal effects and orthotic solutions are presented in Table 16.6.

Insoles
Insoles may be accommodating or corrective. Accommodating insoles do not attempt to realign the foot fully but attempt to provide an improved weight-

Table 16.6 Common foot and ankle postures and potential proximal effects.

Foot & ankle posture	Proximal effects	Correction	Orthosis
Excessive plantar flexion, equinus deformity	Knee hyperextension, potential hip retraction	Limit plantar flexion or accommodate equinus	Rigid polypropylene AFO, hinged AFO with plantar-flexion stop and/or heel raise to accommodate equinus
Excessive dorsiflexion and lack of plantar flexion	Excessive knee and hip flexion	Limit dorsiflexion	Fixed polypropylene AFO
Pronation	Internal tibial and hip rotation	Prevent over pronation	Medial heel wedge, medial arch support, appropriate AFO (ankle foot orthosis)
Supination	External tibial and hip rotation	Prevent supination	Lateral heel wedge, appropriate AFO (ankle orthosis)

AFO, ankle foot orthosis.

bearing surface. In the sagittal plane, this may be in the form of a heel raise in a fixed equinus position. Accommodating insoles can provide stability and reduce pain and proximal compensations, and tend to be used for fixed deformities.

Corrective insoles are used in mobile feet where correction is possible. When correcting the foot and associated joints, the insole is shaped or angled to offer corrective force in weight bearing. Medial wedging will tend to resist eversion while lateral wedging will resist inversion. The dynamic insole offers support to the dynamic arches of the foot and may be of benefit to neurologically impaired patients by offering a more stable base and greater weight-bearing surface for the foot.

Special footwear

These may be needed when normal footwear cannot accommodate foot deformities and/or the insoles required to manage them. It may be possible to provide special orthotic extra depth footwear but in extreme cases it may be necessary to provide made-to-measure or made-to-plaster-impression footwear.

Supra malleoli ankle foot orthoses (ankle braces)

There are many types of ankle foot orthoses (AFOs). Those termed ankle braces have limited leverage at both the ankle and subtalar joint but allow for more control than offered by insoles (Figure 16.2). They give some limitation to foot

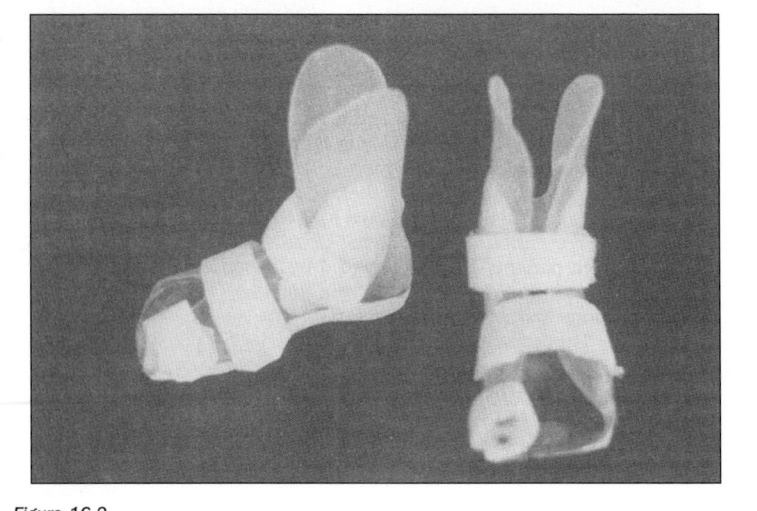

Figure 16.2
Supramalleolar ankle foot orthosis (AFO).

drop if corrective forces required are minimal. Generally they are used to provide stability to the subtalar joint where inversion or eversion is problematic if the deforming forces are large, e.g. due to increased tone.

Ankle foot orthoses (AFOs)

These orthoses potentially offer maximum control to the ankle and subtalar complex. It is important to give careful consideration to the demands and expectation of the orthosis, as depending on design and stiffness, it can have considerable influence in both swing and stance phase of gait in both the sagittal and coronal plane. More flexible designs will have less impact on stance phase while rigid designs can be a powerful tool in modifying proximal alignment. A rigid AFO is influenced considerably by shoe design and especially heel height (Figure 16.3).

It is often assumed that callipers of the metal frame design are old fashioned but they offer practical alternatives to the thermoplastic design. Generally,

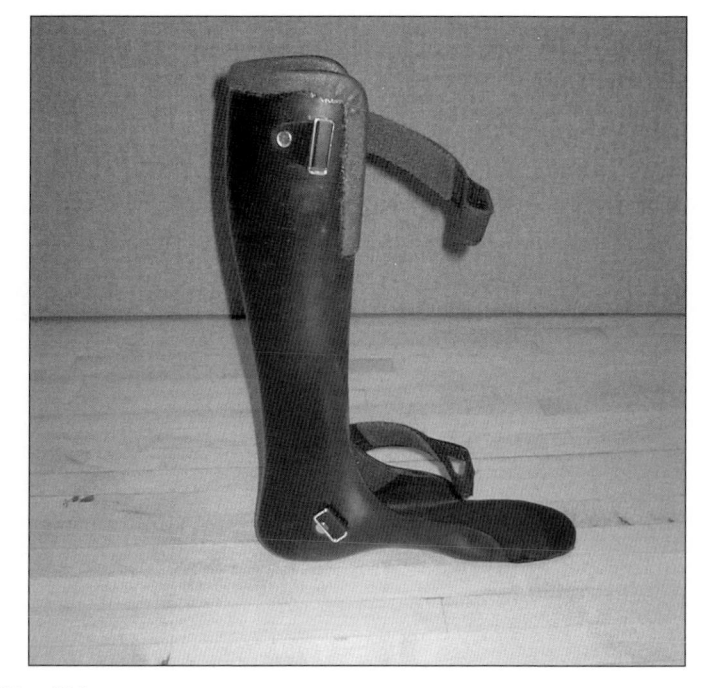

Figure 16.3
Rigid polypropylene ankle foot orthosis (AFO).

thermoplastic orthoses are more accurate and offer better control with reduced weight while conventional metal callipers allow a degree of adjustment and accommodation.

Knee ankle foot orthoses (KAFOs)

In neurorehabilitation, knee problems commonly occur in combination with control challenges at the ankle, so both problems can be resolved with one orthosis (KAFOs). If only the knee is addressed, then problems at the ankle are highlighted due to the close relationship between the two joints. There are, however, some presentations where the knee is the prime problem and a knee orthosis is appropriate. The challenge of knee orthoses (KO) is the relatively high forces and short levers, so when used they should be as long as possible (Figure 16.4).

KAFOs offer maximum control at the knee and ankle and can help with hip extension in stance. Control will depend on design, most commonly KAFOs are used to provide knee stability in stance in the presence of poor extension; however they can be provided purely for medial, lateral or hyperextension control. Prior to provision of a KAFO, it may well be worth assessing by use of a back slab and AFO to ensure functional effect and patient compliance, as KAFOs are relatively expensive.

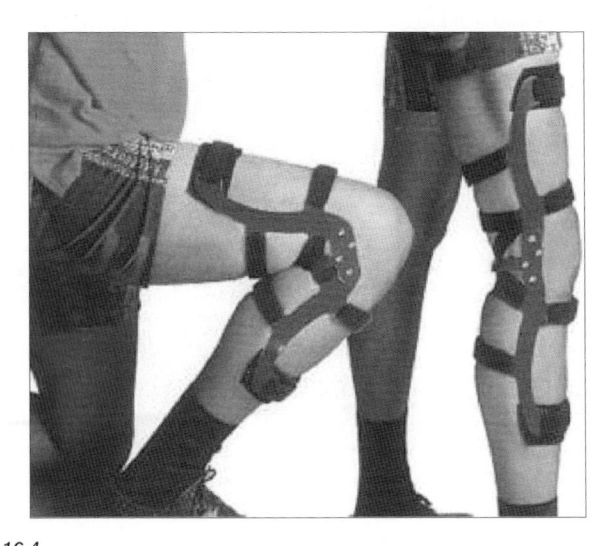

Figure 16.4
Long hinged knee orthoses (KO) for control of hyperextension.

16

Shoulder orthoses

There are many orthoses advertising ability to reduce shoulder subluxation. Those holding the humerus by a cuff are likely to have a limited effect due to lack of a bony fix. In sitting the problem is probably best managed by supporting with pillows or more permanent attachment simply to support the weight of the arm.

Hand and wrist orthoses

Good alignment of the wrist in some degree of extension is essential for effective control of the hand and fingers. An orthosis to hold the wrist in such a position will be functional. Resting orthoses to maintain range are important to maintain function and facilitate hygiene in situations where increased tone closes the hand in a fist. Where the force required to oppose increased tone is such that application of an orthosis is difficult and painful, spasticity management in whatever form may be required to make orthotic management viable.

Orthoses may offer proprioceptive input rather than mechanical stability to the benefit of some patients. Soft close-fitting materials such as silicone and Lycra orthoses may be of some benefit.

COMPLIANCE, CHOICE AND COMPROMISE

The least effective orthosis is the one that is never used. By involving the patient in their treatment and clinical reasoning, compliance may improve. If the effect of the orthoses is simulated and objectives explained, this may help. However, some patients will reject orthotic intervention on the grounds of cosmesis, comfort and taste in footwear. These considerations must form part of assessment and a less intrusive compromise may have to be reached. Some patients reach a point whereby they can manage well over short distances or within safe environments but may only wear an orthosis when they fatigue or are in unfamiliar surroundings.

Tyson & Thornton (2001) sought the views of hemiplegic patients wearing hinged polypropylene AFOs and found that even large cumbersome orthoses can be well tolerated if there is perceived functional benefit.

ACCESSING AN ORTHOTIC SERVICE

Orthotic service delivery to the NHS in the UK is widely variable. Most hospitals contract in the service. To provide optimum orthotic intervention, a close working relationship is required between the treating therapist and orthotist, including joint assessments. As well as clinical work, it can be very useful to input training and developments between professions to best understand and benefit from each discipline's abilities.

References

Baker K, Charlton P 2005 The effect of physiotherapy and orthotic intervention 40 years after stroke. Physiotherapy Research International 10:169–175.

Butler PB 1997 Improvement of gait parameters following late intervention in traumatic brain injury: a long term follow up report of a single case. Clinical Rehabilitation 11:220–226.

Butler PB, Major RE 1992 The learning of motor control: biomechanical considerations. Physiotherapy 78:1–6.

Butler PB, Thompson N, Major RE 1992 Improvement of walking performance of children with cerebral palsy: preliminary results. Developmental Medicine and Child Neurology 34:566–567.

Condie E 2004 A report on a consensus conference on the orthotic management of stroke patients. ISPO, ISBN 87-89-809-14-9.

de Wit DC, Buurke JH, Nijlant JMM et al 2004 The effect of an ankle foot orthosis on walking ability on chronic stroke patients: a randomised control trial. Clinical Rehabilitation 18:550–557.

Edwards S, Charlton P 2002 Splinting and the use of orthoses in the management of patients with neurological disorders. In: Edwards S (ed) Neurological physiotherapy; a problem-solving approach, 2nd edn. Churchill Livingstone, London, pp 219–253.

Franceschini M, Massucci M, Ferrari L, Paroli C 2003 Effects of an ankle foot orthosis on spatiotemporal parameters and energy cost of hemiparetic gait. Clinical Rehabilitation 17:368–372.

Hesse S 2003 Rehabilitation of gait after stroke: evaluation, principles of therapy, novel treatment approaches, and assistive devices. Topics in Geriatric Rehabilitation 19(2):109–126.

Hesse S, Leucke D, Jahnke MT 1996 Gait function in spastic hemiparetic patients walking barefoot, with firm shoes and with ankle foot orthosis. International Journal of Rehabilitation Research 19:133–139.

Hesse S, Werner C, Matthias K 1999 Non velocity related effects of a rigid double stopped ankle foot orthosis on gait and lower limb muscle activity of hemiparetic subjects with an equinovarus deformity. Stroke 30:1855–1861.

ISO 8549-1 1989 Prosthetics and orthotics – Vocabulary – Part 1: General terms for external prostheses and orthoses.

Leung J, Moseley A 2002 Impact of ankle foot orthoses on gait and leg muscle activity in adults with hemiplegia. Systematic literature review. Physiotherapy 89(1):39–50.

Shumway-Cook A, Woollacott MH 2001 Motor control. Theory and practical applications. Lippincott Williams and Wilkins, Baltimore.

Training Council of Orthotists 1976 Classification of orthoses. HMSO, London.

Tyson SF, Thornton H 2001 The effect of a hinged ankle foot orthosis on hemiplegic gait: objective measures and users opinions. Clinical Rehabilitation 15:53–58.

Further reading and key web sites

British Asssociation of Prosthetists and Orthotists (BAPO): www.BAPO.org.

International Society for Prosthetics and Orthotics: www.ISPO.org.uk.

16

Charlton P, Ferguson D 2001 Orthoses, splinting and casting. In: Barnes M, Johnson G (eds) Upper motor syndrome and spasticity clinical management and neurophysiology. Cambridge University Press, pp 142–165.

Kent RM, Gilbertson L, Geddes JML 2004 Orthotic devices for abnormal limb posture after stroke or non-progressive cerebral causes of spasticity. The Cochrane Library Issue 2, Chichester, UK.

APPENDICES

Neurological investigations

Christopher Kennard

INTRODUCTION

There are a wide variety of neurological investigations which can be used to confirm or refute a clinical diagnosis or differentiate between a range of possible diagnoses, made on the basis of taking a neurological history and carefully examining the patient. It is therefore essential that the most appropriate investigations are ordered and in a logical sequence – a blunderbuss approach to investigations is to be frowned upon. It is also important to plan investigations which provide the maximal amount of information about the patient's illness but which will result in the least possible discomfort and risk.

The principal investigations for diagnosing brain and spinal cord disease are computed tomography (CT) scanning, magnetic resonance imaging (MRI), evoked potentials (EP) and electroencephalography (EEG), and for peripheral nerve and muscle disease electromyography (EMG) and nerve conduction studies.

BRAIN AND SPINAL CORD IMAGING INVESTIGATIONS

To make the most of imaging the brain and spinal cord it is essential that the focus of the imaging is directed at the correct area of the neuraxis. The symptomatology of the patient and any abnormal physical signs combined with a reasonable knowledge of neuroanatomy should prevent scanning the incorrect area of the neuraxis. Occasionally it is necessary to image the whole neuraxis when signs are present which could arise from lesions both in the brain and/or the spinal cord. Imaging techniques are summarized in Table Ap.1.1.

ELECTRODIAGNOSTIC TESTS

These tests involve the amplification and recording of the electrical activity of the brain and peripheral nerves, which may be either spontaneous or induced by appropriate simulation (Table Ap.1.2, p. 281).

Table Ap.1.1 Brain and spinal cord imaging.

Test	Description of technique	What it tells us	Presentation of common problems
Plain radiology of the skull	Routine X-rays of the skull. Usually both lateral and antero-posterior views are taken.	Reveals the presence of bone abnormalities which may be intrinsic e.g. skull fractures or bone tumours, or due to extrinsic lesions in the brain impinging on the bone e.g. enlargement of the pituitary fossa due to a pituitary tumour or opacity of the sinuses (frontal and maxillary) due to sinusitis.	Mainly used for patients presenting with mild to moderate head injuries to rule out skull fractures. Of no use in patients presenting with headaches only.
Plain radiology of the spinal column	Routine X-rays of the spine usually taken in lateral and antero-posterior views.	Reveals the bony vertebrae but not the intervertebral discs or the spinal cord. Can reveal spinal fractures following trauma, and collapse of vertebrae resulting from osteomyelitis, Paget's disease, and neoplasia (usually secondary deposits), which may result in cord repression. X-rays of spine will reveal evidence of osteo-arthrosis.	Useful investigation in patients with new severe cervical or lumbar back pain to help to exclude secondary deposits. Also important investigation in patients after head and neck trauma to exclude fractures.

Computed tomography (CT) scanning	The first imaging technique which provided images of slices through the brain. The X-ray beam passes through the brain and is blocked to varying degrees by tissues of differing density. The resulting X-rays are recorded using crystals. This tissue density is measured across several tomographic horizontal levels, and computers construct images of slices of the brain. Different structures in the brain can be revealed. Enhancement of the images, produced by the intravenous injection of a contrast medium, may add precision to the diagnosis.	CT scanning shows the brain tissues and the size and shape of the ventricular system. It reveals cerebral haemorrhage and infarction, brain tumours, abscesses and enlargement of the ventricles, hydrocephalus (see Fig. Ap.1.1).	In patients presenting with stroke a CT scan is essential to exclude haemorrhage before treatment with thrombolytic therapy. Useful test in patients with new headache to exclude a brain tumour but depending on availability, MRI scanning provides a more detailed scan.
Magnetic resonance imaging (MRI)	Similar to CT scanning producing 'slice' images of the brain in any plane, but of higher resolution and without the need to use ionizing radiation. The patient's head is placed in a powerful magnetic field, which causes temporary physical changes in the atoms of the brain. This results in the production of radiofrequency energy which is picked up and is then subjected to computer analysis from which images are constructed.	Produces exquisite images of the brain with differentiation of grey and white matter. Particularly good for identifying abnormalities of the white matter such as demyelination and for defining the spinal cord with clear visualization of cervical and lumbar roots. Gradually superseding CT scanning.	Useful in patients presenting with monophasic neurological symptoms and signs such as optic neuritis, sensory disturbance in one limb or unilateral ataxia. If the MRI reveals evidence of demyelination this supports the diagnosis of multiple sclerosis (see Fig. Ap.1.2). Vascular lesions, such as aneurysms, can also be visualized (Fig. Ap.1.3).

(continued)

Table Ap.1.1 Brain and spinal cord imaging—cont'd.

Test	Description of technique	What it tells us	Presentation of common problems
Cerebral angiography	In cerebral angiography a contrast medium, which is opaque to X-rays, is injected via an intra-arterial catheter into the cerebral blood vessels. This outlines all the extra and intra-cerebral vasculature. In recent years, MR angiography has taken over from cerebral angiography and is preferable because it is non-invasive and does not require ionizing radiation.	The extra and intra-cerebral blood vessels are clearly delineated and any blockage, abnormality e.g. arteriovenous malformation or aneurysm (see Fig. Ap.1.4).	Used routinely to investigate a patient with a sudden onset of a very intense headache suggestive of a subarachnoid haemorrhage in which blood leaks into the CSF usually from a ruptured Berry aneurysm.
Positron emission tomography (PET)	Radioactive isotopes are used to label naturally occurring products, e.g. H_2O and CO_2, or chemical compounds to produce ligands (bonds). These are inhaled or injected into the subject who is then placed in a scanner which contains multiple arrays of detectors. These identify the photons emanating from the decaying isotopes and computers produce maps of the local concentrations of these compounds in different regions of the brain.	PET has mainly been a research tool used to show abnormalities of regional cerebral blood flow and the distribution of certain neurotransmitter receptors e.g. dopamine in Parkinson's disease.	Can be used to show reduced dopamine uptake in the basal ganglia in certain movement disorders and can assist in distinguishing between different diseases in patients presenting with the parkinsonian syndrome. The technique is extremely costly and available in relatively few centres throughout world.

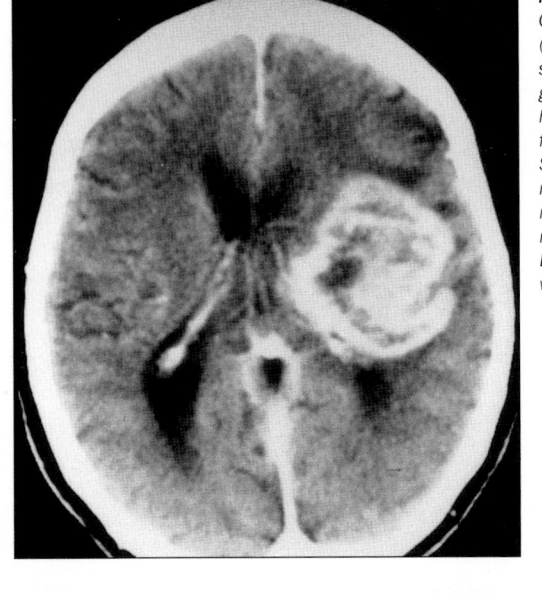

Figure Ap.1.1
Computed tomography (CT) scan of the brain showing a malignant glioma in the right hemisphere. Reproduced from Figure 2.1A in Stokes M (ed) Physical management in neurological rehabilitation, 2nd edn. London: Elsevier; 2004, with permission.

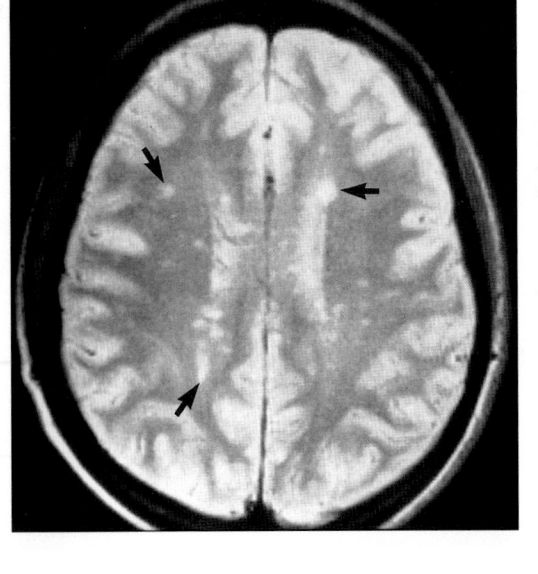

Figure Ap.1.2
Magnetic resonance scans of the brain. Axial section (T2-weighted) through the brain of a patient with multiple sclerosis. The plaques of demyelination appear as areas of high signal attenuation in the white matter (arrowed). Reproduced from Figure 2.2A in Stokes M (ed) Physical management in neurological rehabilitation, 2nd edn. London: Elsevier; 2004, with permission.

Figure Ap.1.3
Coronal section (T2)
through the brain of
a patient with an
aneurysm on the left
internal carotid artery,
lying centrally (arrowed)
and compressing the
optic chiasm.
Reproduced from Figure
2.2C in Stokes M (ed)
Physical management in
neurological
rehabilitation, 2nd edn.
London: Elsevier; 2004,
with permission.

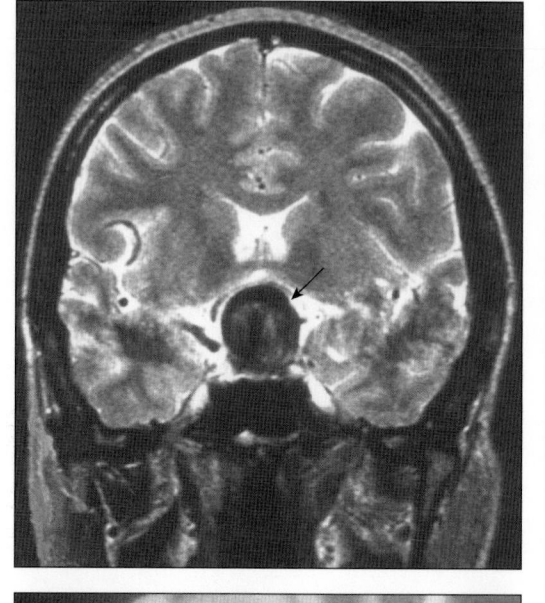

Figure Ap.1.4
A cerebral angiogram
showing a tight stenosis
of the right internal
carotid artery (arrowed)
at its origin from the
common carotid artery.
Reproduced from Figure
2.3C in Stokes M (ed)
Physical management
in neurological
rehabilitation, 2nd edn.
London: Elsevier; 2004,
with permission.

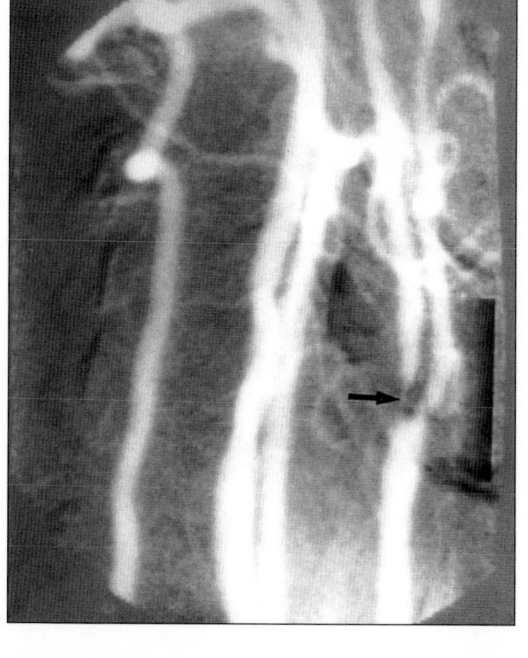

Table Ap. 1.2 Electrodiagnostic tests.

Test	Description of technique	What it tells us	Presentation of common problems
Electro-encephalography (EEG)	A method of recording spontaneous cerebral electrical activity through the intact skull. Electrodes are attached to the skull and the electrical activity is amplified to provide several channels of activity recorded on a chart recorder.	The EEG reveals alterations in brain wave activity as a result of pathological processes.	It is useful in the differential diagnosis of patients with recent altered consciousness, in particular when an encephalitic process is included in the differential diagnosis. It is also used in identifying specific types of epilepsy but is not a useful test in a patient presenting with a single blackout of unknown causation.
Evoked potentials (EP)	Sensory EP's are time-locked electrical activations of specific parts of the brain in response to a stimulus, which may be visual (flashed light or pattern), auditory (a click or tone) or a somatosensory (electrical pulse to the skin) stimulus. The brain activation is recorded using surface electrodes placed over the appropriate sensory receiving station in the cortex. The latency (the delay between the onset of the stimulus and the recorded onset of the response), is measured and provides a measure of conduction along the sensory pathway.	Sensory EP's provide information about the normal conduction along a sensory pathway. If, for example, in multiple sclerosis, there is demyelination in the optic nerve then there will be a delay in the arrival of the response in the visual cortex and the latency is prolonged. However if optic nerve fibres are lost then the response will be of reduced amplitude but normal latency.	These tests are useful in identifying subclinical episodes of demyelination in the various sensory pathways.

(continued)

Table Ap. 1.2 Electrodiagnostic tests—cont'd.

Test	Description of technique	What it tells us	Presentation of common problems
Nerve conduction velocity	The conduction along the sensory or motor component of a peripheral nerve is measured by recording the sensory or motor response downstream from a site of electrical stimulation. The time taken for the action potential to travel along a defined segment of nerve allows the conduction velocity of that nerve to be calculated.	Useful in the diagnosis of entrapment syndromes and different types of peripheral neuropathies or disorders of the neuromuscular junction, for example myasthenia gravis.	In patients presenting with numbness or tingling in the fingers of one hand. Evidence of slow conduction across the median nerve at the wrist confirms a diagnosis compression of the nerve in the carpal tunnel, carpal tunnel syndrome. In a peripheral neuropathy it can be used to distinguish between those that are due to axonal dropout from those due to demyelination.
Electromyogram (EMG)	A recording electrode is inserted into a variety of muscles in different parts of the body and the spontaneous (at rest) and induced (by contraction of the muscle) electrical muscle activity is recorded.	Can be used to differentiate between primary muscle disease and denervation of muscle due to lower motor neurone damage.	In a patient presenting with progressive weakness and wasting of the proximal muscles, EMG can differentiate between diseases such as motor neurone disease, a muscular dystrophy and polymyositis.

LUMBAR PUNCTURE AND THE CEREBROSPINAL FLUID (CSF)

Examination of CSF can be of great importance in the diagnosis of neurological disease, particularly in patients suspected of having meningitis, subarachnoid haemorrhage and inflammatory brain disease (Table Ap.1.3).

A lumbar puncture carries a very small risk if the intracranial pressure is raised due to a unilateral space-occupying lesion such as a tumour. In this situation

Table Ap.1.3 Lumbar puncture.

Test	Description of technique	What it tells us	Presentation of common problems
Lumbar puncture (LP)	After infiltration of local anaesthetic a sterile fine-bore needle is inserted into the L3-L4 interspace until it enters the subarachnoid space and CFS is obtained.	An LP allows the CSF pressure to be measured. The CSF is analysed for its cellular, chemical and bacteriological constituents.	Essential in patients presenting with recent onset of headache, neck stiffness and photophobia in whom a possible diagnosis of meningitis is made. The CSF usually reveals raised numbers of cells and the bacteria can often be identified or grown and identified, ensuring that the correct treatment is given.

Table Ap.1.4 Muscle biopsy.

Test	Description of technique	What it tells us	Presentation of common problems
Muscle biopsy	A biopsy is taken from an affected muscle either using a small needle or by an open operative procedure. The biopsied tissue is then processed for light and electron microscopy. Special staining techniques are used to identify the different muscle fibre types and abnormalities in specific enzyme pathways.	It provides evidence of the normal muscle structure and enzyme pathways and whether or not there are inflammatory processes at play.	Patients with painless proximal muscle weakness often require muscle biopsy to diagnose an inflammatory condition such as polymyositis.

Table Ap.1.5 Other tests for neurological diagnosis.

Test	Description of test	What it tells us	Presentation of common problems
Erythrocyte sedimentation rate (ESR)	Provides a measure of how quickly the red cells settle over a one hour period in a capillary tube.	In inflammatory conditions such as infection or rheumatoid arthritis the ESR is increased.	In any patient over the age of 50 presenting with headache an ESR should be undertaken to exclude temporal arteritis.
Creatine phosphokinase (CPK)	Plasma level of a constituent muscle enzyme.	Raised levels indicate muscle damage.	In patients with proximal weakness, a raised CPK is indicative of polymyositis.
Serum copper and plasma caeruloplasmin	Measurement of the level of caeruloplasmin, a copper transporter protein, combined with the level of serum copper provides evidence of copper metabolism.	If the levels are abnormal this is suggestive of the inherited movement disorder, Wilson's disease.	In patients presenting with unusual movement disorders, such as dyskinesia and dystonia, it is essential to exclude the treatable condition, Wilson's disease.

tonsillar herniation and possible death may ensue. If such a space-occupying lesion is a possibility then a CT scan must be requested beforehand.

MUSCLE BIOPSY

Muscle biopsy can be extremely valuable in the diagnosis of neuromuscular diseases, particularly intrinsic pathology of the muscle (Table Ap.1.4).

OTHER TESTS

Routine haematological, biochemical and serological analysis of blood may sometimes assist neurological diagnosis (Table Ap.1.5).

General reading

Donaghy M 2001 Brain diseases of the nervous system, 11th edn. Oxford University Press, Oxford.

Perkin GD 2002 Neurology, 2nd edn. Mosby, Edinburgh.

Warlow C 2006 The Lancet handbook of treatment in neurology. Elsevier Health Sciences, Oxford.

Drug treatment in neurological rehabilitation

Madhu Khanderia

The majority of neurological disorders are chronic and require multiple drug therapy. This appendix focuses on drugs frequently used for treating and controlling symptoms in such disorders but is not exhaustive. The reader requiring comprehensive information about a particular drug or drugs is referred to the *British National Formulary* (2008) and *Martindale* (2007). For drug uses and side-effects considered relevant to the physiotherapist, see Khanderia (2004).

International non-proprietary, or generic, names (rINN), have been used in this appendix. Proprietary names are marked with asterisks and are those used in the United Kingdom; those used outside the UK may be found in *Martindale* (2007). This appendix does not include unlicensed uses of drugs for clinical or research purposes.

Table Ap.2.1 lists a cross-reference between generic names (rINN), proprietary names and the indication for use of these drugs in neurological conditions. This is not an exhaustive list; some of the most commonly prescribed medications are referred to.

Table Ap.2.1 Generic and proprietary drug names and their use in neurological disorders.

Drug name	Main use/s of drug
Abilify*/Aripiprazole	Schizophrenia
Aceclofenac/Preservex*	Pain and inflammation
Acemetacin/Emflex*	Pain and inflammation
Acetazolamide	Tonic-clonic and partial seizures
Alfuzosin/Xatal*	Urinary retention
Allegron*/Nortriptyline	Depression, neuropathic pain
Almogran*/Almotriptan	Acute migraine

(continued)

Table Ap.2.1 Generic and proprietary drug names and their use in neurological disorders—cont'd.

Drug name	Main use/s of drug
Almotriptan/Almogran*	Acute migraine
Alteplase	Acute ischaemic stroke
Amantadine/Symmetrel*	Parkinson's disease, fatigue in multiple sclerosis (MS)
Amisulpride/Solian*	Schizophrenia
Amitriptyline	Depression, Neuropathic pain, migraine prophylaxis
Anafranil*/Clomipramine	Trigeminal neuralgia, depression
Apomorphine/Britaject*	Parkinson's disease
Arcoxia*/Etoricoxib	Pain, inflammation
Aricept*/Donepezil	Dementia
Aripiprazole/Abilify*	Schizophrenia
Aspirin	Pain, inflammation, acute ischaemic stroke
Atomoxetine/Strattera*	Attention deficit hyperactivity disorder (ADHD)
Avomine*/Promethazine	Vestibular disorders
Avonex*, Rebif*/Beta-1a interferon	MS
Baclofen/Lioresal*	Spasticity
Benzatropine/Cogentin*	Parkinson's disease
Beta-1a interferon/Avonex*, Rebif*	MS
Beta-1b interferon/Betaferon*	MS
Betaferon*/Beta-1b interferon	MS
Betahistine/Serc*	Vertigo, tinnitus
Bethanechol/Myotonin*	Urinary retention
Botulinum A toxin/Botox*, Dysport*	Torticollis, blepharospasm, spasticity
Botulinum B toxin/NeuroBloc*	Torticollis
Britaject*/Apomorphine	Parkinson's disease
Botox*/Botulinum A toxin	Torticollis, blepharospasm, spasticity
Brocadopa*/Levodopa	Parkinson's disease
Broflex*/Trihexyphenidyl (Benzhexol)	Parkinson's disease, tremor, chorea, tics

Table Ap.2.1 Generic and proprietary drug names and their use in neurological disorders—cont'd.

Drug name	Main use/s of drug
Bromocriptine/Parlodel*	Parkinson's disease
Brufen*/Ibuprofen	Pain, inflammation
Buprenorphine/Temgesic*	Pain
Cafergot*/Ergotamine	Migraine
Cabaser*/Cabergoline	Parkinson's disease
Cabergoline/Cabaser*	Parkinson's disease
Carbamazepine/Tegretol*	Seizures, trigeminal neuralgia, bipolar disorders
Cardura*/Doxazosin	Urinary retention
Celance*/Pergolide	Parkinson's disease
Celecoxib/Celebrex*	Pain, inflammation
Chlorpromazine/Largactil*	Schizophrenia and other psychoses, mania and behaviour disturbance
Cinnarizine/Stugeron*	Vestibular disorders
Cipralex*/Escitalopram	Depression, panic disorder, anxiety
Cipramil*/Citalopram	Depression/panic disorder
Citalopram/Cipramil*	Depression/panic disorder
Clomipramine/Anafranil*	Depression
Clonazepam/Rivotril*	Status epilepticus, other forms of epilepsy
Clonidine/Dixarit*	Motor tics, chorea, migraine
Clopixol*/Zuclopenthixol	Psychoses
Clotam*/Tolfenamic Acid	Acute migraine
Clozapine/Clozaril*	Schizophrenia
Clozaril*/Clozapine	Schizophrenia
Co-beneldopa/Madopar*	Parkinson's disease
Co-careldopa/Sinemet*	Parkinson's disease
Codeine	Pain, diarrhoea
Cogentin*/Benzatropine	Parkinson's disease

(continued)

Table Ap.2.1 Generic and proprietary drug names and their use in neurological disorders—cont'd.

Drug name	Main use/s of drug
Comtess*/Entacapone	Parkinson's disease
Copaxone*/Glatiramer acetate	MS
Cymbalta*/Duloxetine	Depression, diabetic neuropathy, stress incontinence
Cystrin*/Oxybutynin	Urinary frequency
Dantrium*/Dantrolene	Spasticity
Dantrolene/Dantrium*	Spasticity
Darifenacin/Emselex*	Urinary incontinence
Decadron*/Dexamethasone	Inflammation
Deltastab*/Prednisolone	Inflammation
Depakote*/Valproic acid	Manic episodes associated with bipolar disorders
Depixol*/Flupentixol	Schizophrenia and other psychoses
Depo-Medrone*/Methylprednisolone	Inflammation
Dexamethasone/Decadron*	Inflammation
Dexamfetamine/Dexedrine*	Narcolepsy, ADHD
Dexedrine*/Dexamfetamine	Narcolepsy, ADHD
Dexibuprofen/Seractil*	Pain, inflammation
Dexketoprofen/Keral*	Pain
DF118*/Dihydrocodeine	Pain
Diamorphine	Pain
Diazepam/Valium*	Status epilepticus, muscle spasm
Diclofenac/Voltarol*	Pain, inflammation
Diconal*/Dipipanone	Pain
Dihydrocodeine/DF118*	Pain
Dimenhydrinate/Dramamine*	Vestibular disorders
Dipipanone/Diconal*	Pain
Disipal*/Orphenadrine	Parkinson's disease, spasticity

Table Ap.2.1 Generic and proprietary drug names and their use in
neurological disorders—cont'd.

Drug name	Main use/s of drug
Distigmine/Ubretid*	Urinary retention
Ditropan*/Oxybutynin	Urinary frequency
Dixarit*/Clonidine	Motor tics, chorea, migraine
Dolmatil*/Sulpiride	Schizophrenia
Domperidone/Motilium*	Vestibular disorders
Donepezil/Aricept*	Dementia
Doralese*/Indoramin	Urinary retention
Dosulepin/Prothiaden*	Depression/sedation
Doxazosin/Cardura*	Urinary retention
Doxepin/Sinepin*	Depression/sedation
Dramamine*/Dimenhydrinate	Vestibular disorders
Duloxetine/Cymbalta*	Depression, diabetic neuropathy, stress incontinence
Durogesic*/Fentanyl	Pain
Dysport*/Botulinum toxin	Torticollis, blepharospasm
Ebixa*/Memantine	Dementia
Edronax*/Reboxetine	Depression
Efexor*/Venlafaxine	Depression
Eldepryl*/Selegiline	Parkinson's disease
Eletriptan/Relpax*	Acute migraine
Emflex*/Acemetacin	Pain and inflammation
Emselex*/Darifenacin	Urinary incontinence
Entacapone/Comtess*	Parkinson's disease
Etoricoxib/Arcoxia*	Pain, inflammation
Epanutin*/Phenytoin	Seizures, status epilepticus
Epilim*/Sodium valproate	Seizures
Ergotamine/Cafergot*, Migril*	Migraine

(*continued*)

Table Ap.2.1 Generic and proprietary drug names and their use in neurological disorders—cont'd.

Drug name	Main use/s of drug
Escitalopram/Cipralex*	Depression, panic disorder, anxiety
Ethosuximide/Zarontin*	Seizures
Exelon*/Rivastigmine	Dementia
Faverin*/Fluvoxamine	Depression
Feldene*/Piroxicam	Pain, inflammation
Fenbufen/Lederfen*	Pain, inflammation
Fentanyl/Durogesic*	Pain
Flavoxate/Urispas*	Urinary frequency
Flomaxtra XL*/Tamsulosin	Urinary retention
Fluoxetine/Prozac*	Depression
Flupentixol/Depixol*	Schizophrenia and other psychoses
Fluphenazine/Modecate*	Schizophrenia and other psychoses
Fluvoxamine/Faverin*	Depression
Flurbiprofen/Froben SR*	Pain, inflammation
Froben SR*/Flurbiprofen	Pain, inflammation
Frovatriptan/Migard*	Acute migraine
Gabapentin/Neurontin*	Seizures
Gabitril*/Tiagabine	Seizures
Galantamine/Reminyl*	Dementia
Gamanil*/Lofepramine	Depression
Glatiramer acetate/Copaxone*	MS
Glycopyrronium bromide/Robinul*	Drying secretions
Haldol*/Haloperidol	Schizophrenia and other psychoses, mania and behaviour disturbance
Haloperidol/Haldol*, Serenace*	Schizophrenia and other psychoses, mania and behaviour disturbance
Hydrocortisone/Hydrocortistab*	Inflammation
Hydrocortistab*/Hydrocortisone	Inflammation

Table Ap.2.1 Generic and proprietary drug names and their use in neurological disorders—cont'd.

Drug name	Main use/s of drug
Hyoscine/Kwells*, Scopaderm*	Reduce secretions
Hypovase*/Prazosin	Urinary retention
Hytrin*/Terazosin	Urinary retention
Ibuprofen/Brufen*	Pain, inflammation
Imigran*/Sumatriptan	Migraine
Imipramine/Tofranil*	Depression, neuropathic pain
Imodium*/Loperamide	Diarrhoea
Inderal*/Propranolol	Essential tremor, migraine
Indocid*/Indometacin	Pain, inflammation
Indometacin/Indocid*	Pain, inflammation
Indoramin/Doralese*	Urinary retention
Isocarboxazid	Depression
Kemadrin*/Procyclidine	Parkinson's disease
Keppra*/Levetiracetam	Seizures
Keral*/Dexketoprofen	Pain
Ketoprofen/Alrheumet*/Orudis*/Oruvail*	Pain, inflammation
Kwells*/Hyoscine	Reduce secretions
Lamictal*/Lamotrigine	Seizures
Lamotrigine/Lamictal*	Seizures
Largactil*/Chlorpromazine	Schizophrenia and other psychoses, mania and behaviour disturbance
Larodopa*/Levodopa	Parkinson's disease
Lederfen*/Fenbufen	Pain, inflammation
Levetiracetam/Keppra*	Seizures
Levodopa/Brocadopa*, Larodopa*	Parkinson's disease

(continued)

Table Ap.2.1 Generic and proprietary drug names and their use in neurological disorders—cont'd.

Drug name	Main use/s of drug
Lioresal*/Baclofen	Spasticity
Lisuride/Revanil*	Parkinson's disease
Lithium/Priadel*	Mania, bipolar disorders, depression
Lofepramine/Gamanil*	Depression
Lomotil*/Diphenoxylate and atropine	Diarrhoea
Loperamide/Imodium*	Diarrhoea
Lumiracoxib/Prexige*	Pain, inflammation
Lustral*/Sertraline	Depression
Lyrica*/Pregabalin	Neuropathic pain, partial seizures
Madopar*/Co-beneldopa	Parkinson's disease
Manerix*/Moclobemide	Depression
Maxalt*/Rizatriptan	Acute migraine
Maxolon*/Metoclopramide	Vestibular disorders
Meclozine/Sea-legs*	Vestibular disorders
Mefenamic acid/Ponstan*	Pain, inflammation
Meloxicam/Mobic*	Pain, inflammation
Memantine/Ebixa*	Dementia
Meptazinol/Meptid*	Pain
Meptid*/Meptazinol	Pain
Methocarbamol/Robaxin*	Spasticity
Methylphenidate/Ritalin*	ADHD, narcolepsy
Methylprednisolone/Depo-Medrone*	Inflammation
Methysergide/Deseril*	Migraine
Metoclopramide/Maxolon*	Vestibular disorders
Migard*/Frovatriptan	Acute migraine
Migril*/Ergotamine	Migraine

Table Ap.2.1 Generic and proprietary drug names and their use in
neurological disorders—cont'd.

Drug name	Main use/s of drug
Mirapexin*/Pramipexole	Parkinson's disease
Mirtazapine/Zispin SolTab*	Antidepressant, essential tremor
Mobic*/Meloxicam	Pain, inflammation
Mobiflex*/Tenoxicam	Pain, inflammation
Moclobemide/Manerix*	Depression
Modafinil/Provigil*	Daytime sleepiness
Modecate*/Fluphenazine	Schizophrenia and other psychoses
Molipaxin*/Trazodone	Depression
Motilium*/Domperidone	Vestibular disorders
Morphine/MST Continus*, Oramorph*	Pain
MST Continus*/Morphine	Pain
Myotonin*/Bethanechol	Urinary retention
Mysoline*/Primidone	Essential tremor, seizures
Nabumetone/Relifex*	Pain, inflammation
Naprosyn*/Naproxen	Pain, inflammation
Naproxen/Naprosyn*/Synflex*	Pain, inflammation
Naramig*/Naratriptan	Acute migraine
Naratriptan/Naramig*	Acute migraine
Nardil*/Phenelzine	Depression
NeuroBloc*/Botulinum B toxin	Torticollis
Neurontin*/Gabapentin	Seizures
Nimodipine/Nimotop*	Subarachnoid haemorrhage (SAH)
Nimotop*/Nimodipine	SAH
Nitoman*/Tetrabenazine	Chorea
Nootropil*/Piracetam	Myoclonus
Nortriptyline/Allegron*	Depression, Neuropathic pain
Olanzapine/Zyprexa*	Schizophrenia

(*continued*)

Table Ap.2.1 Generic and proprietary drug names and their use in neurological disorders—cont'd.

Drug name	Main use/s of drug
Oramorph*/Morphine	Pain
Orap*/Pimozide	Schizophrenia and other psychoses
Orphenadrine/Disipal*	Parkinson's disease, spasticity
Orudis*/Ketoprofen	Pain, inflammation
Oruvail*/Ketoprofen	Pain, inflammation
Oxcarbazepine/Trileptal*	Seizures
Oxybutynin/Cystrin*, Ditropan*	Urinary frequency
Panadol*/Paracetamol	Pain
Paracetamol/Panadol*	Pain
Paracetamol and metoclopramide/Paramax*	Migraine
Paramax* Paracetamol and metoclopramide	Migraine
Parlodel*/Bromocriptine	Parkinson's disease
Parnate*/Tranylcypromine	Depression
Paroxetine/Seroxat*	Depression, obsessive-compulsive disorder, panic disorder, anxiety
Pergolide/Celance*	Parkinson's disease
Perphenazine	Vestibular disorders
Pethidine	Pain
Phenelzine/Nardil*	Depression
Phenergan*/Promethazine	Vestibular disorders
Phenobarbital	Status epilepticus, other forms of seizures
Phenol	Spasticity
Phenytoin/Epanutin*	Status epilepticus, seizures
Pimozide/Orap*	Schizophrenia and other psychoses
Piracetam/Nootropil*	Myoclonus
Piroxicam/Feldene*	Pain, inflammation
Pizotifen/Sanomigran*	Migraine

Table Ap.2.1 Generic and proprietary drug names and their use in neurological disorders—cont'd.

Drug name	Main use/s of drug
Ponstan*/Mefenamic Acid	Pain, inflammation
Pregabalin/Lyrica*	Neuropathic pain, partial seizures
Prazosin/Hypovase*	Urinary retention
Prednisolone/Deltastab*	Inflammation
Pramipexole/Mirapexin*	Parkinson's disease
Preservex*/Aceclofenac	Pain, inflammation
Priadel*/Lithium	Mania, bipolar disorders, depression
Primidone/Mysoline*	Essential tremor, seizures
Probanthine*/Propantheline	Urinary frequency
Prochlorperazine/Stemetil*	Vestibular disorders
Procyclidine/Kemadrin*	Parkinson's disease
Promethazine/Avomine*, Phenergan*	Vestibular disorders
Propantheline/Probanthine*	Urinary frequency
Propiverine/Vesicare*	Urinary frequency and incontinence
Propranolol/Inderal*	Essential tremor, migraine
Prothiaden*/Dosulepin	Depression/sedation
Provigil*/Modafinil	Daytime sleepiness
Prozac*/Fluoxetine	Depression
Quetiapine/Seroquel*	Schizophrenia
Rasagiline/Azilect*	Parkinson's disease
Rebif*/Beta-1a interferon	MS
Reboxetine/Edronax*	Depression
Relifex*/Nabumetone	Pain, inflammation
Regurin*/Trospium	Urinary frequency and incontinence
Relpax*/Eletriptan	Acute migraine
Reminyl*/Galantamine	Dementia

(*continued*)

Table Ap.2.1 Generic and proprietary drug names and their use in neurological disorders—cont'd.

Drug name	Main use/s of drug
Requip*/Ropinirole	Parkinson's disease
Revanil*/Lisuride	Parkinson's disease
Rilutek*/Riluzole	Motor neurone disease
Riluzole/Rilutek*	Motor neurone disease
Risperdal*/Risperidone	Acute and chronic psychosis
Risperidone/Risperdal*	Acute and chronic psychosis
Ritalin*/Methylphenidate	ADHD, narcolepsy
Rivastigmine/Exelon*	Dementia
Rivotril*/Clonazepam	Status epilepticus, other forms of epilepsy
Rizatriptan/Maxalt*	Acute migraine
Robaxin*/Methocarbamol	Spasticity
Robinul*/Glycopyrronium bromide	Drying secretions
Ropinirole/Requip*	Parkinson's disease
Rotigotine/Neupro*	Early Parkinson's disease
Sabril*/Vigabatrin	Seizures
Sanomigran*/Pizotifen	Migraine
Scopaderm*/Hyoscine	Reduce secretions
Sea-legs*/Meclozine	Vestibular disorders
Selegiline/Eldepryl*	Parkinson's disease
Seractil*/Dexibuprofen	Pain, inflammation
Serc*/Betahistine	Vertigo, tinnitus
Serdolect*/Sertindole	Schizophrenia
Serenace*/Haloperidol	Schizophrenia and other psychoses, mania and behaviour disturbance
Seroquel*/Quetiapine	Psychoses
Seroxat*/Paroxetine	Depression, obsessive-compulsive disorder, panic disorder, anxiety
Sertaline/Lustral*	Depression, obsessive-compulsive disorder

Table Ap.2.1 Generic and proprietary drug names and their use in neurological disorders—cont'd.

Drug name	Main use/s of drug
Sertindole/Serdolect*	Schizophrenia
Sinemet*/Co-careldopa	Parkinson's disease
Sinepin*/Doxepin	Depression/sedation
Sodium valproate/Epilim*	Seizures
Solian*/Amisulpride	Schizophrenia
Stelazine*/Trifluperazine	Schizophrenia and other psychoses, anxiety
Stemetil*/Prochlorperazine	Vestibular disorders
Strattera*/Atomoxetine	ADHD
Stugeron*/Cinnarizine	Vestibular disorders
Sulpiride/Dolmatil*	Schizophrenia
Sumatriptan/Imigran*	Migraine
Surgam SA*/Tiaprofenic acid	Pain, inflammation
Surmontil*/Trimipramine	Depression/sedation
Symmetrel*/Amantadine	Parkinson's disease, fatigue in MS
Synflex*/Naproxen	Pain, inflammation
Tamsulosin/Flomaxtra XL*	Urinary retention
Tegretol*/Carbamazepine	Seizures, trigeminal neuralgia, bipolar disorders
Temgesic*/Buprenorphine	Pain
Tenoxicam/Mobiflex*	Pain, inflammation
Terazosin/Hytrin*	Urinary retention
Tetrabenazine/Nitoman*	Chorea
Tiaprofenic acid/Surgam SA*	Pain, inflammation
Tigabine/Gabitril*	Seizures
Tizanidine/Zanaflex*	Spasticity
Tofranil*/Imipramine	Depression, neuropathic pain
Tolfenamic acid/Clotam*	Acute migraine
Tolterodine/Detrusitol*	Urinary frequency

(continued)

Table Ap.2.1 Generic and proprietary drug names and their use in neurological disorders—cont'd.

Drug name	Main use/s of drug
Topamax*/Topiramate	Seizures, essential tremor
Topiramate/Topamax*	Seizures
Tramadol/Zydol*	Pain
Tranylcypromine/Parnate*	Depression
Trazodone/Molipaxin*	Depression
Trifluperazine/Stelazine*	Schizophrenia and other psychoses, anxiety
Trihexyphenidyl (Benzhexol)/Broflex*	Parkinson's disease, tremor, chorea, tics
Trimipramine/Surmontil*	Depression/sedation
Trileptal*/Oxcarbazepine	Seizures
Trospium/Regurin*	Urinary frequency and incontinence
Ubretid*/Distigmine	Urinary retention
Urispas*/Flavoxate	Urinary retention
Valium*/Diazepam	Status epilepticus, spasticity
Valproic acid/Depakote*	Manic episodes associated with bipolar disorders
Venlafaxine/Efexor*	Depression
Vesicare*/Propiverine	Urinary frequency and incontinence
Vigabatrin/Sabril*	Seizures
Voltarol*/Diclofenac	Pain, inflammation
Xatral*/Alfuzosin	Urinary retention
Zuclopenthixol/Clopixol*	Psychoses
Zanaflex*/Tizanidine	Spasticity
Zarontin*/Ethosuximide	Seizures
Zispin SolTab*/Mirtazapine	Antidepressant, essential tremor
Zoleptil*/Zotepine	Schizophrenia
Zolmitriptan/Zomig*	Acute migraine

Table Ap.2.1 Generic and proprietary drug names and their use in neurological disorders—cont'd.

Drug name	Main use/s of drug
Zomig*/Zolmitriptan	Acute migraine
Zotepine/Zoleptil*	Schizophrenia
Zydol*/Tramadol	Pain
Zyprexa*/Olanzapine	Schizophrenia

* Denotes brand (proprietary) name.

References

British national formulary 55, March 2008, published by BMJ Publishing and RPS Publishing, London.

Khanderia M 2004 Drug treatments in neurological rehabilitation. In: Stokes M (ed) Physical management in neurological rehabilitation, 2nd edn. Elsevier Mosby, London.

Martindale: the complete drug reference, 35th edn 2007. Pharmaceutical Press, London.

Abbreviations

AAC augmentative and alternative communication

ABG arterial blood gas

ABI acquired brain injury

ACA anterior cerebral artery

ACP American College of Physicians

ACPIN Association of Chartered Physiotherapists Interested in Neurology

ACSM American College of Sports Medicine

ADL activities of daily living

AFO ankle foot orthosis

ALS amyotrophic lateral sclerosis

ANS autonomic nervous system

AR associated reaction

ARDS adult respiratory distress syndrome

ASIA American Spinal Injury Association

BBS Berg balance score

BG basal ganglia

BOS base of support

BP blood pressure

CAOT Canadian Association of Occupational Therapists

CC cerebrocerebellar circuit

CBST corticobulbarspinal tract

CDH congenital dislocation of the hip

CIMT constraint-induced movement therapy

CK creatine kinase

CNS central nervous system

COM centre of mass

COPM Canadian Occupational Performance Measure

CP cerebral palsy

CPAP continuous positive airway pressure

CPG central pattern generator

CPK creatine phosphokinase

CPM continuous passive movement

CPP cerebral perfusion pressure

CRPS complex regional pain syndrome

CSF cerebrospinal fluid

CSP Chartered Society of Physiotherapy

CT computed tomography

CVA cerebrovascular accident

DM1 dystrophic myotonica (myotonic dystrophy)

DMD Duchenne muscular dystrophy

DoH Department of Health

DVT deep vein thrombosis

EBP evidence-based practice

ECG electrocardiogram

EEG electroencephalography/electroencephalogram

EMG electromyography/electromyogram

ENS enteric nervous system

EP evoked potentials

ES electrical stimulation

ESR erythrocyte sedimentation rate

FAM Functional Assessment Measure

FBC full blood count

FES functional electrical stimulation

FIM Functional Independence Measure

fMRI functional magnetic resonance imaging

FiO_2 fraction of inspired oxygen

FRC functional residual capacity

FSH fascioscapulohumeral muscular dystrophy

FVC forced vital capacity

GABA gamma-aminobutyric acid

GBS Guillain–Barré syndrome

GCS Glasgow Coma Scale/Score

HD Huntington's disease

HEP home exercise programme

HO heterotopic ossification

HR heart rate

HSP hemiplegic shoulder pain

ICF International Classification of Functioning

ICP integrated care pathway (Ch 12)

ICP intracranial pressure (Chs 1, 10.1, 13)

IPPB intermittent positive-pressure breathing

ISO International Standards Organisation

ITU intensive therapy unit

KAFO knee ankle foot orthosis

KO knee orthosis

LACI lacunar infarcts

LL lower limb

LMN lower motor neurone

LMNL Lower motor neurone lesion
LOC level of consciousness
LP lumbar puncture
MAP mean arterial blood pressure
MAS Modified Ashworth Scale
MCA middle cerebral artery
MCS motor control system
MD muscular dystrophy
MDT multidisciplinary team
MEP motor evoked potential
MHI manual hyperventilation
MND motor neurone disease
MNDA Motor Neurone Disease Association
MP motor programme
MRC Medical Research Council
MRI magnetic resonance imaging
MS multiple sclerosis
NHS National Health Service
NICE National Institute for Clinical Excellence
NIV non-invasive ventilation
NMJ neuromuscular junction
NSF National Service Framework
NTD neural tube deficit
OCD obsessive-compulsive disorder
OSA obstructive sleep apnoea
OT occupational therapy
PACI partial anterior circulation infarcts
$PaCO_2$ partial pressure of carbon dioxide
PaO_2 partial pressure of oxygen
PCA posterior cerebral artery
PCS post concussion symptoms
PD Parkinson's disease
PET positron emission tomography
PFC prefrontal cortex
PMC premotor cortex (Ch 4)
PMC primary motor cortex
PMH past medical history
PNS peripheral nervous system
PNS parasympathetic nervous system
POP plaster of Paris
POCI posterior circulation infarcts

PPC posterior parietal cortex
PPS post-polio syndrome
PTA post-traumatic amnesia
RAMP restore, adapt, maintain, prevent (Figure 8.2)
RHBD right hemisphere brain disorder
rINN recommended international non-proprietary name
ROM range of movement
RR respiratory rate
RST reticulospinal tract
RT rubrospinal tract
SAH subarachnoid haemorrhage
SCI spinal cord injury
SCOPA Scales for Outcomes in Parkinson's disease
SLR straight-leg raising
SLT speech and language therapist
SMA spinal muscular atrophies (Ch 6)
SMA supplementary motor area (Ch 4)
SMART Framework goals – specific, measurable, achievable, realistic, timed
SNS sympathetic nervous system
SOAP Notes – subjective, objective, assessment, plan
SOM standardized outcome measure
TACI total anterior circulation infarcts
TBI traumatic brain injury
TENS transcutaneous electrical nerve stimulation
TIA transient ischaemic attack
TT tilt table
UKABIF UK Acquired Brain Injury Foundation
UL upper limb
UMN upper motor neurone
UMNL upper motor neurone lesion
VAS visual analogue scale
VC vital capacity
VIM ventral intermediate nucleus
WCPT World Confederation for Physical Therapy
WHO World Health Organization

Glossary of terms

For definitions of common neurological conditions, please see relevant sections of Chapter 6.

Acidosis: increased acidity of blood.

Afferent nerve: transmits impulses centrally from tissues towards the brain and spinal cord (sensory nerve).

Agnosia: inability to recognize objects.

Akinesia: inability to initiate movement due to difficulty selecting and/or activating motor pathways in the central nervous system. Common in severe Parkinson's disease.

Allodynia: meaning 'other pain'. Exaggerated response to non-noxious stimuli. Can be either static or mechanical.

Aneurysm: a localized, blood-filled dilatation (bulge or ballooning) of a blood vessel (usually of an artery) caused by disease or weakening of the vessel wall.

Anoxia: complete deprivation of oxygen supply.

Aphasia: inability to communicate. Either a receptive or expressive problem affecting the understanding and use of correct words (content) in speech or writing.

Apnoea: cessation of breathing (see OSA).

Apraxia: loss of ability to carry out learned purposeful movements, despite having the desire and physical ability to perform movements. A disorder of motor planning.

Assessment: process of understanding a measurement in a specific context.

Ataxia: disturbance of movement co-ordination. Occurs with disorders of the cerebellum or its brainstem connections, e.g. multiple sclerosis, Friedreich's ataxia, posterior fossa tumours.

Atelectasis: collapse of part or all of a lung.

Autonomic dysreflexia/hyperreflexia or sympathetic hyperreflexia or paroxysmal hypertension: an overactivity of the ANS in response to an irritating stimulus below the level of spinal cord injury, such as an overfull bladder. The stimulus sends nerve impulses to the spinal cord which are blocked by the lesion at the level of injury, activating a reflex that increases activity of the sympathetic portion of the ANS. This results in spasms and increased blood pressure. Nerve receptors in the heart and blood vessels detect this rise in blood pressure, which cannot be regulated due to the spinal lesion. Occurs predominantly in patients after spinal cord injury at T5 level and above. Can develop suddenly and become a possible emergency situation. If not treated promptly and correctly, it may lead to seizures, stroke, and even death.

Autonomic nervous system (ANS) or visceral nervous system: the part of the peripheral nervous system that acts as a control system, maintaining homeostasis in the body. Primarily operates without conscious control or sensation. The ANS regulates body functions including: blood pressure, heart rate, respiration rate, bowel and bladder emptying, perspiration, pupil diameter in the eyes, salivation, digestion. The ANS has three components: the sympathetic nervous system, parasympathetic nervous system and enteric (gut) nervous system.

Ballismus: violent, large amplitude involuntary movements of limbs. Sometimes affecting one side of the body – *hemiballismus*. Occurs in Huntington's disease.

Bradycardia: heart rate below 60 beats per minute (bpm).

Bradykinesia: slowness in execution of movement.

Cardiovascular accident (CVA): see 'Stroke'.

Central nervous system (CNS): brain and spinal cord.

Chorea: brief, irregular contractions that are not repetitive or rhythmic, but appear to flow randomly from one muscle to the next. Occur in basal ganglia disorders, e.g. Huntington's disease.

Client-centred practice: an approach to rehabilitation that seeks to respect clients' right to autonomy – ability to act on choices and be in control of one's own life.

Clinical hypertonicity: increase in tone that occurs during voluntary movement resulting from e.g. insufficient trunk control during a task or compensatory training patterns. May be fluctuating or persistent.

Clinical practice guidelines: represent the consensus opinion of experts based on explicit and objective reviews of the scientific literature.

Continuity of care: refers to patients experiencing some form of transition or transfer of care.

Contracture: shortening of a muscle or tendon.

Critical appraisal: the process of methodically examining research evidence to assess its validity, importance and applicability to clinical practice.

Decerebrate posture/rigidity: abnormal body posture with arms extended by the sides, legs extended and toes pointing downward and backward arching of the head – usually indicates brainstem damage.

Decorticate posture/rigidity: abnormal body posture with arms flexed and turned inward towards the body, hands clenched into fists held on the chest and legs extended. Indicates damage to the corticospinal tract (pathway between brain and spinal cord).

Demyelination: immune-mediated destruction of the myelin sheath insulating nerve fibres. Characteristic of some neurodegenerative disorders, such as multiple sclerosis and Guillain–Barré syndrome.

Diplopia: double vision. Simultaneous perception of two images of a single object.

Dynamometer: apparatus for measuring force, torque or power of skeletal muscles.

Dysaesthesia: uncomfortable sensation, often described as burning, tingling, or numbness.

Dysarthria: motor disorder of speech, characterized by poor articulation. Difficulty in producing or sustaining the range, force, speed and coordination of movements needed to achieve appropriate breathing, phonation, resonance and articulation for speech.

Dysphagia: difficulty with swallowing due to disruption in the swallowing process.

Dyskinesia: an involuntary movement distinguished by the underlying cause e.g. myoclonus, chorea, ballismus, dystonia, tic, tremor. The term hyperkinesia also used but is misleading, as it implies movements are faster but this is not the case.

Dysphasia: impaired ability to communicate, usually used synonymously with aphasia but the latter is a total inability to communicate.

Dystonia: movement disorder characterized by involuntary and repetitive contraction of muscle groups, resulting in twisting movements, unusual postures and possible tremor. (Previously known as athetosis.)

Efferent nerve: transmits impulses away from the central nervous system to a muscle (motor neurone) or organ.

Enteric nervous system (ENS): directly controls the gastrointestinal system. It is capable of autonomous functions such as the coordination of reflexes but receives considerable innervation from the autonomic nervous system and thus is considered a part of it.

Evidence-based practice: a systematic process for finding, appraising and applying current best evidence to inform clinical practice.

Fasciculation: or 'muscle twitch' is a small, local, involuntary muscle contraction (twitching) visible under the skin arising from the spontaneous discharge of a bundle of skeletal muscle fibres. Fasciculations have a variety of causes, the majority of which are benign, but can also be due to disease of the motor neurones.

Fatigue: describes a range of abnormal functions or states, varying from a general state of lethargy to a specific work-induced sensation in muscles. Fatigue can be both physical and mental. *Physical fatigue* is the inability to continue functioning at the level of one's normal abilities. *Mental fatigue* manifests as somnolence (drowsiness). Physiological classification of *neuromuscular fatigue*: central and peripheral. *Central fatigue* occurs in the brain or spinal cord; *peripheral fatigue* occurs at or distal to the anterior horn cell, at the neuromuscular junction or muscle cell membrane.

Goniometry: measurement of joint angles to assess range of movement.

Hemianopia: visual field defect – blindness or reduction in vision in one half of the visual field due to damage of the optic pathways in the brain.

Hemiplegia: the paralysis of muscles on one side of the body affecting the arm, trunk, face and leg (contralateral to the side of the lesion in the brain).

Heterotopic ossification (HO): development of bone in abnormal areas, usually in soft tissues, particularly muscles, around joints or long bones. Results from traumatic injuries, commonly spinal cord injury.

Hydrocephalus: abnormal accumulation of cerebrospinal fluid (CSF) in the ventricles of the brain. May cause increased intracranial pressure (ICP).

Hypercapnia/hypercarbia: levels of carbon dioxide increased in the blood.

Hyperesthesia: increased sensitivity.

Hypertonia: increased muscle tone – spasticity and rigidity.

Hypocapnia: state of reduced carbon dioxide in the blood. Usually results from deep or rapid breathing, known as hyperventilation.

Hypokinesia: slowness in initiation of movement.

Hypotonia: reduced muscle tone, occurs in central or peripheral nervous system disorders.

Hypoxaemia: reduced oxygen level in the blood.

Hypoxia: deprived of adequate oxygen (whole or part of body).

Impairment: a problem in body function or structure such as a significant deviation or loss.

Incidence: probability that a patient without disease develops the disease during an interval, referring only to new cases e.g. incidence of stroke for people aged 55 years or more ranges from 4.2 to 6.5 per 1000 population per annum.

INVOLVE: a government supported organization that aims to improve patient, carer and public involvement in research (www.invo. org.uk).

Ischaemia: restriction in blood supply resulting in damage or dysfunction of tissue.

Kyphosis: spinal curve that results in an abnormally rounded upper back, either due to bad posture or a structural abnormality of the spine.

Labyrinth: vestibular sense organ in the inner ear. See 'Proprioception'.

Measurement: application of standard scales or instruments to variables, giving a numerical score, which may be combined for each variable to give an overall score.

Micturition: bladder emptying.

Motor learning: the process of improving motor skills, the smoothness and accuracy of movements. Motor re-learning (adaptation): regaining motor performance.

Motor skill: ability to use skeletal muscles effectively in a goal-directed manner, as a result of practice of specific tasks. Indicator of quality of performance.

Myoclonus: brief shock-like jerks of a limb or body part.

Myometer: instrument for measuring skeletal muscle contraction force.

Neurological weakness: loss of central ability to produce and sustain muscle force.

Neuromuscular junction (NMJ): the synapse (junction) between a nerve fibre and muscle tissue. The axon terminal of the motorneurone joins with the motor end plate (highly excitable region of the muscle fibre membrane responsible for initiation of action potentials), causing the muscle to contract. The signal passes through the NMJ via the neurotransmitter acetylcholine.

Neurone (nerve cell): electrically excitable cell in the nervous system that processes or transmits information. Neurones are the core components of the brain, spinal cord and peripheral nerves.

Nystagmus: rapid, repetitive movement of the eye in one direction, alternating with a slower movement in the opposite direction.

Obstructive sleep apnoea (OSA): cessation of airflow during sleep preventing air from entering the lungs caused by an obstruction.

Oedema: swelling. Increase of insterstitial (intercellular) fluid in any tissue or organ.

Orofacial paresis: partial paralysis of the muscles of facial expression. Leads to problems with drooling, swallowing and feeding.

Orthosis: an external device used to correct deformity or assist/improve function by modifying the structural or functional characteristics of the neuromusculoskeletal system.

Paralysis: complete loss of muscle function for one or more muscle groups. Often includes loss of feeling in the affected area. Caused by damage to the central (brain or spinal cord) or peripheral (nerve cells or fibres) nervous systems.

Parasympathetic nervous system (PNS): regulates actions that do not require immediate reaction, complimenting the actions of the sympathetic nervous system. The PNS is concerned with conservation and restoration of energy, as it causes a reduction in heart rate and blood pressure, and facilitates digestion and absorption of nutrients, and consequently excretion of waste products. The preganglionic outflow of the PNS arises from cranial nerves III, VII, IX and X in the brain stem and the 2nd–4th sacral segments of the spinal cord, known as the cranio-sacral outflow. The PNS uses only acetylcholine (ACh) as its neurotransmitter.

Paresis: partial loss of movement or impaired movement.

Paresthesias: abnormal sensations, including numbness, tingling ('pins and needles'), burning, prickling and increased sensitivity, or hyperesthesia.

Peripheral nervous system (PNS): extends outside the central nervous system to serve the limbs and organs. The PNS is divided into the somatic nervous system and the autonomic nervous system.

pH: measure of acidity or alkalinity.

Plasticity: ability to permanently change or deform. *Neuroplasticity or neural plasticity* – any enduring changes in neurone structure or function to better cope with the environment. When an area of brain is damaged, another area may take over the same function. *Synaptic plasticity* – a property of a neurone or synapse to change its internal parameters in response to its history. *Muscle plasticity* – adaptability. Ability to change to accommodate specific stressors.

Positive reinforcement: method for improving behaviour employing praise, rest breaks, positive social attention and meaningful (tangible) rewards.

Prevalence: probability of disease in the entire population at any point in time, e.g. prevalence of stroke is 500–800 cases per 100 000.

Proprioception: sensory modality that provides feedback on the status of the body internally for self-regulation of posture and movement. Feedback originates in receptors embedded in the joints, tendons, muscles and labyrinth.

Prosopagnosia: inability to recognize faces.

Ptosis: drooping eyelids.

Quadraparesis/tetraparesis: weakness of all four limbs.

Rehabilitation: a process of learning to live well with an impairment in the context of one's own environment.

Reliability: extent to which measurement is consistent and free from error.

Rigidity: increase in muscle tone, leading to resistance to passive movement throughout the range of motion. Common in Parkinson's disease.

SMART framework: goals are specific, measurable, achievable, realistic and timed.

Somatic nervous system: the part of the peripheral nervous system associated with voluntary control of body movements and with reception of external stimuli, which helps keep the body in touch with its surroundings (e.g., touch, hearing and sight).

Spasticity: velocity-dependent increase in resistance to passive (stretch reflex hyperactivity) of a muscle, with exaggerated tendon reflexes.

Spondylosis: spinal degeneration and deformity of the joint(s) of two or more vertebrae that commonly occurs with aging. Can involve compression of nerve roots and, less commonly, direct pressure on spinal cord.

Stroke: a rapidly developed loss of cerebral function of presumed vascular origin and of more than 24 hours' duration. Also termed cardiovascular accident (CVA).

Subarachnoid haemorrhage (SAH): bleeding into the subarachnoid space, usually from ruptured aneurysm at or near the Circle of Willis.

Sympathetic nervous system (SNS): responsible for automatic regulation of many homeostatic mechanisms in the body. The SNS enables the body to be prepared for fear, flight or fight. Sympathetic responses include: increased heart rate, blood pressure and pupil size, contraction of sphincters. The cell bodies of the preganglionic fibres are in the lateral horns of the spinal cord at T1–L2, the so called thoraco-lumbar outflow. The preganglionic fibres enter the sympathetic ganglia, arranged in two paravertebral chains lying anterolateral to the vertebral bodies, called the sympathetic ganglionic chains. Several transmitter substances are involved in the SNS, including adrenaline, noradrenaline, acetylcholine.

Talipes equinovarus: or club foot. Heel is elevated, the foot inverted and the person appears to be walking on their ankle.

Tenodesis grip: wrist actively extended, fingers and thumb pulled into flexion to produce a functional 'key-type' grip.

Tetraparesis/quadraparesis: weakness of all four limbs.

Thrombolysis: breakdown of blood clots by pharmacological means (thrombolytic drugs e.g. alteplase, a tissue plasminogen activator). Early treatment for ischaemic stroke.

Titubation: 1. head tremor or nodding; 2. staggering, bobbing, stumbling or ataxic gait – cerebellar in origin.

Tracheostomy or trachiotomy: surgical procedure on the throat to create a direct airway through an incision in the trachea.

Transcranial magnetic stimulation: noninvasive method to excite neurones in the brain, used to study the circuitry and connectivity of the brain.

Transient ischaemic attack (TIA): a stroke-like syndrome in which recovery is complete within 24 hours.

Tremor: an unwanted, rhythmic, sinusoidal movement of a limb or body part, classified according to the situation in which it occurs. Types include: *resting tremor* (when limb relaxed and fully supported, occurs in Parkinson's disease); *action tremor* (during movement) associated with cerebellar dysfunction and includes *postural tremor* (when limb is held against gravity), *kinetic tremor* (during any type of movement) and *intention tremor* (worsens at the end of a goal-directed movement).

Urinary incontinence: inability to hold urine in the bladder due to loss of voluntary control over the urinary sphincters resulting in the involuntary, unintentional passage of urine.

Validity: ensures a test measures what it is intended to measure.

Valsalva's manoeuvre: forced exhalation (strain) against a closed airway (closed lips and pinched nose) forcing air into the middle ear.

Vasovagal response/syncope (fainting): characterized by the common faint, resulting from 'vagally' mediated cardioinhibition and vasodepression. Caused by excessive venous pooling (commonly from prolonged standing or upright sitting) that paradoxically results in vasodilatation and bradycardia rather than the appropriate physiologic responses of vasoconstriction and tachycardia. The resulting bradycardia reduces cerebral blood flow to a level inadequate to maintain consciousness.